Color Atlas of
Endodontics

Color Atlas of
Endodontics

J. J. Messing BDS, FDS, RCS
Emeritus Reader in Operative Dental Surgery,
University College, London, England

C. J. R. Stock BDS, MSc,
Senior Clinical Lecturer (part-time)
Eastman Dental Hospital, London, England

The C. V. Mosby Company
St. Louis · Washington, D.C. · Toronto

Copyright © J. J. Messing, C. J. R. Stock, 1988
Published by Wolfe Medical Publications Ltd, 1988
Printed by Toppan Company(s) Pte. Ltd., Singapore
ISBN 0-8016-5303-7

Distributed in the United States by
The C. V. Mosby Company
11830 Westline Industrial Drive
St. Louis, Missouri 63146
U.S.A.

Distributed in Canada by
The C. V. Mosby Company, Ltd.
5240 Finch Avenue East
Scarborough, Ontario
Canada M1S 5A2

Contents

Chapter		Page
	Introduction	6
1	Radiography	9
2	Histology of the pulp	31
3	Diagnosis and treatment planning	38
4	Anaesthesia	59
5	Basic instruments and materials	64
6	Rubber dam	84
7	Treatment of the emergency patient	96
8	Access cavities	108
9	Root canal anatomy	119
10	Preparation of the tooth	133
11	Preparation of the root canal	141
12	Filling the root canal	153
13	Calcium hydroxide	170
14	Primary dentition	184
15	Surgical endodontics	
	1) apicectomy	194
	2) replantation and hemisection etc	211
16	Endo perio lesion	225
17	Root resorption	237
18	Removal of root canal obstructions	249
19	Bleaching	257
20	Restoration of the treated tooth	260
21	The way ahead	272
	References	274
	Trade references	275
	Index	277

Introduction

The purpose of this Atlas is to provide a simple description, liberally illustrated, of the modern concept of endodontics together with the techniques and materials currently in use. It is directed at the undergraduate student and at the general dental practitioner to introduce them both to the practical, rather than the theoretical, approach to treatment.

Endodontics has become established as an important discipline in dentistry with a predictably high success rate. The recent rapid growth in interest has been matched by the large amount of research into the subject. During its history endodontics had a serious setback. In 1911 Hunter's theory of oral sepsis castigated the dental profession by placing the blame on restorative dentistry as the cause of many medical diseases, although not mentioned in the paper, root canal therapy was completely discredited as a form of dental treatment. The theory of oral sepsis was denounced some twenty-five years later but the effect on endodontics was devastating. Dental schools insisted that root canal therapy could be completed only after a negative culture had been obtained. This involved attempts to sterilise the root canal using powerful bactericides; silver nitrate, sulphuric acid, iodoform, various phenolic derivatives and arsenical compounds were all used. Periapical radiolucent areas were considered to be a serious threat to a patient's health and the offending teeth were extracted; indeed, many dentists condemned all pulpless teeth whatever their condition.

A gradual change in the rationale of endodontics has taken place, stimulated by research and demand by both the patient and the profession to retain rather than extract teeth. It is no longer considered necessary in routine cases to use a culture technique. Intra-canal medication should be non-toxic to the periapical tissues so that healing is promoted, not delayed. Many operators use no medication in the root canal between appointments. The most important aspect of root canal therapy is the removal of the contents of the root canal(s) so that the cause of irritation is eradicated. The walls of the root canal are then flared to allow the complete preparation and obturation of the root canal system. The root filling material should be non-irritant and insoluble. The commonest cause of failure is incomplete obturation of the root canal which allows toxic products to leak out of the tooth into the periapical tissues. It is not sufficient to provide an apical seal, as leakage may occur through lateral canals which may be found anywhere along the length of the root canal and which are present in approximately 50 per cent of all teeth.

Gutta Percha has remained the root canal filling material of choice, despite the introduction of several other materials. Silver points, introduced 50 years ago, have two faults. If not correctly sealed so that leakage occurs, they tend to corrode and the corrosion products are toxic; secondly, root canals are not round in cross section, so the silver point relies on a sealer to complete the obturation and all sealers are soluble. It is not possible to fill the root canal completely if only a paste or sealer is used as a root filling material. Manufacturers have introduced many different types of sealer, some of them containing medicaments likely to cause tissue irritation — paraformaldehyde has been the active ingredient of many sealers. One of the problems in root canal therapy is that no matter which technique or material is used a relatively high rate of success will be achieved. The classical technique requiring extensive and thorough mechanical debridement and complete obturation is exacting, time consuming and in general receives poor remuneration. An extract from an editorial in 'Dental Cosmos' (1899) proves that the argument is not a new one:

'It is far less difficult to seal a pellet of mummifying paste into a cavity, complete the operation in a short single sitting, and collect the fee upon its completion, than it is to do a thorough canal operation, and the very ease which this short-cut through an essentially difficult operation to the fee for it confers, is a dangerous temptation to degrade the high standard of dental work which should always be maintained.' Some eighty years later, the conflict has still not been resolved. Evidence in the form of longitudinal studies on the success rate of the mummification technique has not been published; on the other hand, research has raised serious doubts about the efficacy of using paraformaldehyde in root canal therapy.

The rationale concerning endodontic surgery has also undergone some change. The treatment of choice is root canal therapy. If this cannot be carried out, then apicectomy with retrograde filling may be the answer. There is no place in endodontics for periapical curettage or apicectomy without retrograde filling. Large periapical radiolucencies do not necessarily indicate a need for periapical surgery. The objective in root canal therapy is to prevent leakage of toxic products from the root canal system. In apicectomy the objective is the same, and this will be achieved by sealing all communication between the canal(s) and the periapical tissues.

There are several different numbering systems for teeth. The most common ones are the Universal, Quadrant and F.D.I. Two Digit. In the authors' view, the F.D.I. Two Digit system will become generally accepted in a few years' time. In order to avoid any confusion, it was decided to identify teeth throughout this Atlas by referring to them in full, thus 'maxillary right first molar' or 'lower left second premolar'.

By the time a book has been written and published some of the text inevitably must be out of date, particularly in a rapidly growing subject such as endodontics. The past two-three years have seen changes in the techniques available for both the preparation and filling of the root canal. In addition, the current climate has dictated that dental personnel with patient contact should wear gloves. Despite this, some illustrations are shown where the operator is without gloves although the authors are well aware of the need for such protection.

Acknowledgements

The authors would like to thank Mrs A. Christie, who prepared the line drawings, and Mr A. Johnson from the Photographic Department of the Eastman Dental Hospital for the majority of the non-clinical photography. The authors are also indebted to the staff of the Department of Conservative Dentistry at the Eastman for helping to provide some of the clinical material. Finally, thanks are due to Mr F.J. Harty, Mr L.J.J. Searson, Mr D. Cohen and Mr A.H. Croysdill for allowing their material to be published.

The author of chapter 14 thanks Professor G.B. Winter for providing pictures 732, 735, 736, 752, 755, 767; Mr. J.F. Roberts for 737, 739, 740, 742, 745, 746, 747, 748, 751; Mr. D.C. Rule for 758, 760, 763, 764, 768, 769, 770; Professor G.B. Winter and Mr. F.J. Hill for 753, 754 (from *Paediatric Dentistry,* 2nd ed., Ed. Braham & Morris, published by Williams & Wilkins Co., Baltimore).

1 Radiography C J Stock

Endodontics is one of the few branches of dentistry in which both diagnosis and treatment depend largely on the radiograph. It is therefore well worth studying the equipment, materials, and techniques involved in producing the best possible periapical radiographs.

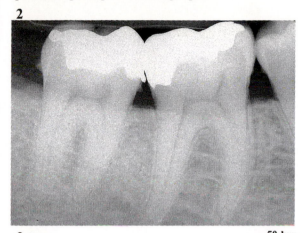

50 kvp

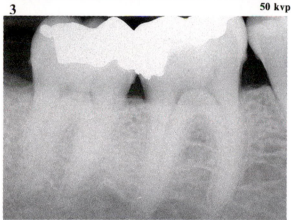

65 kvp

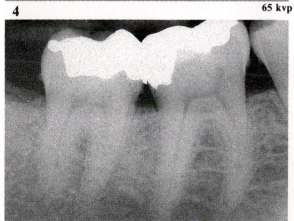

90 kvp

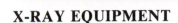

X-RAY EQUIPMENT

1 The X-Ray machine The quantity and quality of X-Rays produced depends respectively on the milliamperage and kilovoltage used by the machine. The kilovoltage controls the wavelength of the X-Rays produced and hence their penetrating power. Dental machines vary from 50 to 100 kvp (kilovolt peak). Most machines have a fixed kvp value. The higher the milliamperage the faster the X-Rays which are produced and so the shorter the exposure time necessary. In dental machines the range will be between 5 and 15 milliamps and the machines usually have a fixed value.

2, 3, 4 Density and contrast Density is the degree of blackness of a film, and contrast is the difference in the degrees of blackness between adjacent areas. Generally speaking the higher the kvp the greater the number of shades of grey will be recorded. This will tend to show early pathological changes in bone. The lower kvp values are more pleasing to the eye as they appear crisper showing mainly black or white and few shades of grey. A 65 kvp machine will be adequate for most dental purposes. The 3 radiographs illustrate the differences between 50, 65 and 90 kvp.

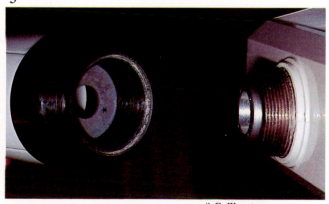

* Collimator

5 Collimation The X-Ray tube produces a divergent beam of X-Rays. The Collimator is a lead diaphragm with a circular aperture which removes the divergent rays, allowing only the more parallel beam to be emitted. Only those rays which are parallel or nearly parallel to the central ray are desirable for image formation because they cause the least distortion.

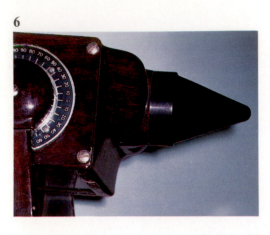

6

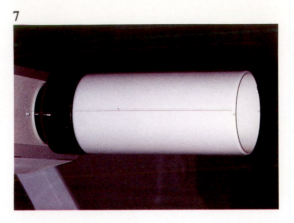

7

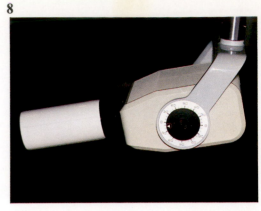

8

6, 7   Closed cone or open cylinder   The pointed closed cone (**6**) was designed originally as an aiming device but the plastic material deflects and scatters X-Rays, producing secondary radiation. The open ended cylinder (**7**) is advised for both bisecting and paralleling techniques.

8   Long or short cone   There are several lengths of cone which may be fitted to the X-Ray machine eight, twelve or sixteen inches. The purpose of the cone is to extend the distance between the X-Ray source and the film (focal film distance or ffd) which will produce a more parallel beam. The optimum distance for the ffd is between eight and sixteen inches. Most modern machines are now designed with the tube at the rear of the head which extends the ffd and means that an eight inch cone is satisfactory for most purposes (**8**).

9, 10   Film holders   These are designed to hold the film in a flat plane at right angles to the X-Ray beam to reduce distortion. The need is greater in the maxilla than the mandible due to the curve of the palate. If no holder is available cotton wool rolls placed alongside the maxillary teeth will help to prevent the film being bent by the patient's finger (**9**). In the mandible Spencer Wells clipped on to the film will make it simpler to place more accurately in the mouth and it is easier for the patient to hold (**10**).

Films   Several different makes and sizes are available but in endodontics periapical films are the ones most often used — DF-54, a children's film 34 mm. x 22 mm.; DF-57 for adults 40 mm. x 30 mm., which contains two films; and DF-58 containing a similar-sized single film. The children's size is useful for anteriors and small mouths in adults.

9

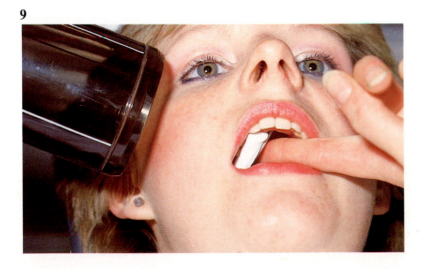

10

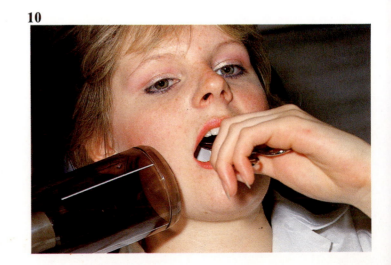

11 Three simple film holders are shown (**11**) a modified Spencer Wells; Snap-a-Ray[1] which is used for anteriors with a pre-set bisecting angle, the other end being used for posteriors; on the right, the Eggin[2] holder with a plastic section to hold the film and allow the patient to bite, the metal strip acting as an aiming device.

12 A more sophisticated device is the Rinn XCP[3] with localising ring. Two rings, a posterior (illustrated) and an anterior, are required for endodontics.

13, 14 The Masel[4] precision paralleling instrument is illustrated. A set of three are required, two posterior and one anterior.

For trade references (eg Snap-a-Ray[1]) see page 275.

11

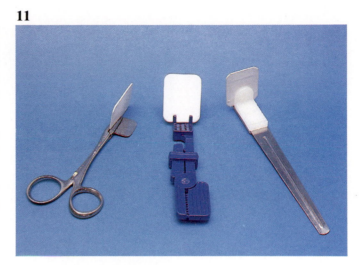

12

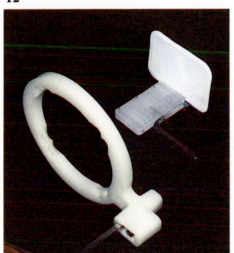

13

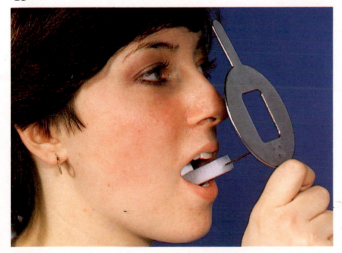

14

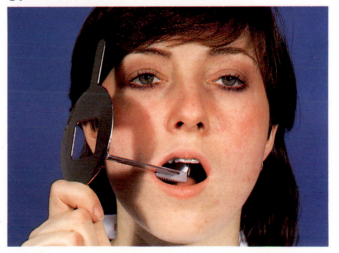

X-Ray processors In endodontics it is essential to have a quick method of processing films in the surgery. There are two types of processing, manual and automatic.

15 Manual A quick simple system is illustrated in the Super X30[1]. The film is enclosed in a white light-proof plastic container which includes two pull tabs to release developer and fixer into the container. Development takes place in 80 seconds. A Super X30 is shown processed (**16**).

The plastic box with a viewing panel (Westone Manumatic)[2] (**17, 18**) contains four baths, one developer, one fix and two water. A film may be processed in 45 seconds for viewing but will require further fixing and washing. The processor is sited in the surgery which is an obvious advantage as no darkroom is needed.

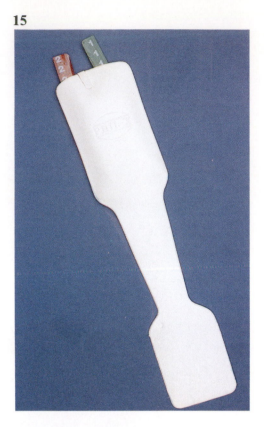

15

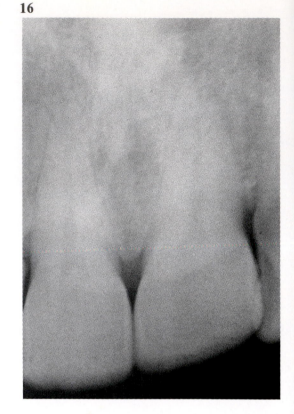

16

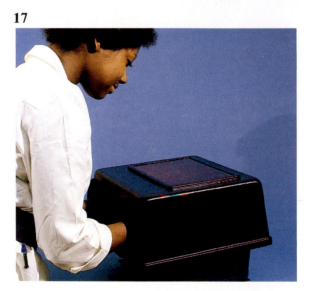

17

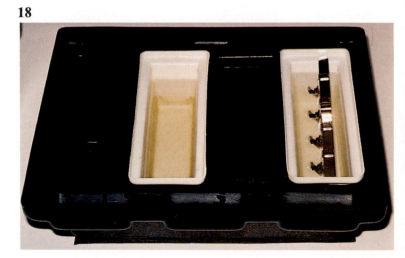

18

19

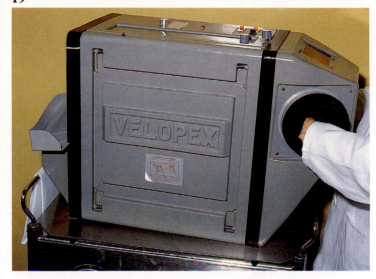

20

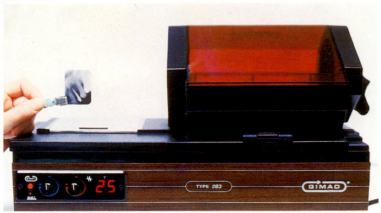

19, 20 Automatic A variety of machines are available. Some of them contain a heated blower. Although few processing faults should occur, these machines take considerably longer to develop and fix, usually about five minutes. An example at (**19**) is the Velopex[1] Automatic processor which takes all sizes of X-Ray films from children's to full skull X-Rays. Its advantage is that it includes a drying unit so that radiographs may be placed directly into the patient's records.

A recent addition to the range of automatic processors is the Gimad 283[2] (**20**). The advantage of this processor is that it develops, fixes and places the film in the water bath ready for viewing in 90 seconds.

21, 22 Viewers As much extraneous light should be removed as possible when viewing radiographs. This point is illustrated using the same radiograph with the background blacked out in (**22**).

21

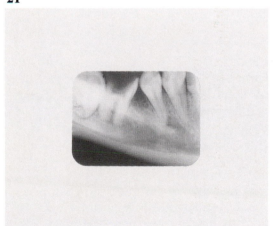

22

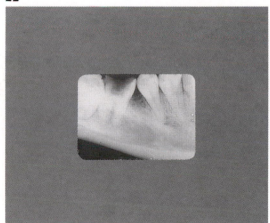

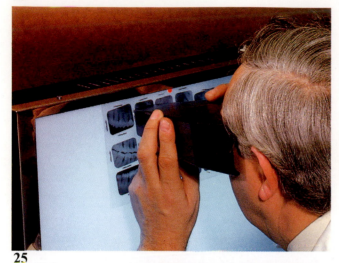

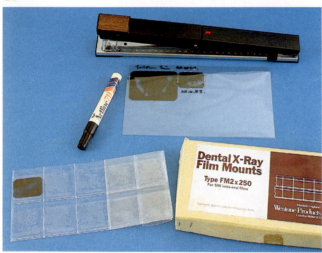

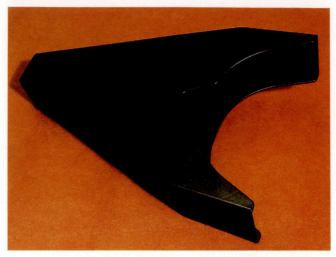

23, 24 A simple commercial viewing device which also magnifies is illustrated.

25 Mounts Radiographs must be kept with the patient's record and a method of mounting for easy viewing which also protects the film should be selected. Two methods are illustrated. One involves placing the film between two sheets of acetate[1] and stapling around but not through the film. A black permanent felt pen is used to record the patient's name and film date. The second method is simpler as the radiograph is merely placed into the pouch[2]. Each pouch is a single unit and may be torn from the roll, or a series may be kept together.

XERORADIOGRAPHY

Xeroradiography is a new technology using the Xeroradiographic copying process to record images produced by dental X-rays. Xeros is from the Greek word meaning dry which differentiates Xeroradiography from the conventional photochemical system which requires a dark room. Instead of an X-ray film, dental Xeroradiography uses a rigid aluminum photo-receptor plate. The plate is electrically charged, placed in a light-proof plastic cassette, positioned in the mouth and exposed to X-rays. The entire technique of image processing is fast, requiring only 25 seconds for a dry permanent image. The plates may be reconditioned, recharged and used repeatedly.

The Xeroradiograh may be viewed either by reflected or transilluminated light. The image gives a range of greys rather than the conventional X-ray film which exhibits optical densities from black through grey to white. However, the Xeroradiograph has the property of edge enhancement of all imaged boundaries, the result is an image which is superior in depicting small structures. The endodontic studies conclude that Xeroradiography provided better visualisation of metallic instrument tips and root apices, allowing more accurate length measurements. It appears to be a valuable addition to the endodontist's diagnostic armamentarium.

SAFETY

The dangers arising from excessive radiation to the patient, operator and staff may be reduced to a minimum providing simple precautions are observed. The first basic rule is that one radiograph is too many if it is not necessary. Concerning the patient there is no maximum dose for radiographic examinations needed for diagnosis and treatment. The benefit from dental radiography ordinarily outweighs the risks if radiographic examinations and techniques are properly chosen and executed. Safety in dental radiography may be divided into three areas, the patient, operator and staff, and the X-Ray equipment.

The patient The methods used to produce the minimum radiation dose to the patient are as follows:
1. The X-Ray cone should be pointed or the patient's head positioned so that the beam does not unnecessarily irradiate the body, in particular the gonads. Scattered radiation may reach the reproductive organs when any dental X-Rays are taken and for this reason a protective apron equivalent to 0.25

mm of lead is recommended. The patient shown is wearing a gonad protector (**26**).

2. Dental treatment which requires radiography during pregnancy should be postponed if possible until after the confinement. If radiography is necessary the most favourable time is in the middle trimester. Any dental radiography taken when the patient is pregnant should be done with the patient wearing a full protective apron (**27**).

3. Film holders and bite wing films should be used so that the patient does not hold the film packet with his hands.

4. Only those persons whose presence is essential should remain in a room during a radiographic exposure.

The operator and staff All those involved with taking radiographs should understand the danger of excessive radiation and be conversant with the safety precautions.

There are several units of measurement for radiation. There is a distinction between radiation exposure and dose. Exposure is the quantity of radiation in an area to which the patient is exposed. Dose is the amount of radiation absorbed per unit mass of tissue at a particular site.

Roentgen. This is a unit of exposure and is the amount of X-rays needed to produce one electrostatic unit in one cc of air in standard conditions.

rad. The radiation-absorbed dose is defined as 100 ergs of energy per gram of absorber.

rem. The roentgen equivalent in man is the dose of radiation that will produce the same biologic effects in man as are produced by the absorption of 1 R (Roentgen) of X-radiation or gamma radiation.

In Europe the unit of measurement for dose equivalent in the Sievert or in the old units is 100 rems.

The annual maximum permitted whole body dose is 50 msv (millisieverts).

Exposure to radiation can be checked by a film badge (**28**). Practitioners using X-Rays are strongly urged to obtain tests for themselves and their staff. It is considered unnecessary to monitor staff continuously when the radiation dose is unlikely to exceed 30 per cent of the maximum level permitted. An appropriate procedure would be for all staff concerned to wear a dosemeter for six separate four-week periods. Provided these doses are neither high nor extremely variable, the radiation check on staff should be continued by wearing a dosemeter for periods of four weeks every six months.

Persons under the age of 16 must not be allowed to assist in work with ionising radiations.

The radiation dose to the operator will be reduced by observing the following rules:

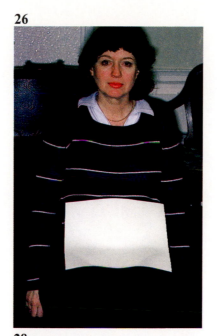

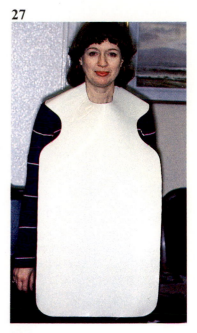

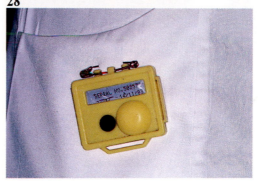

1. The operator should not stand in the direct beam during exposure.

2. The operator should stand at least 1.5 metres from the patient and the X-Ray tube during exposure. This distance should be increased to two metres if the X-Ray machine is higher than 70 Kv.

3. A protective barrier is only necessary if more than 300 periapical films are taken per week, providing all other safety rules are followed.

4. The tube housing the cone or the film must not be held by the operator or staff.

The equipment Periodic checks should be made on X-Ray equipment to ensure that there is no radiation leakage and that the timer is working correctly. The following points should be noted concerning safety:

1. The fastest X-Ray film should always be used.

2. If an extra-oral radiograph is required an intensifying screen must be used to reduce the exposure time.

3. For X-Ray machines up to 70 Kv a filter is required.

PROCESSING RADIOGRAPHS

Meticulous attention to the correct concentration of chemicals, their temperature and the right immersion times for the film must be observed.

A correctly processed radiograph is shown (29).

Operators must be aware of the various faults which may occur and their prevention:

1. Bent film The dark lines across the corners of the radiograph (30) are due to bending the film prior to insertion into the mouth.

2. Distortion The distortion occurs when the patient's finger pushes the film and adapts it to the shape of the curve of the dental arch or palate (31, 32).

3. Scratches When the film is wet after processing the emulsion is easily damaged causing a white scratch (33). A dark mark on the radiograph is due to damage to the film before it is developed (34). A common cause is pressure from a fingernail while removing the film from the packet for processing.

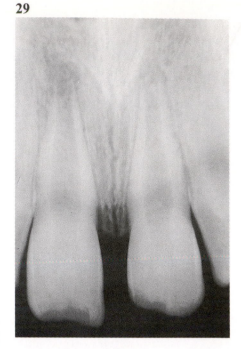

29

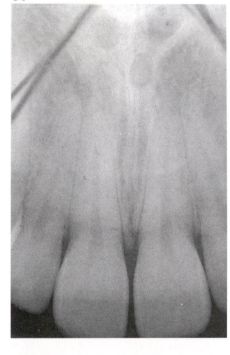

30

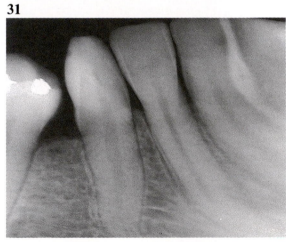

31

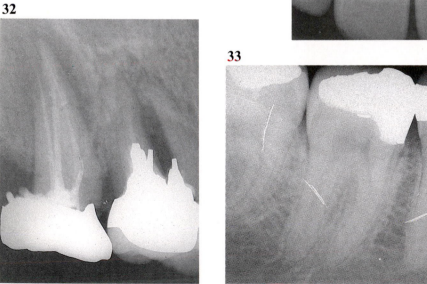

32

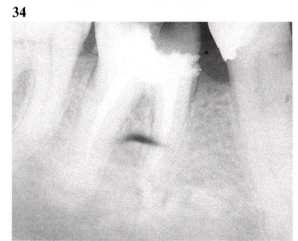

33

34

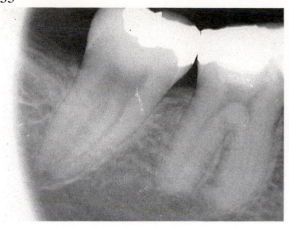

35

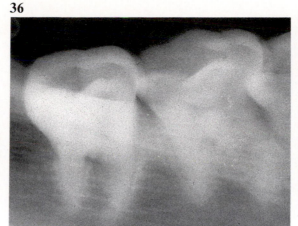

36

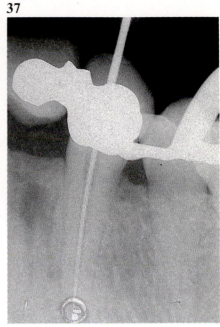

37

4. Partial image   Referred to as 'coning off'. If the X-Ray cone is not pointing towards the centre of the film part of the X-Ray beam may miss the film, leaving a curved white portion on the radiograph (35).

5. Blurred image   The radiographic image will be blurred if there is movement by the patient, film or the X-Ray tube (36).

6. Film clip   Care should be taken to place the film clip at or near the dot on the film. The radiograph shown (37) had the clip placed over the apex, making the film useless for estimating canal length.

7. Obstructions   All extraneous radiopaque objects must be removed from between the X-Ray cone and the film. Examples are a saliva ejector (38) and a radiopaque rubber dam frame (39). Sometimes spectacle frames which have metal inserts may be superimposed on the image.

38

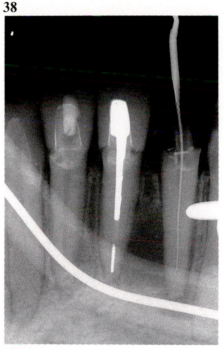

39

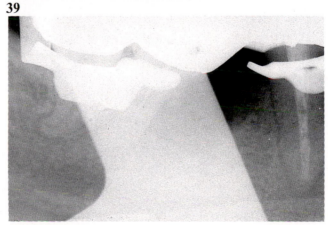

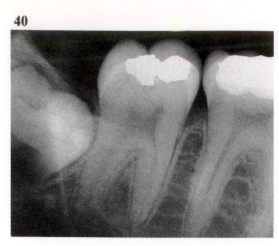

40

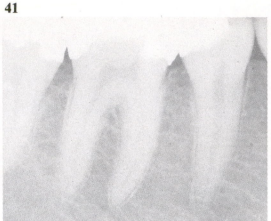

41

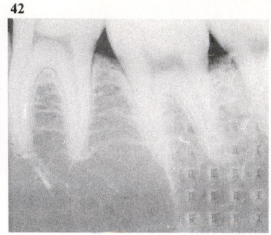

42

8. Dark Film (40) This may be due to:

Prolonged exposure time

Prolonged development time

Temperature of developer too high

Developer too concentrated

9. Light Film (41) This may be due to:

Insufficient exposure time

Insufficient development time

Developer exhausted

Developer temperature too low

Developer concentration too weak

10. Reversed film A film that has been exposed in the mouth the wrong way around appears light and also displays a pattern shown here (42) on the right hand side.

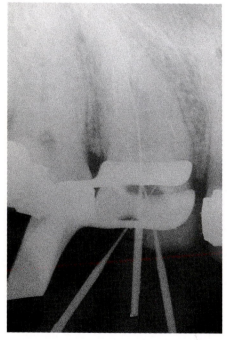

43

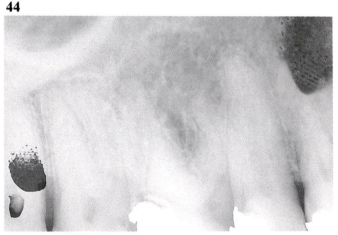

44

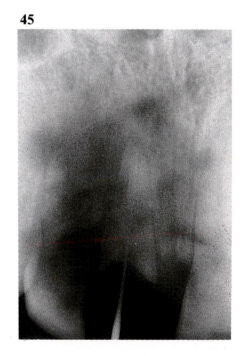

45

11. Fogging (43) This may be due to:

Prolonged or incorrect storage of film

Extraneous X-radiation before or after exposure

Exposure to daylight before fixing

Faulty safe light

12. Spots, streaks, browning and encrustations Meticulous attention to clean processing and thorough fixing and washing in running water will prevent most of these faults from occurring. The illustrations show fix marks (44) and poor fixing (45).

13. Blank Film. This may be due to:

X-Ray machine not switched on

An unexposed film was inadvertently developed

The film was placed directly into the fix

14. Black film. This is caused by exposure to light before developing.

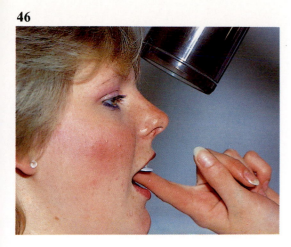

46

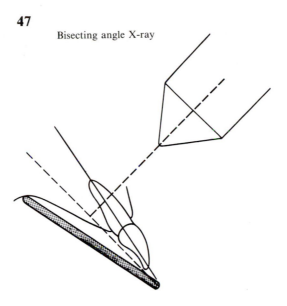

47

Bisecting angle X-ray

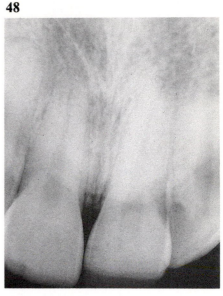

48

PERIAPICAL RADIOGRAPHIC TECHNIQUES

Two methods of taking periapical radiographs are the bisecting angle and the parallel techniques.

Bisecting angle technique   (BA) The film is positioned close to the lingual or palatal surface of the tooth. The X-Ray cone is directed at right angles to a line bisecting the plane of the film and the long axis of the tooth (**47**). The illustration (**46**) shows a bisecting angle radiograph being taken of the central incisors. Note the acute angle of the tube.

The bisecting angle radiograph is shown (**48**).

Paralleling technique   The film is positioned in the mouth parallel to the long axis of the tooth. To achieve this in the maxillary arch the film must be held away from the tooth. The X-Ray cone is then directed along a line at right angles to the film. The X-Ray tube must be positioned further from the patient than in the BA technique (increased ffd) to reduce the magnification of the image by allowing only the more parallel X-Rays to reach the film (**50**). An extended cone is often used to help direct the X-Ray beam accurately and it is this which has given rise to the term long cone, which is incorrect. The method should be referred to as the paralleling technique.

A paralleling radiograph is shown (**49**) being taken of the central incisors using a Rinn holder and localising ring. The resultant radiograph is shown (**51**).

51

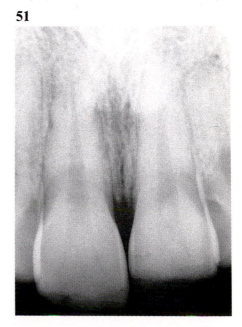

49

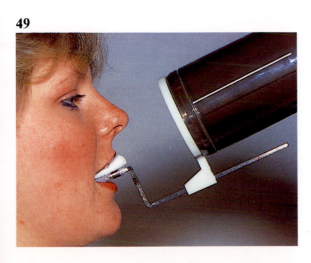

50

Parallel X-ray

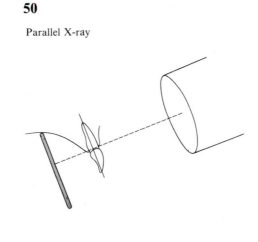

ADVANTAGES AND DISADVANTAGES OF THE BISECTING ANGLE AND PARALLELING TECHNIQUES

Bisecting Angle

1. Quick and easy to use.

2. Relatively easy and comfortable for the patient.

3. Will produce distorted radiographs.

4. May be used in all mouths.

5. Simple to use with rubber dam in place.

6. Zygomatic arch frequently superimposed over apices of maxillary molar teeth.

7. Difficult to reproduce a radiograph on recall for comparison.

8. No additional equipment required.

9. Possible to have partial image by coning off.

10. Difficult to take same tooth from different angles without severe distortion.

Paralleling

1. Inexpertly used it takes longer but with regular use it is as easy, quick and produces more reliable results.

2. Often uncomfortable for the patient.

3. Almost distortion free radiographs produced.

4. Difficult to take in small mouths or patients with shallow flattened palates.

5. Difficult to take with a rubber dam in place.

6. Apices lie below Zygomatic arch on radiograph.

7. Easily reproducible mandatory for comparing periapical radiolucencies and bone levels on recall.

8. Film holder required.

9. Coning off is unlikely to occur providing localising ring used.

10. Simple and useful to view tooth undistorted from several angles.

11. RADIATION DOSE IS SIMILAR FOR BOTH TECHNIQUES

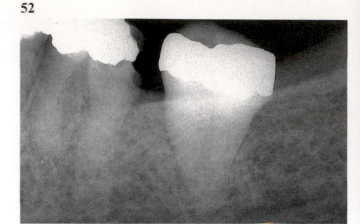

52 Bisecting angle. The patient complained of pain from the lower left first molar. No cause is visible from this radiograph.

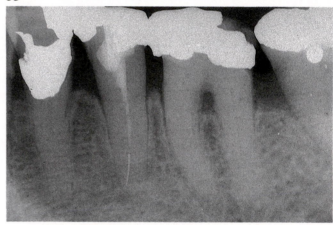

53 Paralleling Technique. The lower left first molar is in the correct relation to the bone level. Furcation involvement is apparent.

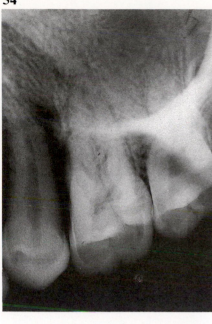

54 Bisecting angle. The Zygomatic arch is superimposed over the tooth of both first and second maxillary molars. The bone level is indistinct.

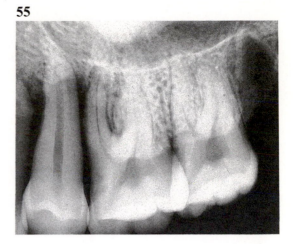

56, 57, 58 Below are three radiographs taken from different angles of a post which has perforated the central incisor. The diagrams explain the changes in position of the post and root on the radiographs.

55 Paralleling Technique. The molar root formation is visible and the teeth are in their correct relationship to the antrum and bone levels.

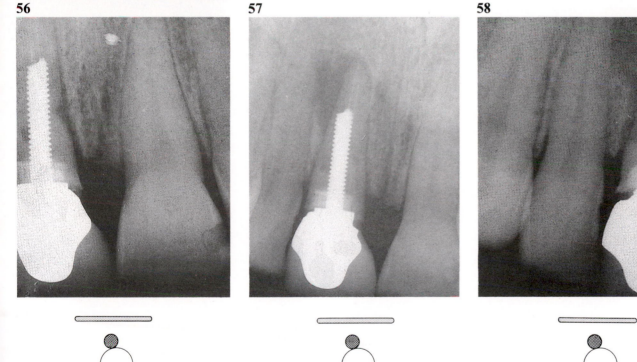

The paralleling technique is useful in the maxilla, particularly in the molar region. In the mandible it is of limited use because the anatomy allows the film to be placed alongside the tooth and parallel to its long axis.

In endodontics it is recommended that a paralleling technique is used for the pre-operative and postoperative radiographs. The bisecting angle is used during treatment when the rubber dam is in place. A compromise treatment between the two techniques is achieved with the use of cotton wool rolls between the tooth and the film so that the film is made more parallel to the tooth.

NORMAL RADIOGRAPHIC LANDMARKS

59 Enamel, dentine and cementum Enamel is the most radiopaque structure. Dentine should be uniform in density. In the radiograph note the 'burnt out' appearance around the enamo-dentinal junction. This is observed commonly and may easily be mistaken for caries. Cementum cannot be seen radiographically.

Cancellous bone The bony trabeculae have a coarser pattern in the mandible and tend to run horizontally. Compare **59** with the finer lace-like pattern found in the maxilla (**60**).

Periodontal ligament (pdl) Often referred to as the periodontal ligament space on the radiograph. It should be narrow and even around the whole of the root surface that lies within the bone. Any definite widening of the pdl space suggests the presence of pathology.

Lamina dura Despite the definite appearance of a white line surrounding the roots of teeth within bone, investigation has revealed that there is no increase in mineralisation of the cancellous bone lining the tooth socket. The lamina dura therefore is a radiographic artefact and it would be unwise to place too critical an interpretation on the variation in its appearance in diagnosis.

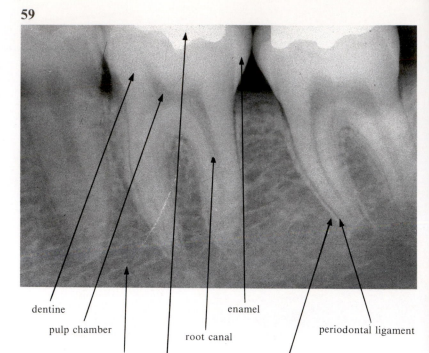

59

dentine · pulp chamber · cancellous bone · metallic restoration · enamel · root canal · lamina dura · periodontal ligament

60 Pulp and pulp stones The pulp chamber and larger canals are readily visible on the radiograph, but finer canals such as those in the disto-buccal canal of the maxillary first molar (**60**) may be more difficult to see. Root canals will never become completely sclerosed in the apical portion of the root. Pulp stones are evident in both molar teeth. Clinically the stones present few problems and their removal is easy from the chamber, although if they become lodged in a root canal they can present difficulties.

61

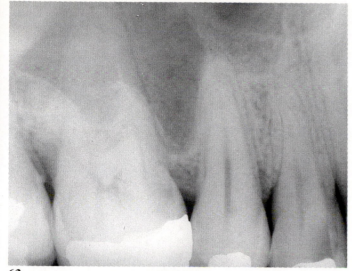

62

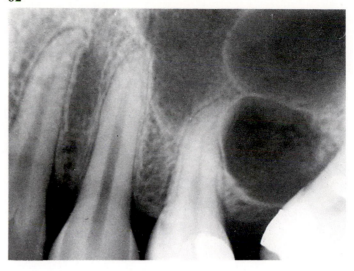

63

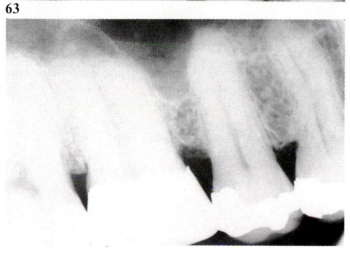

61, 62 Maxillary antrum The antrum may extend from the premolars to the tuberosity. The apices of the second premolar and first molar lie close to or in the antrum. The floor of the antrum may dip between the roots (**61**). The antrum may be loculated giving the appearance of a cyst (**62**).

63 The white line on the radiograph representing the floor of the antrum should be observed carefully. An apparent periapical lesion is shown (**63**) involving the palatal root apex, but on closer examination it is seen to be the continuation of the antral floor.

64 Median suture The median suture of the maxilla appears as a radiolucent line between the central incisors.

Anterior nasal spine The anterior nasal spine appears as a V-shaped radiopacity which lies above or is superimposed on the incisive foramen.

Nasal septum The nasal septum separates the two nasal fossae and is seen as a radiopaque white line.

Nose and lipline The outline of the nose is a definite line across the radiograph. A similar line in both upper and lower anterior radiographs often represents the lip line.

64

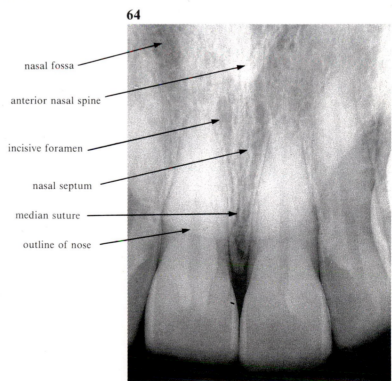

nasal fossa

anterior nasal spine

incisive foramen

nasal septum

median suture

outline of nose

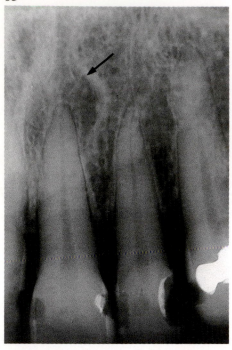

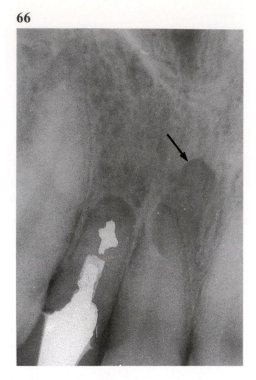

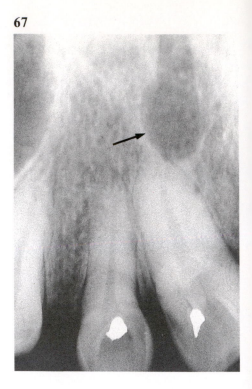

65, 66, 67 Incisive foramen The radiolucent circular shadow of the incisive foramen may be superimposed over the apex of a central incisor and so be mistaken for a periapical lesion. Three examples of incisive foramina are shown (see arrows).

68, 69 Mandibular canal The mandibular canal or inferior dental canal runs from the mandibular foramen in the ramus to the mental foramen. It is seen as a radiolucent band and may lie in close association with the apices of molar and second premolar teeth. Extrusion of medicaments and root canal filling materials may damage the inferior dental bundle.

68

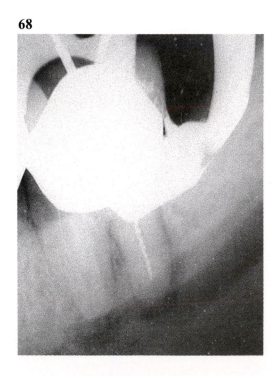

69

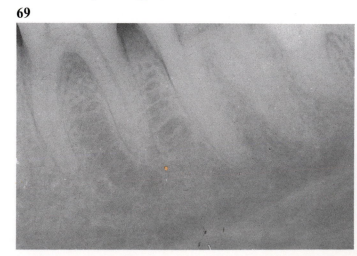

70

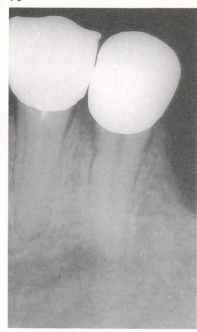

71

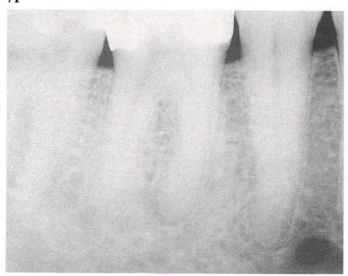

70, 71 Mental foramen The foramen is located below and distal to the apex of the first premolar. This foramen may be mistaken for a pathological lesion when it appears close to the apex of one of the premolars, which is due to the angle at which the radiograph is taken.

72

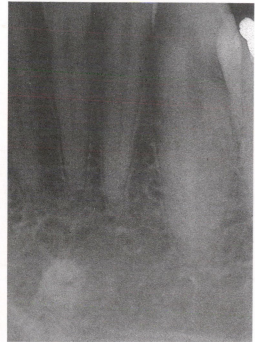

72 Lingual foramen In radiographs of the lower incisor area the lingual foramen may be seen as a white radiopaque area with a small central radiolucent dot.

73

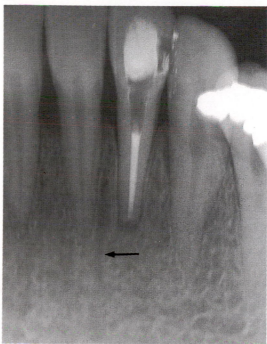

73 Nutrient canal Nutrient canals contain blood vessels supplying the bone and occur in both mandible and maxilla. The nutrient canal illustrated (arrow) lies between the central and lateral incisors as a vertical radiolucent line.

RADIOLUCENCIES OF DENTAL ORIGIN

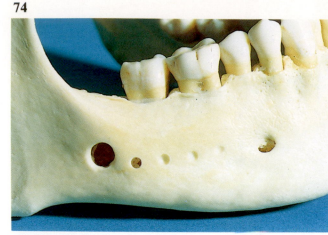

74 Care should be taken in the interpretation of radiolucent areas in the mandible and maxilla. Different angulations of the X-Ray tube can produce different radiographic appearances. Note the succession of bur holes in the buccal cortical plate. The holes become progressively deeper from right to left until a large hole has been cut through the cortical plate.

75

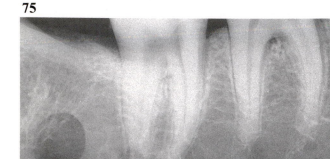

76

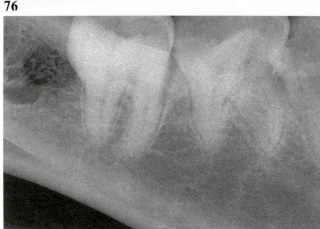

75, 76 These two radiographs were taken of the mandibular area. The first, a parallel radiograph, shows all the bur cavities. The second, a bisecting angle, shows the smaller cavities are no longer visible.

77

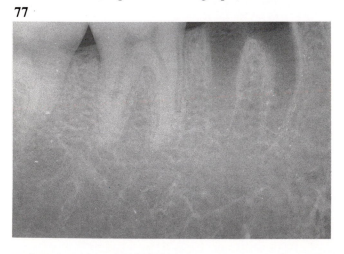

78

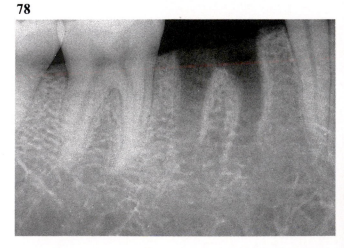

77, 78 A considerable amount of cancellous bone may be destroyed without showing any apparent change in the radiograph. In these two radiographs a tooth was extracted from a dried skull and a radiograph taken. The second radiograph was taken after a No. 8 round bur had been used to remove the apical socket area and a large amount of cancellous bone in the apical area. No difference is apparent on the radiograph.

79

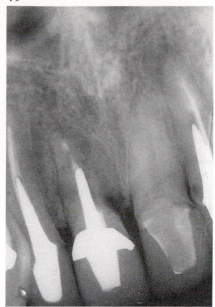

80

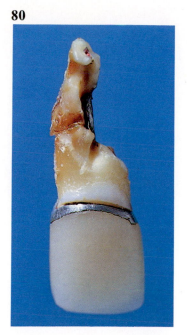

79, 80 It is a consistent clinical finding that the amount of bone or tooth loss is actually greater than shown on the radiograph. The radiograph (**79**) suggests there is a possibility of treatment with the post crowned central. The extracted tooth shows the condition was not treatable.

82

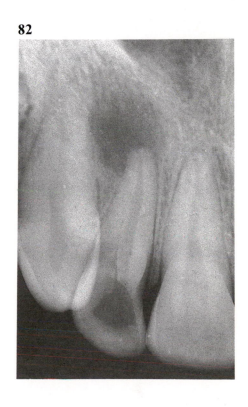

81, 82 Periapical areas The commonest radiolucency found in the jaws is associated with the apices of teeth. It is important in endodontics to be able to interpret early bony changes resulting from pulpal pathology.

Two definite periapical areas are shown in **81** and **82.** In **81** there is a radiopaque line surrounding the area, which usually suggests the lesion is long standing and relatively slow growing. The area in **82** has no radiopaque surround, suggesting a more recent and faster growing lesion. It is not possible to diagnose either of these lesions as cystic from the radiograph.

81

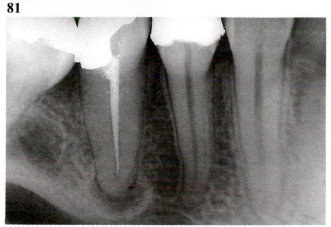

83

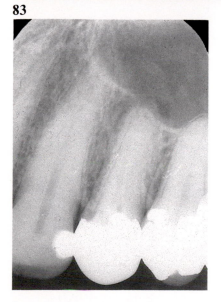

84

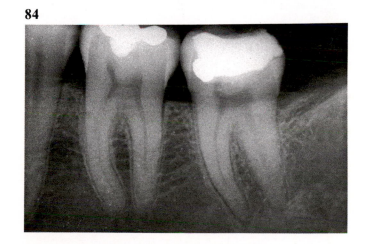

83, 84 Earlier periapical changes are illustrated. The first premolar (**83**) has a definite but discrete area around the apex and the other radiograph shows a definite widened pdl space around the apical third of the mesial root of the distal molar.

85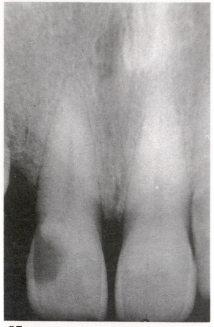

86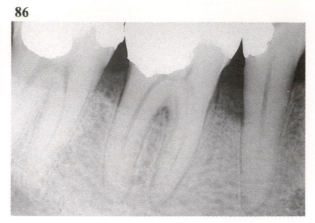

85, 86 Very early periapical change may be seen in the cancellous bone around the apex. An alteration in the pattern of the bony trabeculae which appear to become orientated around the apex. In addition there may be a slight increase in radiopacity. Some of these early changes may be reversible and the vitality of the pulp maintained. The upper right central (**85**) has a large carious cavity and early periapical change. **86** shows a widened pdl space around the mesial root of the first molar and some increase in density of the trabeculae. There is also some furcation involvement with a widened pdl space.

87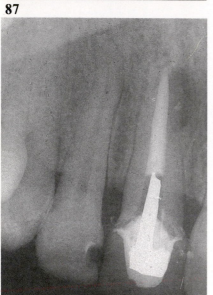

88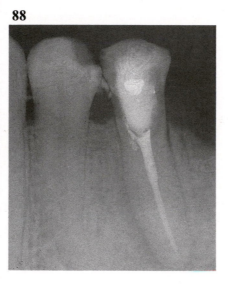

87, 88 Lateral areas The radiographs show a widened pdl space not associated with the apex but still caused by pulpal pathology. Lateral canals are frequently responsible and are visible in both these cases. The radiographs have been taken immediately after treatment.

90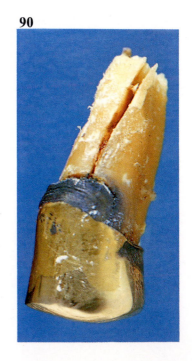

89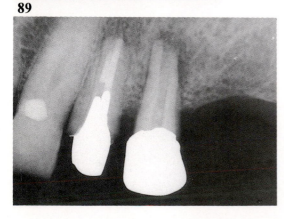

89, 90 Fractured roots may be difficult to diagnose. The second premolar shown (**89**) has an area associated with the apex and also involving the distal aspect of the root. Close examination of the distal wall of the root canal shows a vertical radiolucent line. The photograph of the extracted tooth (**90**) shows the extent of the fracture.

91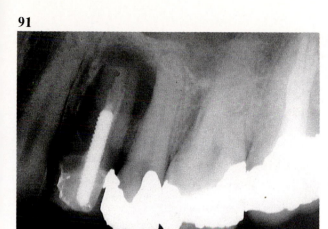

92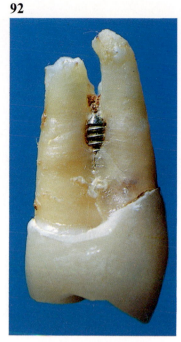

93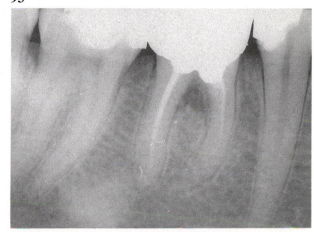

94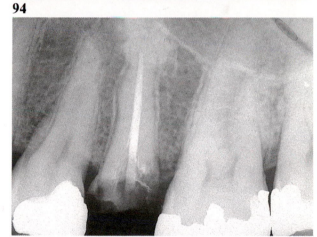

95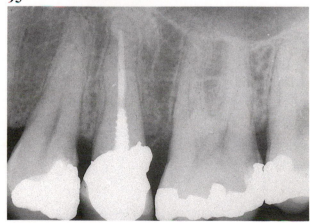

91, 92 Perforations of the lateral wall of the root or furcation will cause rapid bone loss. The cause of the bone loss in the radiograph is self evident when the extracted root is examined.

Condensing osteitis This is not a radiolucency and may or may not be of dental origin. Condensing osteitis is a radiopacity which occurs as a response to some form of injury such as low grade infection or excessive physical stress. The condition is symptomless. Characteristically it is not as radiopaque as enamel.

93, 94 The two examples shown are probably of dental origin. **93** shows condensing osteitis near the distal apex of lower right first molar which has been inadequately root filled.

94 Shows the radiopacity associated with the apex of the upper second premolar. A follow-up one year later (**95**) shows that the condition has remained unchanged.

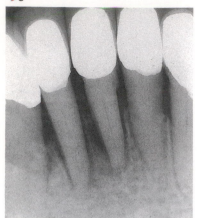

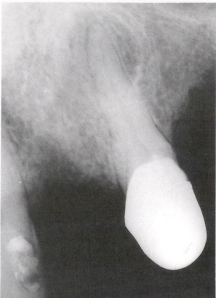

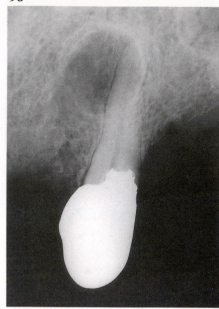

RADIOLUCENCIES NOT ASSOCIATED WITH ROOTS

Advanced periodontal disease will produce bony pockets visible on the radiograph. In this case (**96**) the teeth were vital and the lateral bone loss due to pocketing.

The radiograph (**97**) shows a round radiolucent area superimposed over the apex of a single standing maxillary premolar. The most important aspect is that the pdl space surrounding the root is narrow and even, suggesting that the area is not associated with the root. The second radiograph (**98**) supports this view as it has been taken from a different angle and the area has moved in relation to the root. Vital response to pulp testing further supported the view that the radiolucency was not associated with the premolar.

99 Cementoma stage one Early cementomas present as radiolucent areas, often around the apices of mandibular incisors. They progress over a period of about six years to radiopaque areas. The teeth remain vital to the pulp test and no treatment is required.

100 Cementoma stage two The radiopacity associated with the mesial aspect of lower right first molar is typical of a cementoma stage two. The tooth is vital and the pdl space is continuous around both roots. Cementomas are symptomless and harmless, and so require no treatment.

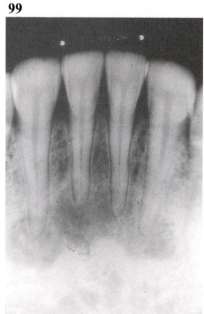

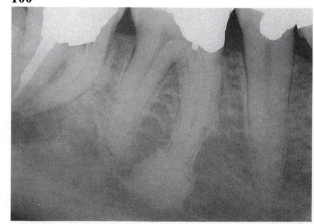

2 Histology of the pulp C J Stock

THE DENTAL PULP

This chapter is intended as a reminder of some of the clinical aspects of histology of the pulp and periapical tissues, namely:

Tooth development
Pulp
Dentine
Pulpal calcifications
Pulpal inflammation
Periapical inflammation

TOOTH DEVELOPMENT

The enamel of a tooth is derived from ectoderm and the pulp and dentine from the ectomesenchyme. During the sixth week of embryonic life tooth formation begins as a localised proliferation of ectoderm associated with the maxillary and mandibular processes. The formation of the tooth germ may be divided into three separate stages, the bud, the cap and the bell.

101   The Bud   This initial stage of tooth development begins with the epithelial cells of the dental lamina which proliferate and produce a bud-like projection called the enamel organ. The dental papilla is first seen at this stage as a proliferation of cells beneath the dental lamina at sites corresponding to the positions of the primary teeth.

102   The Cap   The cells of the dental lamina form a concavity giving a caplike appearance. The outer cells of the cap are cuboidal and constitute the outer enamel epithelium. The cells in the concavity are elongated and form the inner enamel epithelium. Between the two layers is a network of cells referred to as the stellate reticulum. The rim of the enamel organ is called the cervical loop.

101

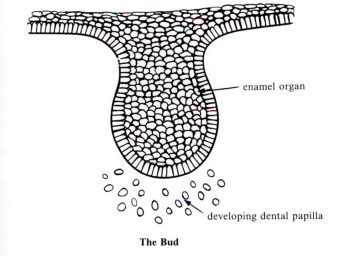

enamel organ

developing dental papilla

The Bud

102

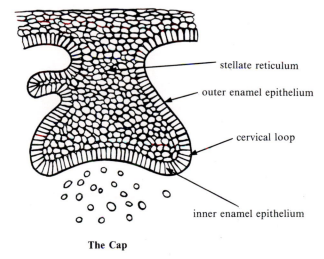

stellate reticulum

outer enamel epithelium

cervical loop

inner enamel epithelium

The Cap

103 The Bell The cells of the cervical loop proliferate and partially enclose the dental papilla, producing a bell shape. A vascular network is developed at this stage in the dental papilla. The condensed ectomesenchyme surrounding the enamel organ and the dental papilla forms the dental sac which develops finally into the periodontal ligament.

The connection between the oral epithelium and the enamel organ is broken by the invasion of mesenchymal cells into the dental lamina. The free end of each dental lamina associated with each primary tooth continues to grow and it is from this structure that the permanent teeth develop.

Differentiation of epithelium and mesenchymal cells into ameloblasts and odontoblasts respectively occurs during the bell stage.

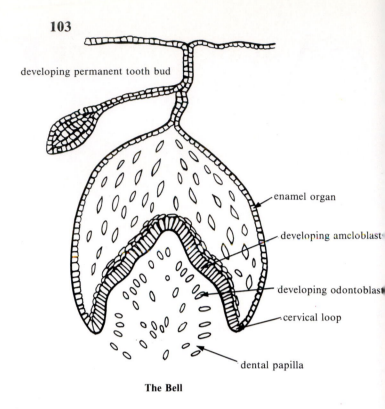

103

developing permanent tooth bud

enamel organ

developing ameloblast

developing odontoblast

cervical loop

dental papilla

The Bell

104 Shows ameloblasts and early odontoblasts. Both types of cell are more fully differentiated at the apex of the bell, the area of the cusp tip, than towards the cervical loop. Although the ameloblasts reach maturity before the odontoblasts, it is the dentine matrix which is formed in advance of the enamel matrix.

The basement membrane gradually disappears as the Von Korff fibres appear. The origin and function of these fibres is unclear.

The developing odontoblasts extend several small processes towards the ameloblasts. The predentine layer is now formed and the odontoblasts start to move away towards the central pulp depositing a matrix. Within the matrix the processes become accentuated and form the odontoblast process. It is around these processes that the dentinal tubules are formed.

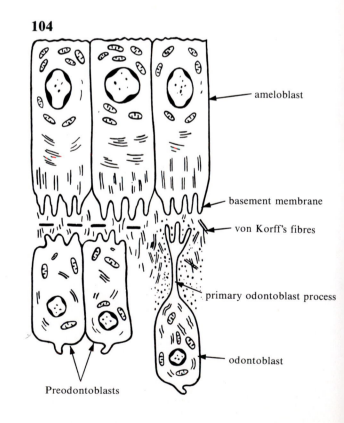

104

ameloblast

basement membrane

von Korff's fibres

primary odontoblast process

odontoblast

Preodontoblasts

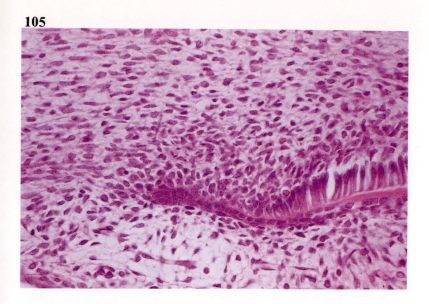

105 Root development Root development starts once the enamel formation is complete. The cervical loop proliferates forming Hertwig's epithelial root sheath, which determines the size and shape of the root or roots of the tooth. Cells in the dental papilla lying close to the enamel epithelium differentiate into pre-odontoblasts and odontoblasts. As soon as the first layer of dentine matrix mineralises gaps appear in the root sheath, allowing mesenchymal cells from the dental sac to contact the newly-formed dentine. These cells then differentiate into cementoblasts and deposit cementum matrix onto the dentine.

Remnants of Hertwig's root sheath persist and are known as cell rests of Malassez. In the presence of chronic inflammation these epithelial cells may proliferate and form a periapical or radicular cyst.

Lateral Canals There are two theories concerning the formation of lateral canals:

(1) During growth of the root sheath a small area fails to form, leaving a gap. Dentinogenesis will not take place opposite the defect. The result is a lateral canal between the dental sac and the pulp.
(2) The lack of dentine formation around a blood vessel which is already present connecting the dental papilla with the surrounding mesenchymal tissue.

PULP

There are several features of the pulp which distinguish it from tissue found elsewhere in the body:

(1) The pulp is surrounded by rigid walls, and so is unable to expand as a response to injury as part of the inflammatory process. Pulpal tissue is therefore susceptible to a change in pressure which will affect the pain threshold.
(2) There is minimal collateral blood supply to pulp tissue, which will reduce its capacity for repair following injury.
(3) The pulp is composed almost entirely of simple connective tissue, yet at its periphery it is a layer of highly sophisticated cells, the odontoblasts. Secondary dentine is gradually deposited as a physiological process which reduces the blood supply and therefore the resistance to infection or trauma.
(4) The innervation of pulp tissue is both simple and complex. Simple in that there are only free nerve endings and consequently the pulp lacks proprioception. Complex because of the innervation of the odontoblast processes which produces a high level of sensitivity to thermal and chemical change.

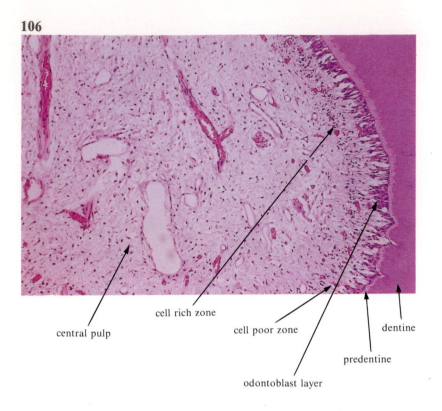

central pulp   cell rich zone   cell poor zone   dentine

odontoblast layer

predentine

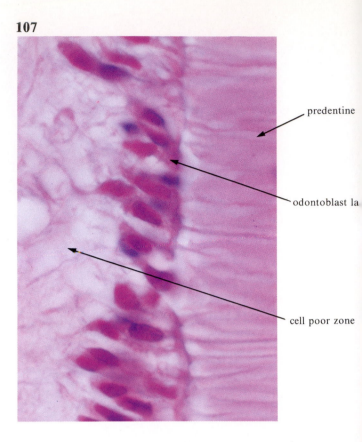

predentine

odontoblast la

cell poor zone

106 Four Zones The mature healthy pulp may be divided into four zones which are illustrated:

Central pulp. The central mass of the pulp contains the larger blood vessels and nerve fibres. The connective tissue cells composed mainly of fibroblasts, together with a network of collagen fibres, are embedded within the connective tissue ground substance.

Cell rich zone. This layer is more prominent in the coronal than the radicular pulp. Apart from fibroblasts the cell rich zone contains a variable number of macrophages, lymphocytes and plasma cells. Odontoblasts that become irreversibly damaged are replaced by cells that migrate from the cell rich zone.

Cell poor zone. The cell poor zone lies immediately beneath the odontoblast layer and is so called because it is relatively free of cells. The zone tends to disappear during periods of cellular activity in a young pulp, rapidly forming dentine and in older pulps where reparative dentine is being formed.

107 Odontoblast layer A higher magnification is shown of this zone. The odontoblastic layer is composed mainly of cell bodies as the odontoblast process lies within the dentine. The layer also contains capillaries and nerve fibres. The odontoblasts vary in height so that their nuclei are not all at the same level, which gives the appearance of a layer several cells in thickness.

There is some disagreement on how far the odontoblast process extends outwards into the dentine. Opinions vary from the mid-dentine to the dentinoenamel junction.

The odontoblast is considered incapable of further division once it is fully mature. Replacements are thought to migrate from the cell rich zone as undifferentiated mesenchymal cells.

108

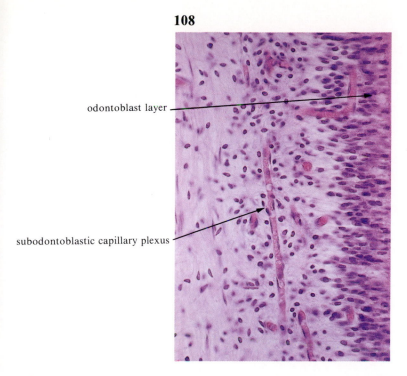

odontoblast layer

subodontoblastic capillary plexus

109

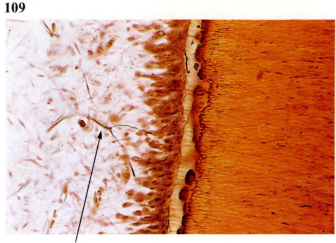

plexus of Raschkow

108 Vascular supply One or more arterioles, branches of the dental artery, enter the tooth via the apical foramen. Smaller vessels may enter through lateral canals. The arterioles pass through the central core of the pulp giving off branches that spread laterally towards the odontoblast layer beneath which they ramify to form an extensive plexus.

The blood passes from the plexus into progressively larger venules, descends through the middle of the pulp and exits through the foramen or foramina. Venules in the pulp have unusually thick walls and are generally larger in diameter than arterioles.

109 Innervation The innervation of the pulp includes both afferent fibres, which conduct sensory impulses, and autonomic fibres which control the micro-circulation.

The nerve fibres enter the foramina alongside the blood vessels and pass through the radicular pulp. In the coronal pulp the nerves send branches to the peripheral pulp where the plexus of Raschkow is formed beneath the cell rich zone. Terminal axons pass beneath the odontoblasts to the predentine, some fibres enter the dentinal tubules and lie in close association with the odontoblast processes.

The sensitivity of the dentine can be explained by the hydrodynamic theory. The theory suggests that when dentine is heated or cooled there is a rapid movement of fluid in the dentinal tubules that mechanically may deform the nerve fibres near the pulpodentinal junction and so induce pain. The arrows in the diagram (**110**) show the direction of movement of dentinal fluid, on the application of A (heat) and B (cold).

Desiccation of exposed dentine during restorative procedures can produce displacement of the odontoblast cell bodies into the tubules presumably due to the hydrodynamic forces. Once displaced the odontoblasts undergo autolysis and disappear from the tubules.

110

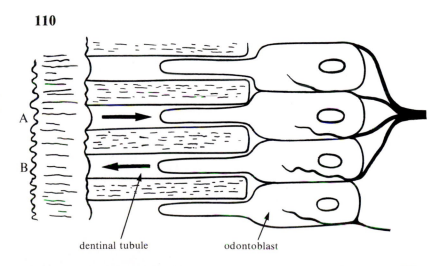

A

B

dentinal tubule   odontoblast

111

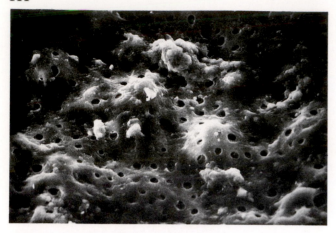

112

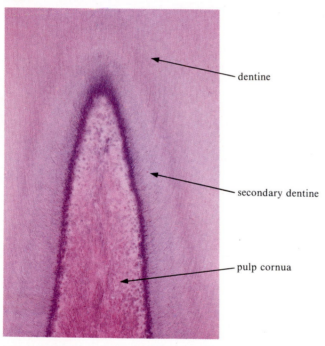

dentine

secondary dentine

pulp cornua

111 Dentine The elasticity of dentine provides a flexible base for the brittle layer of enamel. Dentine (**111**) is composed of mineralised tubules which house the odontoblast processes. The tubules extend from the dentinoenamel junction, DEJ, or the dentino-cemental junction to the pulp. In the coronal dentine the tubules have a gentle 'S' shape as they extend from the DEJ to the pulp. The number of tubules per sq. mm is approximately 29,500. The percentage area occupied by the tubules decreases with age due to the progressive formation of peritubular dentine which narrows their lumen.

This narrowing or sclerosis results in a reduced permeability of dentine which protects the pulp from irritation. Sclerosis is a feature of dentine in the older patient and is recognised by an increase in translucency.

Two types of dentine may be produced in the mature tooth, secondary dentine (**112**) which is a response to age and is laid down slowly throughout the walls of the pulp chamber and canal system. Reparative dentine, the second type, is produced in response to injury and is formed only on the dentinal wall opposite the site of irritation.

Compared to primary dentine reparative dentine is less tubular and the tubules tend to be more irregular with larger lumina. The quality of dentine varies according to the amount of inflammation present, the extent of cellular injury, and the state of differentiation of the replacement odontoblasts.

PULPAL CALCIFICATION

Calcification of pulp tissue is thought to be a pathological condition. The calcifications may be found as pulp stones in the pulp chamber but in the radicular pulp they are more diffuse. Pulp stones will vary in size from microscopic (**113**) particles to filling almost the entire pulp chamber (**114**). The cause of pulpal calcification is unknown. It is also unclear whether pulp stones can cause pain or not as they are a common occurrence.

113

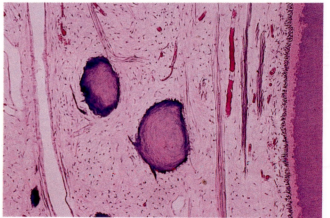

114

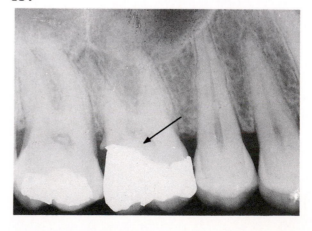

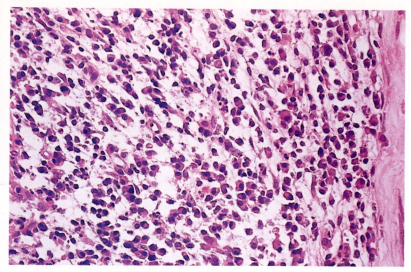

PULPAL INFLAMMATION

The causes of pulpal inflammation may be bacterial, iatrogenic, due to restorative procedures, or traumatic.

The sequence of events in inflammation of the pulp is now relatively well understood. The process is similar to that found in other parts of the body except that it is influenced because it occurs in a confined space with minimum collateral circulation. The initial inflammation starts in the pulp at or close to the site of the insult.

115   Shows an inflamed pulp. There is a large increase in the cellular concentration composed mainly in the acute stage of poiymorphonuclear leucocytes and mononuclear cells.

If the irritation to the pulp is sufficient the following events occur:

(1)   Inflammatory exudate passes through the walls of the blood vessels into the surrounding pulp tissue. Since fluid is not compressible there is a rise in tissue pressure.
(2)   The increase in pressure collapses the thin walls of the venules so that blood flow is interrupted, producing stasis and anoxia. This will lead in time to localised tissue necrosis.
(3)   Necrotic tissue releases chemical mediators which increase the permeability of the vascular walls and also the osmotic pressure in the surrounding tissue. The tissue pressure rises and further blood vessels are affected.
(4)   Once pus appears, forming a micro-abscess, the process is irreversible. The continued spread of local inflammation will gradually involve the entire pulp, producing total necrosis.

PERIAPICAL INFLAMMATION

Periapical inflammation is an extension of the pulpal inflammatory process. The periapical tissues will become involved well before total necrosis of the pulp has occurred. This explains why the pulp may be sensitive in a tooth with a radiolucent area associated with the apex.

As bacteria or their toxins, or breakdown products from the pulp itself, leak through the apical foramina and lateral canals, an inflammatory response is started. The surrounding bone is absorbed and this may be seen radiographically at first as a widening of the periodontal ligament space and later as a radiolucent area. It should be pointed out that periapical disease may be present which does not show radiographically.

Continued inflammation of the periapical tissues may stimulate the dormant epithelial cells found in the periodontal ligament (Cell rests of Malassez) to proliferate. Strands of epithelial cells are commonly found within the granulation tissue around the apex. The reason why in some cases cystic formation occurs with the appearance of epithelial lined cavities is not known.

116   Shows a granuloma attached to the apex of a root.

116

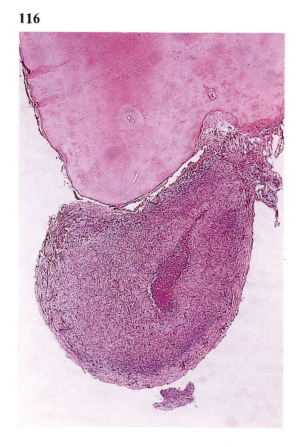

3 Diagnosis and treatment planning C J Stock

The differential diagnosis of facial pain is one of the most difficult problems to confront a dentist. Skill and knowledge is often required to locate, diagnose and finally treat pain of pulpal origin. Some of the difficulties involved are illustrated and some guidelines are suggested.

Diagnosis

CASE HISTORY

Every patient who attends for the first time for treatment should have a case history taken. An example of the front of a patient's folder is shown.

SURNAME ....

C.NAMES...

DATE OF BIRTH ....

M.G.P.'S NAME ....

ADDRESS ....

....

....

TEL. NO. HOME ....

WORK ....

Date of History   Reviewed on

PREVIOUS MEDICAL HISTORY

RHEUMATIC F. (Suspect, confirmed)   YES   NO
    In bed for ...... weeks, months.

HYPERTENSION OR CARDIAC DISEASE   YES   NO

HEPATITIS ....   YES   NO
PREGNANT.....................................   YES   NO
UPPER RESP. TRACT INFECTIONS ....   YES   NO
ALLERGIES TO ....   YES   NO
        ANTIBIOTICS ....   YES   NO
        LOCAL ANAEST. ....   YES   NO
        OTHER DRUGS ....   YES   NO
TAKING ANY DRUGS NOW? ....   YES   NO
        ANTICOAGULANTS ....   YES   NO
        STEROIDS ....   YES   NO
        INSULIN.......................................   YES   NO
        TRANQUILLISERS.......................   YES   NO
        OTHER ....   YES   NO
UNDER TREATMENT BY G.P. OR HOSP.. YES   NO
SERIOUS ILLNESS PAST 3 YRS.   YES   NO

APPOINTMENTS MADE

1. ....
2. ....
3. ....
4. ....
5. ....
6. ....

FURTHER MEDICAL HISTORY

Medical history The medical history should be taken to discover if the patient has any condition, either general or local, that might alter the normal course of treatment. A checklist on the patient's folder gives an easy and accurate record.

There are no medical conditions which specifically contra-indicate endodontics although patients with a history of infective endocarditis should be regarded as a special high risk group and be referred to hospital (Cawson 1983). Antibiotic cover should be considered for certain conditions (Table 1) depending upon the complexity of the procedure and the degree of bacteraemia expected. If it is necessary to provide antibiotic cover or to alter the patient's medication, the patient's medical practitioner (GMP) should be informed and the case discussed, when necessary, before treatment is carried out.

TABLE 1

Some medical conditions relevant to endodontic treatment and the action which should be taken by the dentist.

MEDICAL CONDITION	PRECAUTIONS TAKEN
History of infective endocarditis	Regarded as special high risk group. Patient usually referred to hospital for treatment. Antibiotic cover required.
Congenital cardiac abnormality	Consider antibiotic cover.
Rheumatic fever or Sydenham's Chorea Artificial heart valves Prosthesis for total replacement of a joint	Consider antibiotic cover (see Table 2).
Cardiovascular disease Hypertension	GMP to advise alteration of drug therapy. Non-surgical endodontics preferred. Analgesic to reduce postoperative pain. Appointments not to exceed one hour.
Blood diseases (e.g. haemophilia)	Root canal treatment preferred to extraction. No local anaesthesia if possible. Use of devitalising pastes. Care taken not to lacerate gingivae.
Diabetes	Healing will be retarded. Antibiotic cover if surgery intended or infection present. GMP to advise on drug therapy. No vasoconstrictor in local anaesthetic (Novocain suggested). No general anaesthetic if possible. Glucose kept in surgery.
Hepatitis	Dangers are: 1 Operator contracting disease. 2 Cross-infection via contaminated instruments. GMP to check if patient is carrier. Treat with caution: 1 Rubber gloves, mask and glasses. 2 Low-speed instruments. 3 Dispose of instruments which may pick up micro-organisms, eg files, burs etc. 4 Wash down operating area with 2% glutaraldehyde solution and place all instruments etc. used on patient in the same solution for one hour before sterilisation. 5 Treat at end of day.
Chronic renal failure	Risk of hepatitis cross-infection if patient on kidney machine. Take all precautions as above.
Immunosuppressed states eg patients on corticosteroids or drugs to maintain organ transplants	Antibiotic cover if infection present. Possible corticosteroid supplement by GMP during and after endodontic treatment.
Radiotherapy for malignant disease	Any extractions necessary carried out before radiotherapy to prevent intractable radionecrosis. Root canal treatment preferred to extraction after therapy.
Sexually transmitted disease	Increase in incidence — syphilitic lesion may resemble chronic draining sinus.
Other debilitating diseases, asthma, hay fever and skin rashes	Patients could be sensitive to drugs: only prescribe drugs which patient has taken previously.

TABLE 2

The table shows regimes (*Lancet*, 1982) which are advised currently and may be adopted when antibiotic cover is necessary. Advice on particular regimes is changing constantly: the operator would be well advised to check with current opinion (eg *Journal of Endodontics*, 1986).

ANTIBIOTIC	DOSE
ORAL AMOXYCILLIN	3g one hour before treatment. Children under 10 half the adult dose and under 5 quarter the adult dose. One dose only (dispersable tablets preferred for diabetics).
ORAL ERYTHROMYCIN STEARATE For patients who are allergic to penicillin or who have received a course of penicillin in the preceding month.	1.5g 1-2 hrs before treatment, followed by second dose 0.5g 6 hrs later. Children under 10 half the adult dose and under 5 one quarter the adult dose.
INTRAMUSCULAR AMOXYCILLIN For patients who are having a general anaesthetic.	1g in 2.5ml of 1% lignocaine hydrochloride before induction and a further 0.5g of amoxycillin by mouth 6 hours later. Children under 10 half the adult dose.

Advice should be sought concerning: (1) patients who require a general anaesthetic and are either allergic to the penicillins or have been given amoxycillin in the previous month. (2) patients who have had one or more attacks of infective endocarditis or have a prosthetic valve.

Patient's complaint The patient's complaint should be recorded in his or her own words. It is wise to listen carefully to the patient's description of his problem as it often gives the operator most of the information he needs to make a diagnosis.

Valuable information may be acquired by asking the patient specific questions about the symptoms:

1 How long have you had the pain?
2 Do you know which tooth it is?
3 Does it hurt to bite on the tooth or to touch it?
4 Describe the pain:
  sharp or dull
  throbbing
  mild or severe
  localised or radiating
  getting better or worsening
5 Does it hurt most during the day or at night, and how long does it last?
6 Is the pain started by hot or cold drinks, chewing, sugar, or posture?
7 Have you taken anything to relieve the pain? If so, does it relieve the pain? For how long?

Pulpal pain It is not possible to diagnose the histological state of the pulp from clinical symptoms. The operator can only decide whether the pulp has been irreversibly damaged or not.

Reversible pulpitis is partial pulpitis without necrosis, whereas irreversible pulpitis can be described histopathologically as total pulpitis with necrosis.

The successful diagnosis of reversible and irreversible pulpitis is difficult and depends upon the operator's experience and the severity of the symptoms. Guidelines on differential diagnosis of the two conditions are given in Table 3.

TABLE 3

Guidelines for the differential diagnosis of reversible and irreversible pulpitis

	REVERSIBLE PULPITIS	IRREVERSIBLE PULPITIS
Pain	Momentary — immediate onset. Dissipates quickly after removal of stimulus. Sharp pain.	Continuous — delayed onset. Persists for minutes to hours. Throbbing pain.
Location of Pain	Patient not certain which tooth. Pain is not referred.	Patient is certain which tooth only after the periapex is involved. Referred pain is common.
Lying down	No difference.	Pain increases.
Stimulus	Requires external stimulus, *eg* heat, cold, sugar.	Reacts particularly to heat, also occurs spontaneously. Pain common at night.
EPT	Early response.	Early, late or mixed.
Percussion	Negative.	Negative early stages. Later positive when periapex involved.
Colour	Negative.	Darkening may occur.
Radiography	Negative.	May show slight widening of pdl space and/or alteration of trabeculation around apex.

The pulp does not contain any proprioceptive nerve endings, so that if only the pulp is involved with no periapical irritation, the patient is unable to identify the tooth.

117

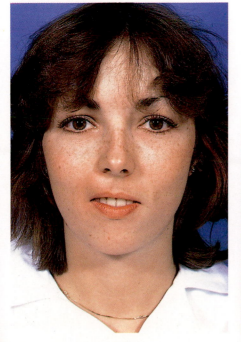

118

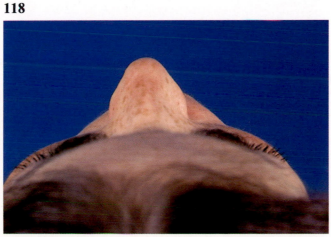

CLINICAL EXAMINATION

A brief clinical examination is carried out before any diagnostic tests.

Facial asymmetry Any facial swelling due to pathology or trauma should be noted. Facial swelling is best viewed from above the patient, as may be seen from the two views (**117, 118**).

119

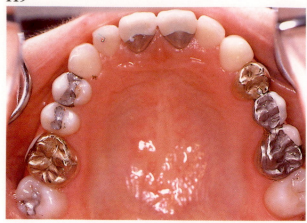

120

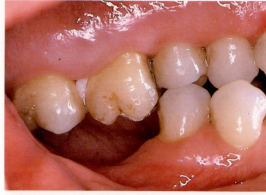

General dental state An examination of the patient should be made to assess:

1 Amount and quality of restorative work (**119**).

2 Missing and unopposed teeth (**120**).

121

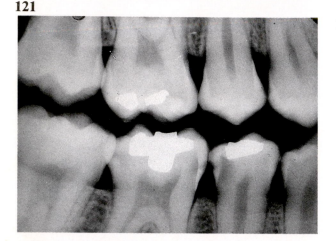

122

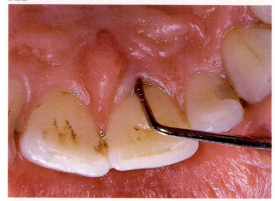

3 Incidence of caries (**121**).

4 General periodontal condition (**122**).

124

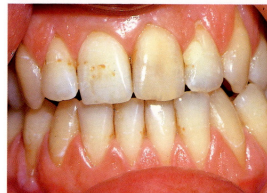

123

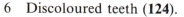

5 Standard of oral hygiene (**123**).

6 Discoloured teeth (**124**).

7 Tooth wear and facets (**125**).

125

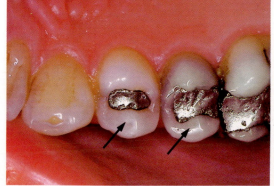

It must be emphasised that problems are not to be dealt with in isolation, and any treatment plan must take the entire mouth and the patient's general medical condition and attitude into consideration.

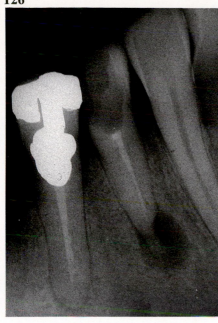

126

DIAGNOSTIC TESTS

The diagnostic tests available at present are relatively crude and none of them is reliable (Chambers, 1982). No one test, no matter how positive, is sufficient to make a definite diagnosis of reversible or irreversible pulpitis.

Doubt has been cast on comparative tests with the corresponding teeth on the other side of the midline.

The diagnostic tests available are illustrated.

Radiography Assessment of any endodontic problem must always include periapical radiographs. Of all the methods of examination discussed, radiographs are the most reliable. In many cases the radiograph may be the only method of demonstrating the presence of pathology (**126**).

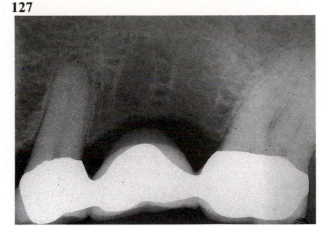

127

The main difficulty in endodontics is that reversible pulpitis and the early stages of irreversible damage are not normally visible on the radiograph. In **127** pain was eventually diagnosed from a pulpitis in the second premolar.

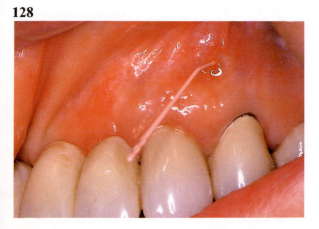

128

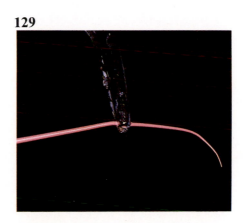

129

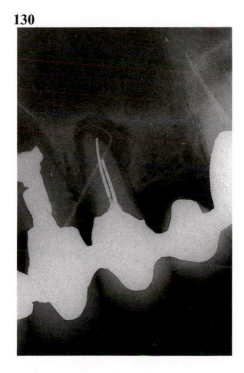

130

Presence of sinus The soft tissues should be inspected for the presence of sinus tracts. These occur usually in the buccal sulcus, but may be present lingually or palatally (**128**). When a sinus is present, a gutta percha point size 20 should be fed into the tract (**129**). The point should track back to the source of the infection and will show on a radiograph (**130**). This will demonstrate which root of a molar tooth is affected and sometimes may point to the adjacent tooth, which was not suspected.

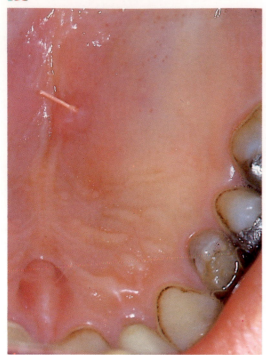

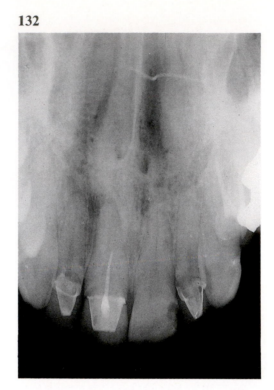

131 The sinus may be remote from the affected tooth. In this case a sinus in the palate was caused by a necrotic pulp in a first premolar (**132**).

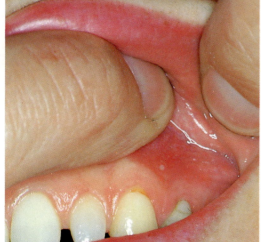

133 Palpation The soft tissues overlying the apices of the teeth are palpated. The patient will report any tender area. Hard and soft swellings will be apparent; if hard, the site and size should be noted on the patient's card; if soft, the swelling should be palpated with two fingers to feel whether it is fluctuant.

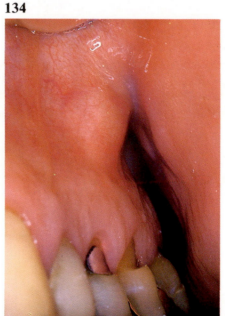

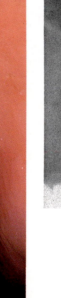

134 A hard bony swelling in the buccal sulcus was treated by conventional root canal therapy on the first molar. **135** shows a radiolucent area associated with the mesiobuccal root.

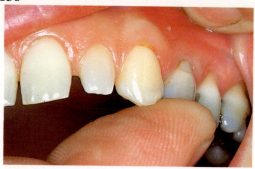

136

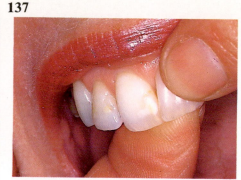

137

137 Mobility Mobility is assessed by placing a finger on either side of the tooth and pressing with one finger to judge the amount of movement.

Mobility may be graded as follows:

1 Slight mobility, which is considered normal.
2 Moderate mobility.
3 Extensive movement in a lateral or mesiodistal direction, combined with vertical displacement in the alveolus.

136 Percussion Gentle tapping with a finger is all that is necessary to elicit tenderness. This should be done in both a vertical and lateral direction on the crown of the tooth.

Pulp testing

ELECTRIC PULP TESTING (EPT)

The electric pulp tester is an instrument which uses gradations of electric current to excite a response from the nervous tissue within the pulp; either an alternating or a direct current is used. Most of the pulp testers manufactured today are monopolar.

Pulp testers should only be used to assess vital or non-vital pulps. They do not quantify disease nor measure health, and should not be used to judge the degree of pulpal disease.

Two examples of pulp tester are illustrated.

138 The Greenwood pulp tester[1] This type of pulp tester requires an assistant to control the increase in current. There is also no indication when electrical contact has been established, or broken, with the tooth.

139 The analytic technology pulp tester[2] The output stimulus is produced in bursts of ten high frequency pulses of negative polarity. The power source is four 1.5V AA penlight batteries. The EPT is turned on automatically when the probe tip touches the tooth (**140**) and turns off when tooth contact is broken after a delay of 15 seconds. The digital display reads from 0-80 and the only control on the EPT is the rate of increase of the electrical stimulus.

Pulp testing technique

The teeth to be tested should be dried and isolated with cotton wool rolls. A conducting medium must be used and the one most readily available is toothpaste. The pulp tester is applied to the gingival third of the tooth avoiding contact with the soft tissues, and any restorations. Electric pulp testers should not be used on patients who have a pacemaker because of the possible electrical interference.

138

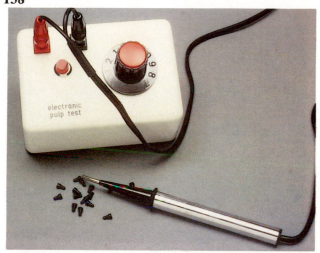

139

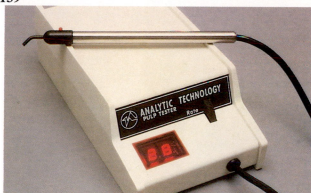

140

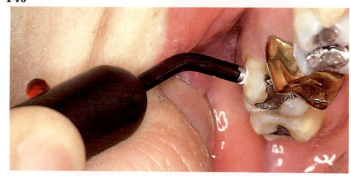

141

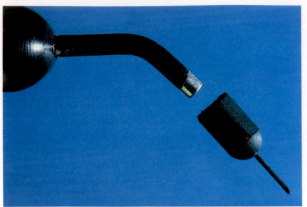

142

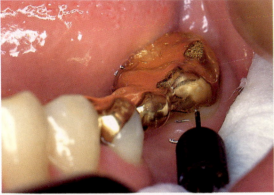

143

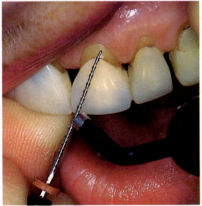

144

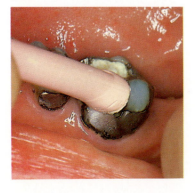

Pulp testing of crowned teeth may be achieved provided that there is a small area of dentine or enamel which can be contacted without touching the gingival tissue. A special end fitting for the analytic technology EPT (**141**) is being used in **142**.

If a different EPT is used contact may be made with the tooth using a hand instrument with a plastic handle (**143**). The other alternative, with little to commend it, is to cut a window through the crown and apply the EPT to the exposed dentine.

There are several disadvantages of EPT. These are:

1   No indication is given of the state of the vascular supply which would give a more reliable measure of the vitality of the pulp. Nerve tissue will respond for some time after the vascular supply has degenerated.
2   False positive readings may be due to stimulation of nerve fibres in the periodontium.
3   Readings taken from posterior teeth may be misleading since some combination of vital and non-vital root canal pulps may be present.

Thermal pulp testing

This involves either heating or removing heat from a tooth. Neither test is reliable, both producing false positive and negative results, but generally cold is considered a better test than heat.

Heat   3.0 mm of the end of a stick of pink gutta percha is heated in a flame for 2 seconds and applied to the suspect tooth (**144**). Two precautions should be taken against the patient receiving sudden acute pain. The tooth surface is lightly coated with vaseline to prevent the GP sticking, and a local anaesthetic is to hand. Another method is to use the heat generated from a rubber wheel in a standard handpiece.

Hot water   In some cases the patient reports a reaction to hot drinks but no reaction to heated gutta percha. Also the patient may have one or more porcelain bonded crowns protecting the natural tooth surface. Hot water is sipped from a cup and held first over the mandibular quadrant on the affected side; if that does not elicit a response the maxillary quadrant is included. If there is a response, a local anaesthetic is given alongside the suspect tooth and the heat reapplied in the same way. A negative response confirms that the tooth with pulpitis has been identified.

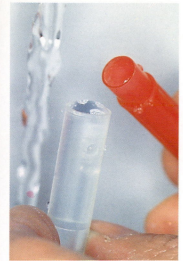

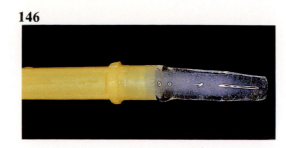

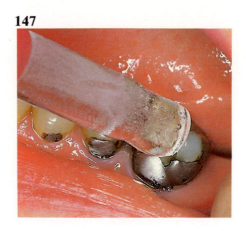

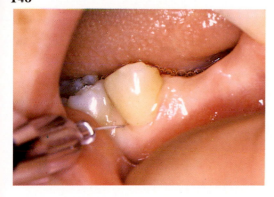

Cold An ice stick is made by filling the plastic protective covers for hypodermic needles with water and freezing (**145**). To make them ready for use one end is removed by warming it slightly in the hand (**146, 147**). An alternative method is to soak a pledget of cotton wool with ethyl chloride and apply to the tooth with tweezers.

Local Anaesthetic

When the patient presents in pain or the pain can be provoked by applying a thermal test, an infiltration injection of local anaesthetic may be used to identify the tooth. The intraligamental injection is particularly useful for this test, because individual teeth in both the maxilla and mandible may be anaesthetised (**148**).

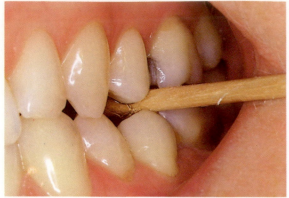

149 **Wooden stick** Incompletely fractured teeth are one of the most difficult conditions to diagnose in endodontics. When a patient presents with a pain related to chewing and there is no evidence of periapical inflammation, then a fracture may be suspected. Biting on a wooden stick may elicit pain, usually on release of biting pressure.

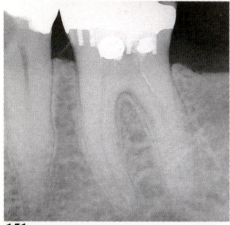

150 The patient had complained of pain from the 6 on eating. The tooth had been re-root treated and the root filling again removed to no avail. The radiograph shows a slight thickening of the periodontal ligament space in the furcation. Transmitted light demonstrated a hairline fracture passing across the floor of the pulp chamber in a buccolingual direction.

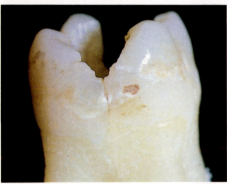

151 **Fibreoptic light** A powerful light is useful for transmitting through teeth to show interproximal caries, and, of particular interest in endodontics, a fracture. The light does not pass across the fracture line so that the part of the tooth nearest to the light is bright and beyond the fracture remains dark. Extraneous light is reduced and the fibreoptic light is placed alongside the neck of the tooth and moved along its surface. **151 and 152** show the difference when a fibreoptic light is used. The fracture is seen as a definite vertical line in **152**.

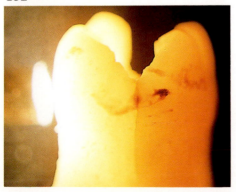

Cutting a test cavity As a last resort a test cavity may be cut in a tooth which is believed to be pulpless. In the author's experience this test is not reliable because a positive response may be obtained from a tooth the pulp of which is necrotic.

Treatment planning

Having taken the case history and carried out the relevant diagnostic tests, the operator has to plan the patient's treatment. Clear-cut options will be considered first and then the problem areas in endodontic planning.

INDICATIONS FOR ENDODONTICS

All teeth with pulpal or periapical pathology are candidates for endodontics. In addition situations arise in which elective endodontics is the treatment of choice.

153 Post space When a tooth has lost the majority of coronal tissue and a crown is to be constructed, the root canal space may be needed for retention of the post. See the lower right first premolar.

154, 155 Overdenture Preservation of the alveolar bone is of paramount importance in prosthodontics. For this reason retention of the roots particularly in the mandible, is often recommended. These teeth should be root treated.

Pulps with vital doubtful prognosis Teeth with doubtful pulps — vital teeth, which are to be restored with large cast restorations or porcelain — should be assessed endodontically beforehand. If there is doubt about the vitality, for example when no canals are visible, or if the vitality tests are indefinite, then root canal treatment should be considered before the restoration is placed. It is often more difficult to carry out root canal therapy later, and may mean the remake of the restoration.

156, 157 The vitality of the upper left first molar was indeterminate. Because the tooth was to be crowned, root canal treatment was carried out beforehand.

153

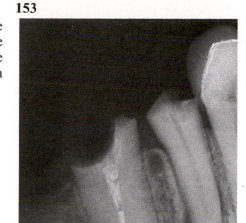

155

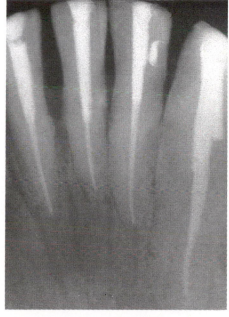

154

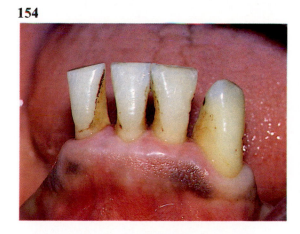

156

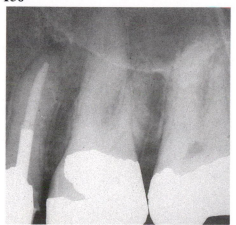

157

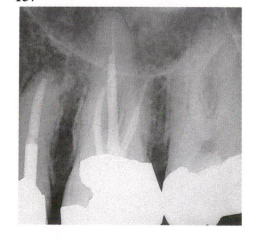

Risk of pulp exposure Cutting bonded crown preparations on teeth in order to reposition them in better alignment with the arch may endanger the pulps. In some cases root canal treatment should be carried out before the preparations are cut.

158 The lower right lateral incisor has been exposed during preparation.

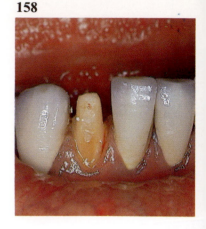

159 Pulpal sclerosis following trauma A tooth may receive a blow which causes secondary or irritation dentine to be laid down. A review of these cases occasionally may show a progressive loss of canal space until the pulp is no longer able to support itself, and eventually dies. When this progressive narrowing of the canal space is seen, it is better electively to root treat the tooth when the canal is still negotiable. Subsequent attempts when symptoms occur can end in perforation.

160, 161, 162 Pulpotomy The purpose of pulpotomy is to preserve healthy radicular pulp in immature teeth, so that the roots may complete their development (**160, 161**). Following pulpotomy the tooth should be reviewed radiographically at six-monthly intervals. If, as occasionally occurs, the canal becomes sclerosed (**162**) or internal resorption occurs, the tooth should be root filled.

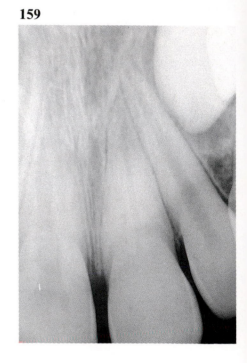

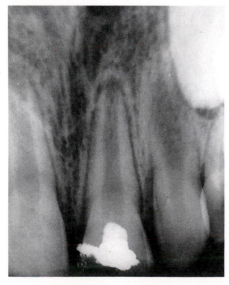

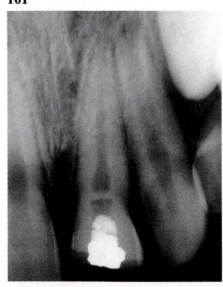

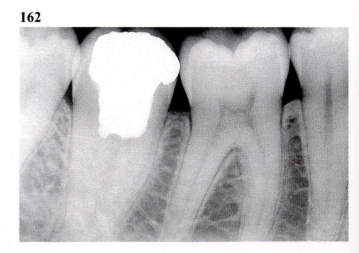

CONTRA-INDICATIONS TO ENDODONTICS

There are no medical contra-indications to endodontics. The conditions requiring special treatment have been listed in Table 1. The contra-indications may be divided into general and local.

General

Small mouth

Access must be sufficient to allow placement of a rubber dam and a clamp. The patient (163) had a restricted opening following mandibular fractures. Treatment was delayed to the fractured second maxillary molar for three months until two fingers could be placed between her incisors (164).

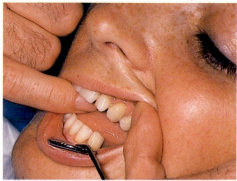
163

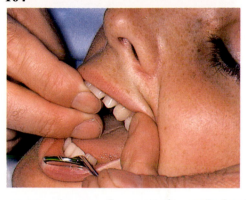
164

An assessment of access for posterior endodontic surgery may be made by retracting the cheek. If the operation site can be viewed directly with ease access is sufficient (165, 166).

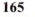
165

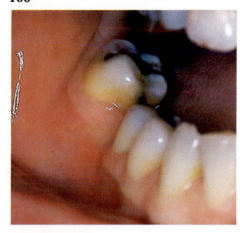
166

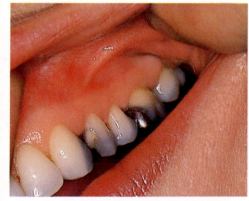
167

Poor oral hygiene (167)

No restorative work, no matter how well it is done, will survive in a patient's mouth unless the oral hygiene standard is adequate. Endodontics should not be carried out unless the patient is able to maintain his mouth in a healthy state or can be taught to do so.

Patient's general medical condition

Some patients' physical or mental condition due to a chronic debilitating disease or old age would not enable them to tolerate endodontic treatment. Similarly, the patient at high risk to infective endocarditis, for example one who has had a previous attack, may not be considered suitable for endodontic treatment.

Patient's attitude

Unless the patient is sufficiently well motivated a simpler form of treatment would be preferable.

Local

Tooth not restorable

It must be possible to restore the tooth to function and health following endodontic treatment. There should be sufficient coronal tooth substance remaining to allow retention for the restoration and a finishing line that may be cleaned by the patient. The finishing line must be supracrestal and preferably supragingival. There is insufficient tooth substance remaining in both the teeth illustrated (**168, 169**).

Insufficient periodontal support

For many years, insufficient periodontal support has been considered a local contra-indication to endodontics. This is no longer accepted. Providing the tooth is functional and the attachment apparatus is healthy or can be made so, endodontic treatment may be carried out (**170**).

Non-strategic tooth

Extraction should be considered for an unopposed distal molar tooth rather than endodontic treatment (**171**). Conversely a single standing molar with the premolar teeth missing should be retained if at all possible. The importance of a particular tooth in the overall treatment plan should be carefully considered.

168

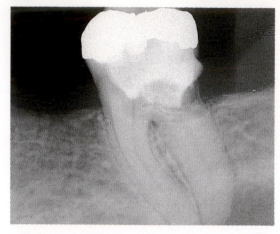

169

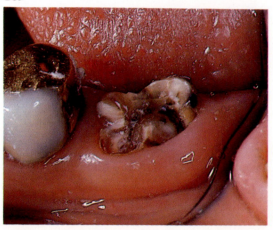

170

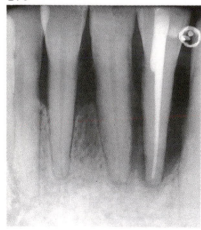

171

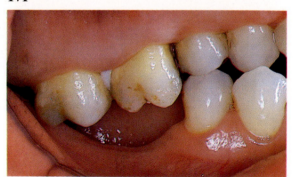

172

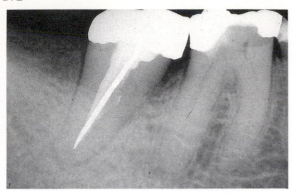

173

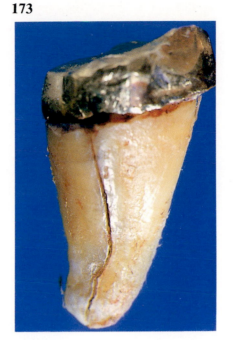

174

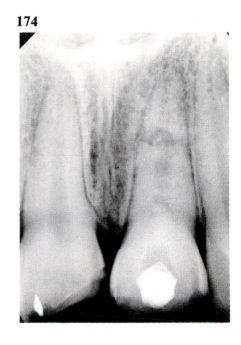

Root fractures

Generally vertical fractures have a poor prognosis and horizontally fractured teeth may often be retained for many years. Horizontal fractures are usually easier to see on a radiograph than a vertical fracture as may be seen from the two cases illustrated (**172, 173, 174**).

Massive internal or external resorption

The radiographic differences between the two types are described in Chapter 17. Both types of resorption when advanced will weaken the root so that fracture and loss of the crown of the tooth are inevitable (**175, 176**).

175

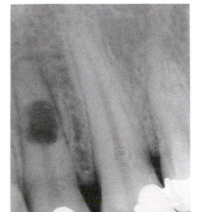

176

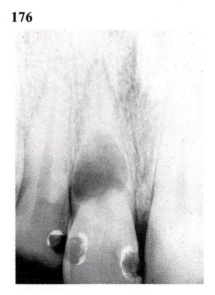

177 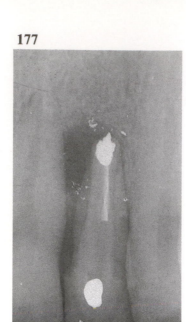   **178** 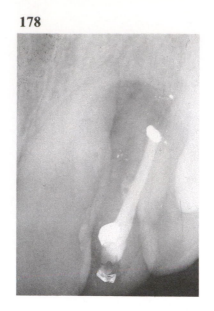   **179**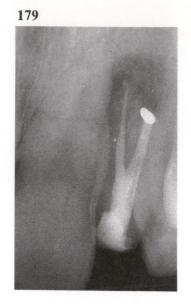

Bizarre anatomy

All teeth may show unusual anatomic variations. Two examples are given. **177** was an upper lateral incisor which had been treated some years previously but had a sinus. It was decided to re-root fill and re-apicect. At operation the canal was re-treated and a new retrograde amalgam placed. The post-operative radiograph (**178**) showed a second root. This was root treated (**179**) but the sinus persisted.

180 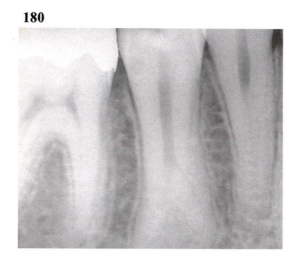   **181** 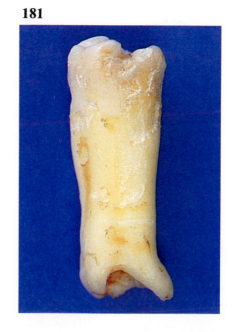   **182**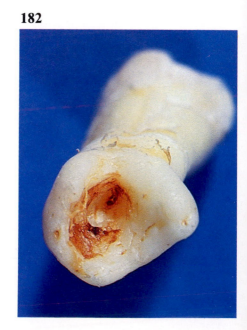

In **180, 181, 182,** a mandibular second premolar shows a widened apical region of the root which would have been difficult or impossible to root fill.

PROBLEM AREAS

This section contains problem areas which frequently confront the operator and pose particular difficulties with treatment planning. These will be divided into different categories but often several may appear together. An example is given (183) of gross caries beneath a crown with a poor root treatment. The mesial canals are not apparent suggesting sclerosis and there is a periodontal problem of the mesial root area which includes the furcation.

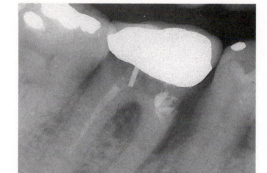

183

Obstructed canals

Sclerosed canals

When the root canals are not visible on the radiograph considerable difficulty may be experienced in locating and negotiating them. The patient should be told that it is not possible to give a prognosis for the tooth until an attempt has been made to locate the canals (184, 185).

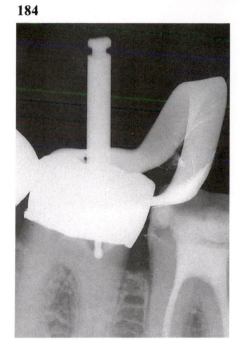

184

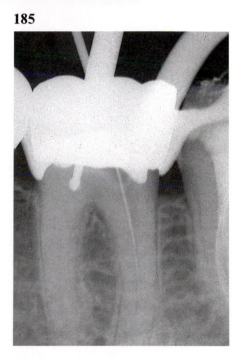

185

Previously root filled teeth

The decision as to whether a tooth should be re-root filled or not can be a difficult one. The criteria the operator should consider when examining an inadequate root filling are given below:

1 Is there any evidence that the old root filling has failed?
  a symptoms from the tooth.
  b radiographic evidence of deterioration.
  c presence of a sinus tract.

2 Does the crown of the tooth need restoring?

3 Is there any obvious fault with the present root filling which could lead to failure?

4 If the root treatment is attempted is it possible to improve on the situation?

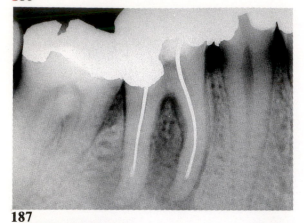

186

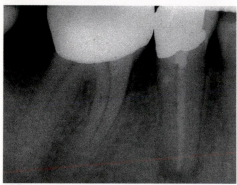

187

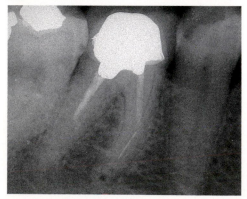

188

189

These criteria are applied to the cases illustrated.

186 Case 1 Mild symptoms from time to time. Tooth is functional with no sinus. Two silver points short of the correct length. Radiolucent area associated with both root apices and the furcation. Previous radiograph shows that the radiolucent area is increasing in size. The restoration requires replacing, as there appears to be a void in the pulp chamber and there is a mesial ledge. It is probable that a mesial canal is unfilled and the distal canal has not been obturated.

There is little doubt that the root filling requires replacing.

187 Case 2 Root filled six years ago. No symptoms, no sinus, tooth is functional. No radiographic deterioration. The restoration is sound. Over-extension of silver points in the mesial canals into the periapical tissues by several millimetres. The silver points could be difficult to remove.

It is suggested that this tooth is not re-root treated.

188 Case 3 Root filled 15 years ago. No symptoms, no sinus and the tooth is functional. Previous radiographs show no change in the periapical area. The tooth requires to be crowned. There is an obvious fault with the root filling which has been poorly obturated probably with a single gutta percha cone. The tooth should be simple to re-root treat.

The correct treatment is to re-root fill the tooth before crowning. If the present restoration had been satisfactory the decision would have been not to root treat.

Fractured instruments

An account of fractured instruments is given in Chapter 18. Unless surgery is considered the only method of dealing with broken instruments in the curved part of a canal is to bypass them or fill the canal up to them. It would not be possible to give the patient an assessment of the prognosis until an attempt had been made to negotiate the canal alongside the fractured instrument. **(189)** As the patient is having symptoms there are three options:

1 extraction.

2 apicectomy with retrograde amalgam seals in both the mesial and distal canals.

3 removal of the crown and an attempt to re-root fill.

Perforations

There are three types of perforation according to their position in the tooth.

Lateral wall of root

The use of engine-operated rotating instruments such as burs or reamers makes perforation of the wall of the root likely. When a lateral perforation is suspected, the site must be established; if it is on the buccal wall surgical correction should be simple, if it is on the palatal it will be extremely difficult.

190

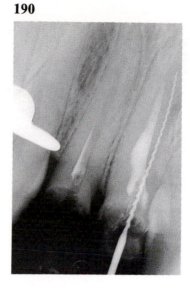

191

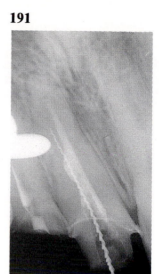

192

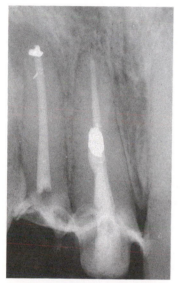

190, 191 show two radiographs, with a diagnostic instrument through the perforation, taken from different angles. The instrument has moved in relation to the root filling and so lies buccal to it. The completed root filling and repair are shown in the final radiograph (**192**).

193

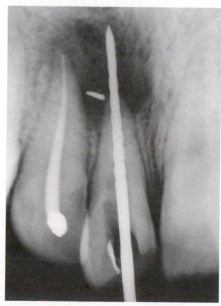

194

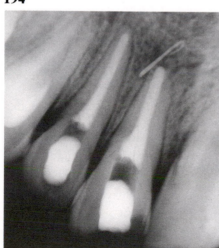

Apex

Over-zealous instrumentation of a canal may result in perforation through the apical foramen. Calcium hydroxide may be used to provide an apical barrier. In **193** there was the additional problem of a foreign body which had been extruded through the apex. This would normally indicate surgery for its removal but in this case healing had occurred, as the final radiograph taken 18 months later shows (**194**).

Floor of the pulp chamber

Perforations through the floor of the pulp chamber quickly become periodontal problems with furcal bone loss and pocketing, unless they are treated immediately. The perforation may be repaired with a material which will provide a good seal. Amalgam, cavit, or gutta percha are commonly used. The larger the perforation and the longer it is left the poorer the prognosis. In certain cases an alternative treatment is the removal of one of the roots. These teeth are difficult to restore and it is also difficult for the patient to maintain a good periodontal condition. In this case (**195**) the patient was advised to have the tooth extracted and a bridge placed.

Perio-endo lesions. These are discussed in Chapter 16. A parallel radiograph must be taken to assess the bone level in relation to the tooth, particularly the posteriors where the furcation may be involved.

ENDODONTIC TIME TABLE

Planning treatment entails arranging the number of appointments required and the time gap between them. Some suggestions are given below.

a   Antibiotic cover   See Table 2. Treatment should be completed in one appointment if possible. If a second appointment is needed it should be within three days so that the antibiotic course is not unnecessarily prolonged. Where more appointments are required a gap of six weeks should be allowed before a further course of antibiotics may be given.

b   Initial restoration of tooth   When it is not possible to isolate a tooth because it is severely broken down, a separate appointment should be given to build the tooth either with a metal band or amalgam restoration. (See Chapters 6 and 10.)

c   Time gap between appointments   The time gap between preparation of the root canals and filling should be not less than one week (except in **a** above) to allow the tooth to become symptomless, and not more than three weeks. Longer than three weeks and there is a danger that the temporary restoration may leak and allow the canal system to become contaminated. Most medicaments would not be effective after three weeks.

d   Long interval between appointments   Long intervals are necessary or unavoidable at times. A good temporary filling, such as IRM or amalgam must be used which will not wear. If there is any danger of fracture, the tooth should be protected with a metal band which is cemented with zinc phosphate.

195

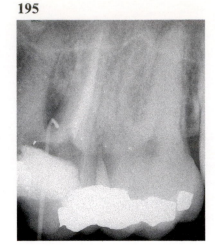

196

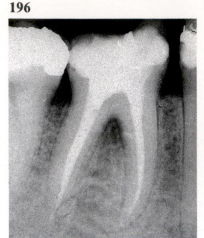

196   The lower right first molar had a radiolucent area in the furcation, due to a lateral canal in the mesial root which shows on the radiograph taken after the root filling had been completed.

197

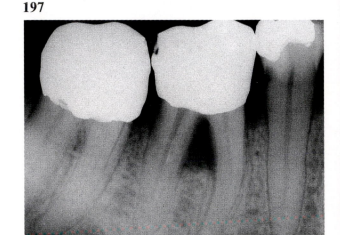

197   The lower right first molar was vital with extensive furcation involvement. Poor oral hygiene and a ledged crown were the cause.

References

Report of a working party at the British Society for Anti-Microbial Chemotherapy. The antibiotic prophylaxis of infective endocarditis. *Lancet* 1982:2:1323-1326.
Cawson, R.A. The Antibiotic prophylaxis of infective endocarditis. *Br. Dent. J.* 1983; 154:183-184.
Wiseman, M.I. American Heart Association revises the antibiotic regimens for the prevention of bacterial endocarditis. *J.Endodont.* 1986; 12:34-35.
Chambers, I.G. The Role and methods of pulp testing in oral diagnosis: A Review. *Int.Endo.J.* 15:1-15.

4   Anaesthesia   J. J. Messing

When it is necessary to alleviate pain occasioned by endodontic procedures, local analgesia by injection of an anaesthetic solution is the usual choice. It is used chiefly for pulpectomy and pulp capping, but when dealing with nervous patients it may be required for the preparation of the canals of pulpless teeth. Similarly, general anaesthesia and sedation techniques will be indicated for children and nervous adults, and for acute soft tissue involvements in which the injection of a local anaesthetic could spread the infection.

ANAESTHETIC SOLUTIONS

Lignocaine hydrochloride is the most commonly used local anaesthetic. Usually it is combined with 1:80,000 adrenaline Hcl as a vasoconstrictor. When adrenaline is contra-indicated on medical grounds, duration of anaesthesia is reduced from approximately 30 minutes to 5-10 minutes. Prilocaine (4%) is effective for only about 5 minutes when infiltrated, or 60 minutes as a regional anaesthetic. Mepivacaine (3%) without vasoconstrictor gives 20-30 minutes of anaesthesia.

As an alternative to adrenaline, when it is contra-indicated, adequate short-term anaesthesia may be provided by Prilocaine (3%), plus Felypressin (.03iu/ml.) in the majority of patients.

In every case, care must be taken to avoid intravascular injection of anaesthetic, through the use of an aspiration technique.

In a small number of cases of acute pulpitis, it may prove impossible to anaesthetize a tooth by infiltration or regional anaesthesia. The simultaneous administration of intravenous Diazepam or the use of general anaesthesia may be considered necessary.

Injection into acutely inflamed tissue can produce a severe spreading infection. Some authorities consider this risk to be nullified by prior administration of a systemic antibiotic drug. The authors feel however, that in such cases, alternative methods of pain control are preferable.

LOCAL ANAESTHESIA

In the absence of tenderness or swelling of the soft tissues, local anaesthesia may be used. Usually in the maxilla, a labial or buccal infiltration is all that is needed, but in the molar region, a palatal infiltration is occasionally required.

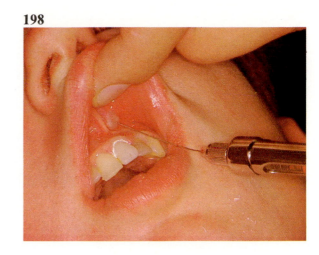

198

Approximately 1.0 ml of anaesthetic solution (2% Lignocaine with 1:80,000 adrenaline or 4% Prilocaine or 3% Prilocaine with Octopressin i.e. Felypressin 0.03 iu/ml.) is infiltrated slowly just beneath the mucosal surface at the periapical level and massaged gently towards the bone (**198**). After a delay of 30 seconds to allow the onset of analgesia, the needle is directed again towards the apex and, insinuating the point beneath the periosteum, a further 0.5 ml of anaesthetic is injected slowly.

INTRAPAPILLARY INJECTION

If this does not produce complete anaesthesia within 2 minutes, an intrapapillary injection (**199**) into the mesial and distal papillae will often be effective. The needle, placed at the base of the papilla, is directed apically at an angle of 45° with the bevel facing the bone and 0.2-0.5 ml is injected very slowly. The papilla is seen to blanche as a result of the pressure engendered by the anaesthetic, which is forced down the periodontal ligament and into the interproximal bone, spreading ultimately to the apical nerve bundle.

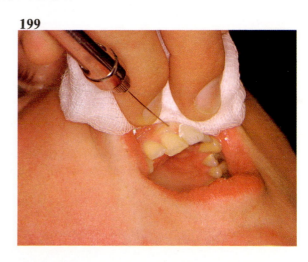

199

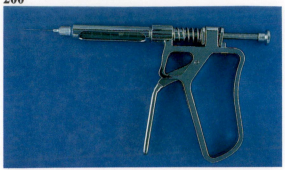

200

INTRALIGAMENTAL INJECTION

As an alternative, the intraligamental anaesthetic technique may be used by injecting directly down the periodontal ligament with a high pressure lever-design syringe (Ligmaject or Peri-press) (**200**). This technique should not be employed in the presence of acute or chronic periodontal disease when used for endodontic or conservative procedures, because of the risk of spreading infection. In all cases, the tissues should be painted with Povidone-Iodine solution before injection. The bevel of the needle is directed towards the bone (**201, 202**). Injections are made mesially and distally into the periodontal ligament and the solution is deposited very slowly. In addition to its use for pulpal anaesthesia it is useful in locating an inflamed pulp by anaesthetizing a single tooth, by means of a buccal injection.

The modus operandi of the intraligamental injection is thought to be a localised, temporary pulpal anoxia.

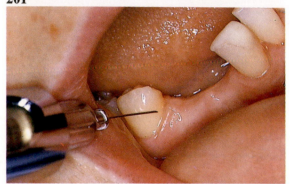

201

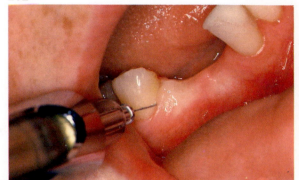

202

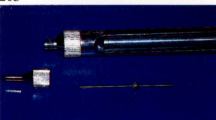

203

INTRA-OSSEOUS INJECTION

This injection, prior to the introduction of the intraligamental technique, was the only certain way of obtaining analgesia when all other injection techniques had failed. However, it is a useful method to keep in reserve. As the name implies, the anaesthetic solution is deposited within the alveolar bone and, in consequence, failure to observe a strictly aseptic technique could lead to serious sequelae.

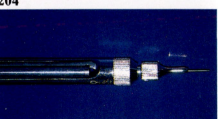

204

Armamentarium

1 Povidone-Iodine 10% solution for disinfection of the mucosa
2 Injection syringe provided with a long hub and short needle (**203, 204**)
3 A root canal reamer slightly wider than the needle
4 A cartridge of local anaesthetic solution.

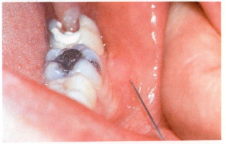

205

205 Technique The need to use intra-osseous anaesthesia usually is established after infiltration or regional anaesthesia has proved inadequate. Hence, the soft tissues already should be anaesthetized. The area is isolated, using a saliva ejector and cotton rolls, and the interdental papilla adjacent to the tooth to be treated, is swabbed buccally with Povidone-Iodine (10%) solution. Illustration shows infiltration of local anaesthetic into the area.

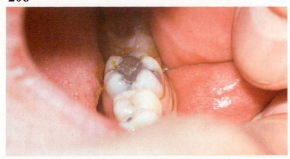

206

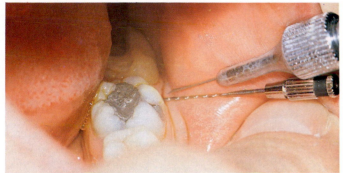

207

The reamer selected is angulated at approximately 45° in the axial plane midway between the teeth and, at the level of the cervical margins, it is inserted through the gingiva into contact with the bone. Using a 90° reciprocating action, the point of the reamer soon pierces the cortical plate when moderate pressure is applied (**206**).

When approximately 3 mm of the reamer is embedded in the jaw, the syringe is brought into position with the needle lying alongside the reamer (**207**). As the reamer is withdrawn, the needle is introduced into the hole until the hub, coming into contact with the gingiva, acts as a washer, preventing back-flow of fluid as the injection is made (**208, 209, 210**).

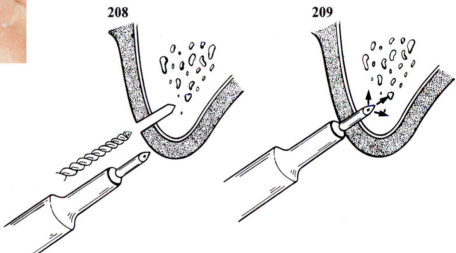

208   **209**

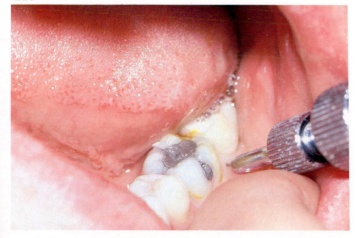

210

The patient is warned to expect a slight increase in heart rate, due to the absorption of some adrenaline from the intra-osseous blood vessels. This can be avoided however, by using a solution without a vasoconstrictor. Approximately 0.5 ml. of anaesthetic thus injected will produce complete anaesthesia for 5-10 minutes in the majority of cases. Usually this will allow sufficient time to extirpate a vital pulp.

After the needle has been withdrawn, the gingiva is once again swabbed with Povidone-Iodine.

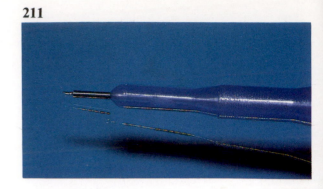

211 The intra-osseous needle A recent development which simplifies the intra-osseous injection is the new tri-bevelled intra-osseous needle. The needle is very fine (30 gauge), and one eighth of an inch in length, and is designed to penetrate bone. It is covered with a mobile sleeve which retracts as the point of the needle is advanced through the tissues, thus conferring resistance to bending or fracture.

The site for injection is first disinfected, using, e.g. Povidone-Iodine, and then rendered insensitive with topical anaesthetic. The point of the needle is pressed into the bone and advanced with an ambi-rotational movement while injecting very slowly. This prevents clogging of the lumen of the needle, which is inserted at the base of the papilla anterior to the tooth to be anaesthetized. Approximately 0.25-0.5 ml. of solution is required to produce deep anaesthesia for about 10-15 minutes. A vasoconstrictor is not required. Anaesthesia develops within one minute and is confined to a single tooth.

Mandibular molars require a further buccal injection at the bifurcation of the roots, the needle guard being restored to its position over the tip of the needle prior to giving the second injection.

ANALGESIA FOR INCISION INTO AN ABSCESS

Incision into an abscess to drain pus should be withheld until it has pointed and fluctuation is demonstrable. At that time, drainage is best established by incision into the most dependent part. The risk of spreading infection contra-indicates the use of injections, although a regional block, in conjunction with intravenous Diazepam may prove satisfactory. The commonly used alternative is a general anaesthetic, but this may not be convenient or possible. The author has frequently employed the following technique with minimum discomfort to the patient.

The surface of the abscess is covered with a layer of cotton wool soaked in 10% Cocaine, which is left in place for at least 5 minutes. This produces good superficial analgesia which can be reinforced by isolating the abscess with gauze and spraying ethyl chloride for a few seconds until the surface frosts over. A number 12 Bard-Parker scalpel blade is now pulled swiftly through the most dependent part of the swelling, the pus and blood are evacuated by aspiration and a rubber drain is inserted.

If an electrosurgical unit is available, an even more pain-free action can be employed, because no pressure is applied when a unipolar electrode is used to incise the swelling and liberate the pus.

FAILURE OF ANAESTHESIA DURING APICECTOMY

Prevention is preferable to cure. The most common causes of inadequate anaesthesia during surgical intervention are insufficient local anaesthetic, incorrect placement of the needle and excessively fast deposition of anaesthetic fluid. It is essential that injection be made slowly so that the vasoconstrictor is given time to become effective before the solution is dissipated over a large area and an inadequate concentration obtained. The anaesthetic should be deposited over the apices of the roots and, in the anterior part of the maxilla, high enough to anaesthetize the floor of the nose. If there is a fenestration, the needle should perforate it, with injection of fluid into the area.

If despite these measures pain is experienced when curetting the periapical bony cavity, a 10% solution of Cocaine on a gauze swab, left in the cavity for about 3 minutes, will provide total anaesthesia for the time required to carry out the curettage.

VITAL REMNANTS OF PULP IN A CANAL

Often, despite thorough debridement and filing at a previous visit when vital pulp was extirpated, some vital remnants cause distress when the canal is being prepared for filling. A careful diagnostic radiograph will ensure the absence of a lateral or foraminal perforation. Copious bleeding from the canal would indicate either a large stump of partly amputated pulp or a perforation. If neither situation exists, residual nerve filaments may be anaesthetized by flooding the canal with 10% Cocaine or 5% Xylocaine (topical) paste. After about two minutes, a file is used gently to pump the fluid or paste up to the apex and, when no further discomfort is experienced, to file out the vital remnants and allow subsequent preparation of the canal.

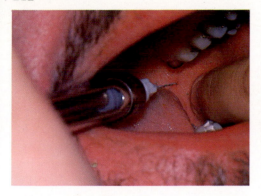

212

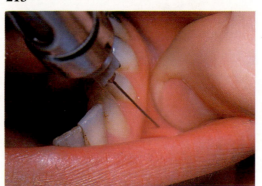

213

THE PROBLEM OF PULPITIC MANDIBULAR TEETH WHICH DO NOT RESPOND TO A NERVE BLOCK

It is not uncommon to encounter pulpitic teeth in which an apparently satisfactory nerve block has failed to provide adequate anaesthesia in a mandibular tooth (212). When this occurs in a mandibular incisor, it is probably due to an element of cross innervation and may be overcome by a), giving intrapapillary injections at mesial and distal aspects of the affected tooth, b) an incisive nerve block on the contra-lateral side (213), c) by an intraligamental injection or d) an intra-osseous injection.

If the pulpitic tooth is a canine, premolar or molar, a long buccal injection should be given, plus a lingual sub-periosteal deposition of anaesthetic at the level of the apices, with the bevel of the needle directed, in the latter injection, towards the tongue. If this does not produce anaesthesia an intraligamental injection should be tried.

In a small number of patients all of these techniques may be of no avail. A final method, short of using general anaesthesia, is the intrapulpal injection. A pledget of cotton is soaked in a 10% solution of Cocaine and placed in the pulp chamber or over the exposed pulp. After a few minutes, an injection of lignocaine is made directly into the pulp. This may be painful for a few seconds but complete anaesthesia is usually obtained. This technique is a useful alternative when a general anaesthetic is contra-indicated, e.g., when an anaesthetist is not available or when the patient has taken food just prior to the visit. There is, however, a potential risk of spreading infection into the periapical bone as a result of the high intrapulpal pressure, hence the technique should be used only as a last resort, and a suitable antibiotic should be given.

Relative analgesia is of value for patients who are unduly nervous or whose teeth prove difficult to anaesthetize. It is used in conjunction with local or regional anaesthesia.

An over-wrought patient is not a good candidate for multiple unsuccessful attempts to obtain anaesthesia. In such cases it is kinder to dress the pulp, either with carbolized resin or a corticosteroid/antibiotic preparation, and to make a further attempt at a subsequent appointment.

DEVITALISING PASTE

An alternative means of producing a relatively fast pulpal necrosis is to place a dressing of devitalising paste over the pulp for 4-7 days. After removal of the dressing, preparation of the pulp canals should be painless. This technique has been supplanted largely by the use of anaesthetic agents, because it tends to cause pain of varying intensity and, should the coronal seal be disturbed between visits, the mixture, which usually contains arsenic or formaldehyde, could enter the oral cavity, producing severe toxic ulceration.

A modified form of this technique however, using a formaldehyde-containing devitalisation paste, is used often for deciduous teeth. (See Chapter 14).

PAIN-FREE TECHNIQUE

Whatever technique is used to produce anaesthesia by injection, every attempt must be made to avoid unnecessary pain and discomfort. The rules for achieving this are as follows:

1 Apply a topical anaesthetic to the injection site. Wait at least 60 seconds before inserting the needle.
2 Use a sharp (disposable) needle.
3 Warm the anaesthetic solution to body temperature (214).
4 Insert the needle with a swift, deft thrust, and infiltrate the fluid very slowly, advancing the needle in stages as the anaesthetic takes effect.
5 Never inject sub-periosteally until the overlying mucoperiosteum has been anaesthetized. A small sub-mucous bulla of anaesthetic is massaged gently towards the bone and, after a delay of about 10 seconds, the needle is carried gently through the periosteum to lie close to the apex of the root, where the solution is deposited slowly.

214

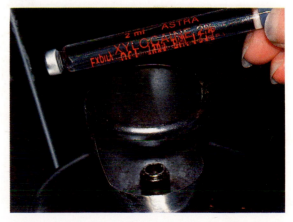

5 Basic Instruments and Materials C J Stock

Space will not permit the inclusion of all endodontic instruments and materials that are commercially available. An attempt has been made to include the basic armamentarium used with emphasis on some of the newer products. It was found necessary for descriptive purposes to include some instruments and materials in later chapters of the book.

215 Instrument pack. Contains the basic instruments which should be available and sterile for root canal treatment. The pack contains (from top to bottom):

Pair of artery forceps — to hold X-Ray films in the mouth	
Sterile cotton wool pledgets and rolls	
Front surface mirror	
Endo locking tweezers	
Briault probe	Ash PRO FT11[1]
Long shank excavator	Ash 141/142[1]
Amalgam plugger	Ash 164[1]
Flat plastic	Ash 156[1]
Canal probe	DG16[2]
Metal ruler	

215

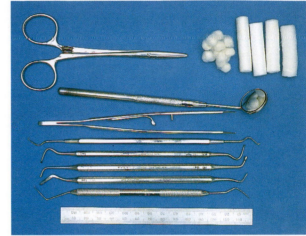

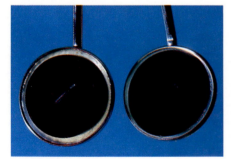

216

216 Mirrors. Front surface reflecting[3] mirrors should be used. The photograph shows two types of mirrors, both of them scratched. The left one is front surface reflecting and in the one on the right the reflecting surface is behind the glass. The image from the back surface reflecting mirror is less clear and any scratches appear double.

217

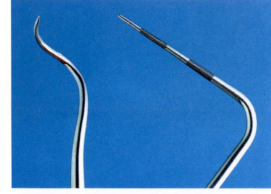

Probes. A canal probe is useful to locate canal entrances in the floor of the pulp chamber. Two probes, although not included in the pack, are suggested to help in periodontal assessment. A pocket measuring probe which has a fine shank with millimetre depth markings and a blunt tip is illustrated. The Marquis[4] (**217** right), is shown.

To probe furcations in posterior teeth a curved instrument is required. The American pattern probe No. 3[5] (**217** left) is shown.

218

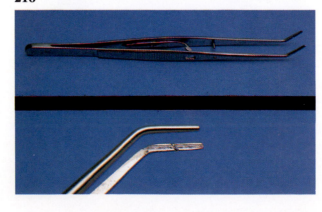

218 Tweezers. Endodontic locking tweezers[6] allow materials such as gutta percha points, paper points or cotton wool pledgets to be carried to the mouth. They are essential for four handed transference between operator and nurse. The tips of the beaks should be blunt and contain grooves.

HAND INSTRUMENTS

Regulations concerning instruments designed to aid in root canal preparation are governed by the International Standards Organisation. Instruments are numbered and colour coded.

The number of each instrument (**219**) refers to the diameter, D_1, of the cutting blade at the tip of the shank. The number is taken from the diameter D_1 in millimetres x 100 e.g. If the diameter at D_1 is 0.25 mm the number of the instrument is 25. D_2 is the diameter of the cutting blade furthest from the tip of the shank. The working part, which lies between D_1 and D_2, is tapered, the degree of taper depending on the type of instrument. Reamers and files have a taper of 0.02 mm per mm of working length.

Colour coding. The International Standards Organisation (ISO) recommends a colour coding system which has now been adopted by the majority of firms manufacturing hand instruments, six colours were chosen in ascending order of size from light to dark. These colours are repeated in each of the 3 groups. The table on the right shows the range of numbered instruments and their allotted colour coding.

Unfortunately not all companies follow the ISO system. Micromega have a different system in which green is replaced by brown and Group 1 starts with 08 as white. The photograph illustrates the difference between the two systems (**220**).

219

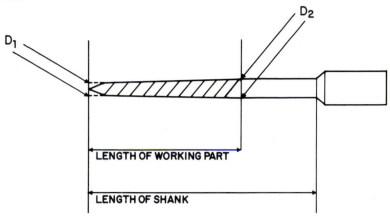

220

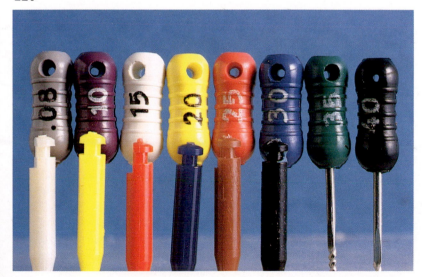

GROUP	NUMBER OF INSTRUMENT	COLOUR CODING
	06	Pink
	08	Grey
	10	Purple
	15	White
	20	Yellow
GROUP 1	25	Red
	30	Blue
	35	Green
	40	Black
	45	White
	50	Yellow
GROUP 2	55	Red
	60	Blue
	70	Green
	80	Black
	90	White
	100	Yellow
GROUP 3	110	Red
	120	Blue
	130	Green
	140	Black

* These sizes are now generally accepted but were not part of the original ISO recommendations.

Instrument lengths. There are four standard lengths manufactured 21 mm, 25 mm, 28 mm, and 31 mm measured from the instrument tip to the base of the handle. These lengths are adequate for the majority of teeth but occasionally longer than 31 mm may be required and these can be ordered specially.

Types of instrument. The various types of instrument in use are illustrated, including several of the more recent designs. Some instruments such as the smooth broach and rat tail files are rarely used and are not described.

221

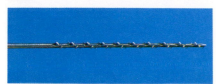

Barbed broach (**221**). These instruments are designed to remove gross pulp tissue. They are made from soft steel and have barbs notched into the shank. They must only be used in the straight part of the canal. The size chosen should fit loosely into the canal to avoid breakage.

Reamer (**222**). The reamer is produced by twisting a square or triangular tapered blank. A reamer will cut only when it is rotated due to the angle of the blade or flute.

K-File (**223, 229**). The K-file received its name from the Kerr Manufacturing Co., who were the first to produce it. The K-file is constructed in the same way as a reamer except that there are 2½ times the number of twists per unit length. The advantage of the file is that it may be used to cut dentine by either a rotary movement or a filing action.

Flex-O-File[2] (**224, 229**). A recent addition, the Flex-O-File is very similar to a K-file but is manufactured with a softer more flexible steel. It does not fracture easily and is so flexible that it is possible to tie a knot in the shank.

K-Flex file[1] (**225, 229**). Another recent addition to the range of hand instruments. It is similar to a K-file except that the shape of the cross section is a diamond. This means that the instrument is more flexible than a reamer or K-file and has a sharper blade.

Hedstroem file (**226, 230**). The instruments are machined from a round tapered blank. A spiral groove is cut into the shank, producing a sharp blade. Because of the angle of the blade the hedstroem file should only be used with a filing action. If a rotary movement is used and the blades engage the dentine there is a danger of the instrument fracturing.

Unifile[3] (**227, 230**). This relatively new instrument is almost identical in appearance to the hedstroem file, but it has two cutting blades instead of one. The grooves cut into the shank of the Unifile remain at the same depth throughout the working part. This increases the stiffness and resistance to fracture in the coronal and middle thirds of the instrument but allows greater flexibility in the apical portion which corresponds to the position of the curve in most roots.

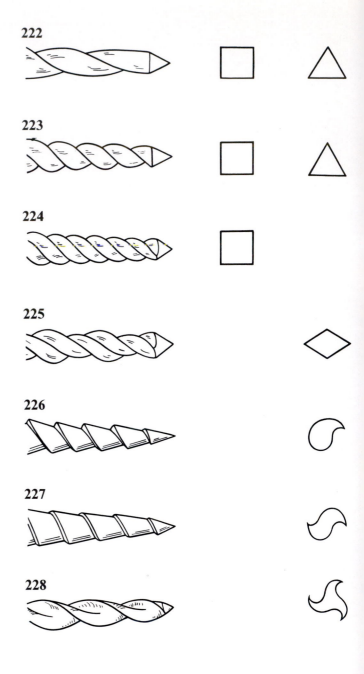

222

223

224

225

226

227

228

Helifile[4] (**228, 238**). The method of manufacture of the Helifile is similar to the Hedstroem and Unifile except that in cross section there are 3 blades. The appearance of the instrument resembles a reamer rather than a Hedstroem file. Little information is available yet concerning their cutting ability or resistance to fracture.

229

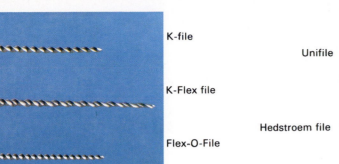

K-file

K-Flex file

Flex-O-File

230

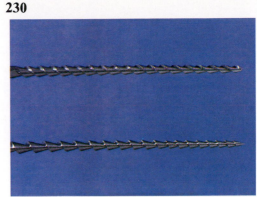

Unifile

Hedstroem file

Instrument Safety and Usage. An ever present danger during root canal preparation is the fracture of an instrument within the canal. This will be unlikely to occur if the following steps are taken.

1 Instruments should be inspected before they are inserted into the root canal (**231**). If there is any sign of the flutes becoming either unwound (B) or overtwisted (A) the instrument should be discarded. Instruments with a sharp bend in the shank should also be thrown away (C). There is no guide to the number of times an instrument should be used as this will depend upon a number of factors. Smaller instruments will be discarded more frequently than larger ones.

2 Never force an instrument into a canal. If an instrument feels tight in the canal short of the working length it should be removed and a smaller size used.

3 Reaming action. All instruments with the exception of the Hedstroem file may be used with a reaming action. The reaming action consists of a quarter to a half turn and withdrawal. An instrument should not be screwed into the canal as this invites fracture. The reaming action produces a rounder hole than filing but should not be used in curved canals as it will produce zipping in the apical portion of the canal.

4 Filing action is carried out by inserting the instrument to the marked depth and then withdrawing it while exerting even pressure on the wall of the canal. The instrument is withdrawn a few mm, reinserted and the movement repeated. The entire wall of the canal is filed by gradually working circumferentially in a clockwise direction.

231

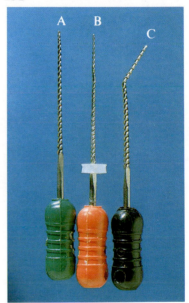

POWER ASSISTED INSTRUMENTS

Several special handpieces are available which take broaches and files to aid root canal preparation. The continuous rotation of the handpiece is transformed into an alternating quarter turn movement. The handpieces are considered a useful addition to the armamentarium in certain circumstances, such as difficult access. Their limitations however should be borne in mind — namely, the increased danger of instrument fracture and excess removal of dentine from the inner curve of the canal. There is no evidence to show that the time required for canal preparation is reduced. Finally tactile sense associated with hand instrumentation is lost with a handpiece.

Root canal preparation should never be attempted with files in a standard handpiece.

232

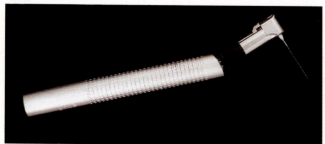

233

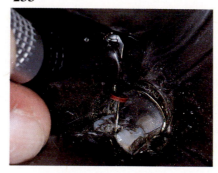

Giromatic[1] (**232, 233**). This alternating handpiece was introduced in 1964 and has gained wide acceptance. It takes latch mounted broaches and Hedstroem files and more recently Heligiro-files. It is generally recommended that the running speed of 3000 rpm advised by the manufacturers be reduced to 1500-2000 rpm.

234

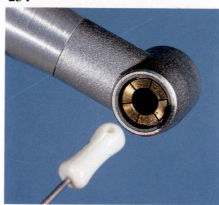

Cursor[2] (**234, 235**). This 4:1 reduction handpiece produces a similar alternating action to the Giromatic but the spring chuck holds standard hand instruments. There are three models available:

1 Holds Maillefer hand instruments.

2 Accepts Kerr, Micromega, Zipperer and several other well known hand instruments.

3 Takes standard latch type instruments.

235

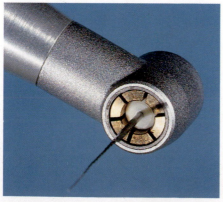

New instruments for alternating handpieces (236, 237, 238).
Recently three new instruments have been designed.

Rispi[1] (**236**). This is a variation on the rat tail file and has a smooth non-cutting tip.

Dynatrak[2] (**237**). A unifile with a non-cutting tip.

Heligiro file[3] (**238**). A Helifile (**228**) with a standard latch type fitting.

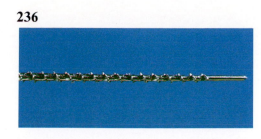

236

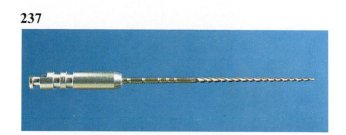

237

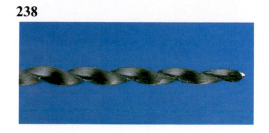

238

SPIRAL ROOT CANAL FILLERS

These are used in a standard handpiece. The size selected must fit loosely in the canal and should not be used around curves in the canal. There are three designs in use. All should be used with care as they are liable to fracture.

1 *Coiled wire.* These are the most likely to fracture. Three are shown in the radiograph in the second molar (**239**).

2 *Twisted blade* (Hawes-Neos[4], **240**). As there is more metal in cross section this type is less prone to fracture.

3 *Coiled wire with safety device* (Micromega)[5]. The wire nearest to the handle is tightly coiled so that it will fracture at this point if the instrument binds, and may be removed easily. All three types are illustrated (**241**).
A   Twisted blade.
B   Coiled wire with safety device.
C   Coiled wire.

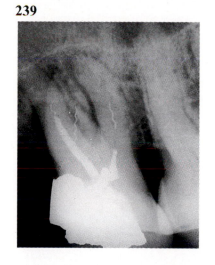

239

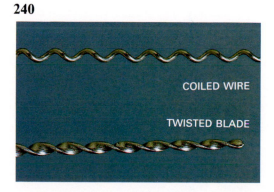

240

COILED WIRE

TWISTED BLADE

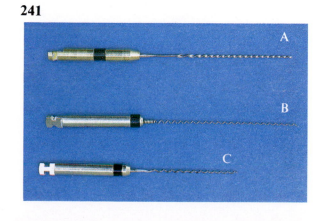

241

A

B

C

BURS

Burs should be used with caution in root canals because of the danger of perforation. There are several burs however which may be required for root canal treatment. **242** shows six varieties of engine burs, from the left:

A   Small standard round bur used occasionally to remove calcified deposits over the entrance to a canal in the pulp chamber floor.

B   16 mm bur for the floor of the pulp chamber. This bur has a shank 3 mm longer than the standard bur.

C   Long shank round bur overall length 23 mm.

D   Goose neck round bur[1]. Both this and the long shank bur are used to locate a partially sclerosed canal. The goose neck has the advantage, because of its extended narrow shank, of not being deflected by the wall of the axis cavity.

E   Peeso reamer[2]. This engine driven instrument has a sharp point and presents a real danger of perforating unless great care is used.

F   Gates Glidden[3]. Both the Gates Glidden and Peeso instruments are used to prepare post holes after the root treatment is complete and to taper the coronal part of the canal during root canal preparation. The Gates Glidden is particularly useful as its tip does not cut which reduces the danger of perforation (**243**).

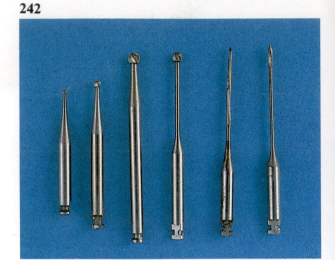

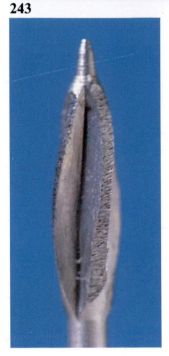

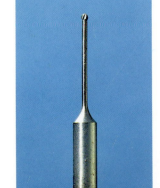

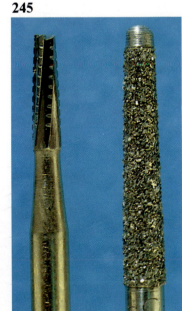

The ½-round long shank pin bur produced by Whaledent[4], which the author has found most helpful in locating canals (**244**).

Access Cavity burs. Two air rotor burs in **245** are used for cutting access cavities.

The Tungsten Carbide[5] 701 tapered fissure is used to obtain initial access through enamel or metal.

The non-end-cutting tapered diamond[6] will produce a smooth finish to the walls of the access cavity without damaging the floor.

STORAGE SYSTEMS

The organisation and storage of endodontic instruments requires some thought and should be tailor-made to the operator's particular requirements. Three different systems will be described.

246

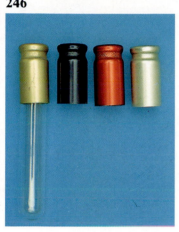

247

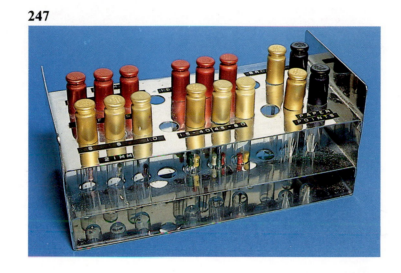

248

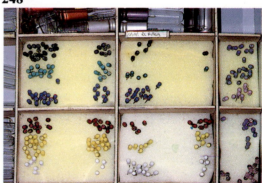

249

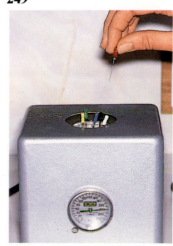

1. Test tubes[1] (**246**). Standard 11 mm wide pyrex test tubes will hold six instruments. The instruments are sterilised in an autoclave inside the test tubes.

The ends of the test tubes are fitted with colour coded aluminium caps[2]. The test tubes may be stored in racks for easy access[3] (**247**). During root canal treatment the cap is removed and the instruments placed on a sterile sponge (see **252**). Artificial sponges are readily available, inexpensive and may be sterilised in an autoclave.

2. Sorter box (**248**). A simpler system is to sterilise the instruments and stick them into a sponge grouped according to their size and length.

When a patient requires root canal treatment the surgery assistant removes the appropriate instruments and resterilises them in a glass bead steriliser (**249**).

250

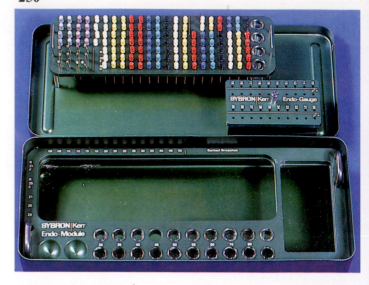

3. Sterile box (**250**). Many types of containers for endodontic instruments are available on the market. A box such as the one shown, Kerr endo-module[1], is chosen and filled with all the instruments that could be required in one day. The box, together with its contents are sterilised in a hot air oven.

The surgery assistant has the box beside her and provides the operator with the necessary instruments. The lid is kept on the box except when removing instruments to keep the contents sterile. At the end of the day or session the used instruments are either discarded or cleaned and returned to the box. Spaces are refilled and the box resterilised.

A disadvantage of this system is that many instruments will be sterilised several times without being used which will reduce their cutting efficiency.

TRAYS

A tray must contain the standard instruments required for root canal treatment and a space for the files or reamers. Two examples are shown (**251, 252**).

RAF Tray[2]. The aluminium tray is divided into four compartments and contains a stand for the files or reamers. The tray measures 28 cm long, 18 cm wide and 3.5 cm deep. The tray has a separate metal lid.

Double Tray (DT)[3]. The plastic tray measures 38.3 cm long by 26.6 cm wide and does not have a cover. It may be adapted by adding a removable sterile sponge cut to fit one of the compartments and retained by pins or screws placed in the compartment walls.

251

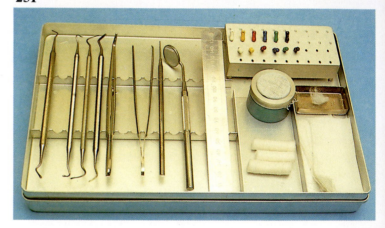

252

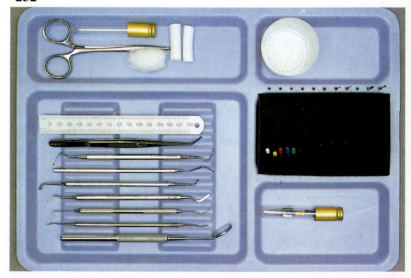

STERILISATION

Sterilisation of all endodontic instruments is important to prevent cross infection. Bacteria, viruses and fungi may contaminate instruments and should be destroyed by chemicals and/or heat. The dangers of cross infection have recently been highlighted by both the AIDS and hepatitis virus. Gloves and masks are now recommended for most dental procedures for both the operator and his chairside assistant. A particular danger facing all dental personnel is stick injuries, either by contaminated needles or instruments and every care must be taken to prevent this type of injury.

Cleaning the instruments. Instruments should be cleaned as soon as possible after use to remove all debris which harbours and protects micro-organisms. Cleaning is carried out by scrubbing with detergent in warm water, or in the case of files and reamers, stabbing them into a sponge. There is little doubt that the best method of removing debris from instruments is to place them in an ultrasonic bath. See the Sonicleaner (**253**)[1]. The expansion and contraction of gas bubbles dislodges the debris from places inaccessible to normal cleaning.

When the instruments are clean they should then be sterilised. There are several methods available:

Chemicals. Numerous chemicals are available to kill micro-organisms although doubt has been raised of the ability of most of them to kill spores. One of the recommended chemicals is Glutaraldehyde because of its efficiency and the indirect evidence that it is effective against the hepatitis virus.

Sporicidin[2] and Cidex[3] are currently two of the most popular methods of chemical disinfection. Both of them are Glutaraldehyde. Sporicidin's active ingredients are:

Glutaraldehyde	2.00%
Phenol	7.05%
Sodium tetra-borate	2.35%
Sodium phenolate	1.20%

Dry heat. Dry heat is the most widely used form of sterilisation. The instruments must be heated to 160°C for one hour. This method is better suited to instruments with sharp cutting edges, paper points, oils and powders. It should not be used for fabrics and rubber products. **254** shows an Elektrohelios[5] hot air steriliser.

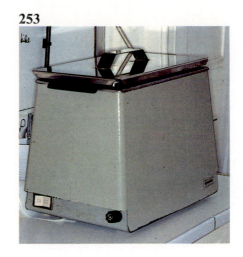

253

Disinfection takes place by immersing instruments for ten minutes at room temperature in a 1 in 16 dilution of the stock solution. Sterilisation will take place in 6¾ hours.

It is not recommended as an overnight holding solution for carbon steel or dental burs. Cases of sensitivity to Glutaraldehyde have been reported in which case Benzalkonium chloride is a viable alternative.

Roccal[4]. Contains one per cent Benzalkonium chloride. The chemical is germicidal for gram positive bacteria and some fungi. The solution is not generally effective against spore forming bacteria or viruses.

If Roccal is used as a holding solution for stainless steel instruments it is recommended to add 2 g Sodium nitrite (or 1 g Sodium nitrite and 2 g Sodium carbonate).

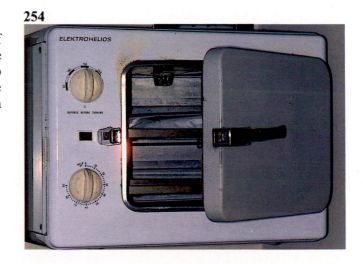

254

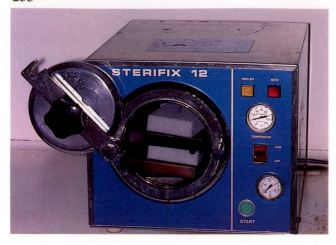

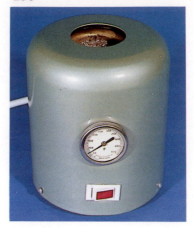

Moist heat (255). Micro-organisms are destroyed at considerably lower temperatures and shorter exposure times when moisture is present because all biologic reactions are catalysed by water.

The instruments are placed in the autoclave for 30 minutes at 15 lb pressure at 121°C (250°F).

Amine compound additives are recommended to reduce corrosion of sharp instruments (e.g. Cyclohexylamine).

Salt or glass bead steriliser[1] **(256).** This is a useful method of sterilising small instruments such as files or reamers by the chairside.

It is wise to select a steriliser which has a temperature gauge so that it can be seen when the working temperature of 218°C (425°F) has been reached. The sterilisation time is 10 seconds.

In the author's opinion, salt is preferred to glass beads as there is a danger that beads may be carried into the root canal on an instrument and produce an obstruction.

Checking Sterilisation. It is possible to check that the inside of the sterilisation chamber has reached the correct temperature for sterilisation. There are two simple methods:

A. *Browne's tubes*[2]. The tubes are used to check dry heat and autoclave sterilisers. The appropriate tube is placed in the steriliser and the colour changes from red to green when the correct temperature and time have been reached. **257** shows a chart below which is a Browne's tube.

B. *Sterilisation bags*[2] *for the autoclave.* Instruments for sterilisation are placed in the bag. One side of the bag is transparent so its contents are visible (**258**). Vertical pale brown stripes on the bag turn to dark brown when the correct temperature is reached. **259** shows the changing colour from (left) to after sterilisation (right).

257

FOR DIRECTIONS SEE LEAFLET					
	UNUSED	UNSAFE		TURNING POINT	EFFECTIVE TREATMENT
		APPROX. TIMES IN MINUTES TO PRODUCE THESE COLOURS AT:				
Tubes Type 1 (Black Spot)	O	12	20	23	25 and over	115°C
	O	8	13	15	16 ,, ,,	120°C
	O	5	9	10	11 ,, ,,	125°C
Tubes Type 2 (Yellow Spot)	O	2	3	3½	4 ,, ,,	130°C
	O	1½	2½	2½-3	3 ,, ,,	135°C

258

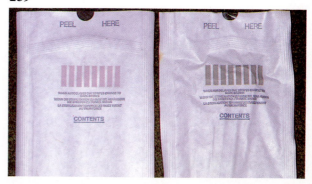

259

MEASURING

The first step in preparation of the root canal is to calculate the working length. The method used must be accurate to within 0.5 to 1 mm. Measurement of the root length may be divided into two steps, calculating the working length and recording it on the instrument shank with a stop.

Calculating working length. The working length is calculated by placing a diagnostic instrument in the root canal and either taking a radiograph or using an electronic device. (See also Chapter 11.)

Millimetre square grid lines on a transparent sheet may be attached to an X-Ray film before exposure. This can be a useful method for straight canals but as can be seen (**260**) it is difficult to measure curved roots.

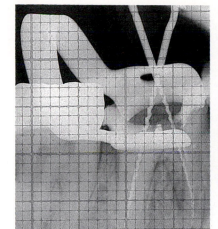

260

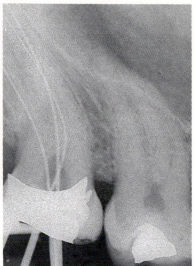

261

Electronic devices. There are many electronic devices currently available. The principle on which they work has been well established and they are capable of accurate measurement. Although they do not replace radiography they will reduce the number of radiographs necessary and provide an accurate check of the working length. The devices are particularly useful in posterior teeth where it may be difficult either to acquire a good radiograph or to interpret the position of the apex (**261**).

262

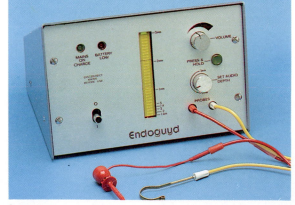

263

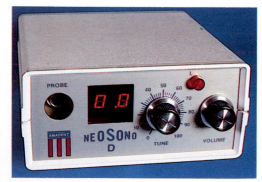

262 and 263 show the Endoguyd[1] and the Neosono D[2]. Both have a display showing the distance of the instrument tip from the apical constriction in millimetres. It is claimed that both instruments will measure accurately in wet canals. As the principle is based on electrical impedance it is obvious that if the root canal contains a dissociating medium such as necrotic debris or sodium hypochlorite the device will give a false reading. Some experience is required to decide if the reading is correct.

264

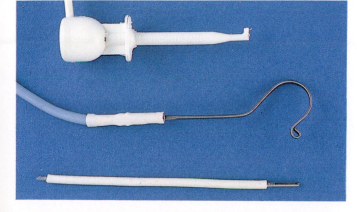

264 shows the accessories required with the Neosono D.

A Spring loaded clip which is attached to the shank of the file.

B Hook which is placed over patient's lip.

C An alternative to the clip. The metal end is placed in contact with the instrument shank.

Recording length on instrument

Having established the working length a stop must be placed at the correct position on the shank of each instrument. It is difficult to understand why so many measuring devices are available as a simple metal ruler is sufficient.

265 shows a ruler which is specifically designed for endodontics[1]. It has a ring attached to the back of a short ruler so that it may be worn on a finger and measurements made and checked.

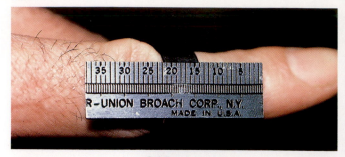
265

Two examples of measuring devices are illustrated.

The Endogauge[2] (266). The endogauge is a metal stand with a platform around a central pillar. The platform is adjusted to the correct height corresponding to the working length. Instruments are placed in the holes in the platform with rubber stops on the shanks and pushed home to the base.

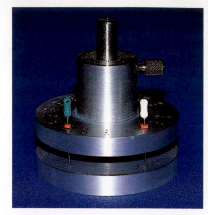
266

A second device (**267**) consists of grooves in a block ranging from 10-30 mm. in length. A whole variety of measuring devices are manufactured, no one in particular being recommended.

Length Stops. There are many ways of marking the correct length on the instrument shank.

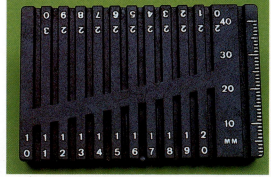
267

Rubber or Silicone Stops[3] These stops must be pierced at right angles through the centre (**268**). Note that the one on the right could result in the inaccurate length preparation. The stops are available in a variety of colours (**269**).

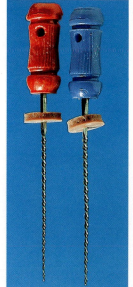
268

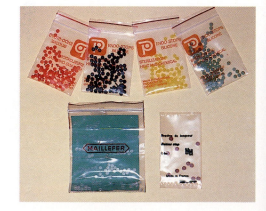
269

Paste. Marking paste may be made from Zinc oxide powder mixed with petroleum jelly. The advantage of paste is that smudging is immediately apparent whereas a rubber stop may be moved along the shank inadvertently and not be noticed.

270

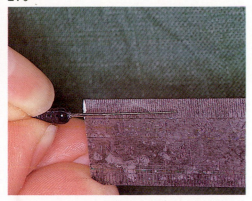

271

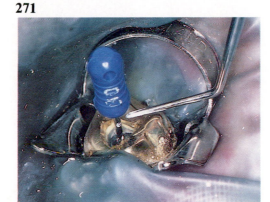

The paste is placed at the end of a ruler as shown (**270**) and the shank of the instrument touched onto the paste at the correct length. **271** shows an instrument placed in the canal and then marking paste placed on the shank with a straight probe opposite the tip of a cusp.

272

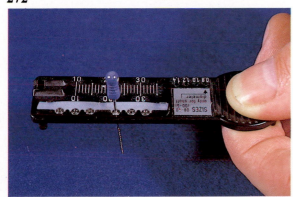

272 Metal stops. These Vari-fix steel stops[1] require 600 g of force to move them and so provide an accurate stable measurement. Although they are now colour coded 4 different diameter holes are required to fit the range of shanks found in a full set of hand instruments.

273

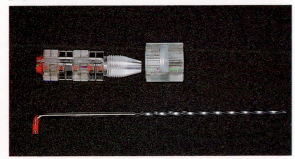

273. Test handle system[2]. These instruments are supplied with a right angle bend at the end of the shank which fits into a special handle. The handle is fitted and clamped tight at the predetermined length. Two lengths of instrument and handle are provided. The one for posterior teeth is adjustable from 16-20 mm and the one for anterior teeth 20-28 mm.

IRRIGATION

The objectives of this important part of root canal preparation are:

Lubrication of root canal instruments.

Dissolution of organic debris.

Flushing out of inorganic debris.

Elimination of micro-organisms.

The irrigating solutions recommended are:

Sterile water

Saline

Local anaesthetic solution

Sodium hypochlorite

Sodium hypochlorite. A 2-2½% solution is favoured. The strength of solution recommended varies from 0.3%-5.5%; the author prefers 2.0% weight per volume. A suitable source for sodium hypochlorite is a standard household bleach. The exact concentration should be ascertained and it must be checked that there are no additives. The strength of household bleaches is usually 5-6% expressed as percentage available chlorine which is equivalent to approximately 14% weight per volume. The solution may be diluted by adding tap water.

Irrigation syringe. The Sodium hypochlorite is injected into the pulp chamber using a disposable syringe and special needle for irrigation. **274, 275**[1] show a standard hypodermic needle (top) and below an irrigation needle and syringe (bottom). Note the side of the needle near the tip is cut away to reduce the risk of forcing the irrigation solution through the apex if the needle became jammed in the canal. Irrigation should be used copiously throughout canal preparation. After completion the canal is dried with paper points.

274

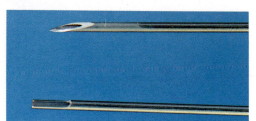

275

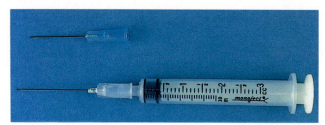

276

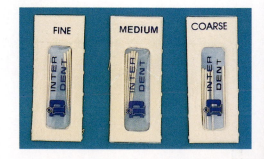

FINE MEDIUM COARSE

Paper points. These are supplied in different sizes which are sterilised or unsterile. The problem with a large box of sterilised points is that once opened the unused points are no longer sterile. A convenient packaging method is to use small packets containing five per packet of pre-sterilised points (**276**)[2].

MEDICATION OF THE CANAL

Research in recent years has shown that the prime objective in root canal preparation is to remove the contents of the canal. In this way the majority of canal debris and micro-organisms is removed. The introduction of powerful bactericides into the root canal may cause pain and delay healing by leaching out into the periodontal areas and damaging normal vital tissue.

Most authorities do not recommend any intra-canal medication except in the following circumstances:

1 To eliminate the few micro-organisms remaining in the root canal system after preparation. The importance of using medication for this reason is open to question. If the canal system is cleaned and obturated any remaining bacteria should be incarcerated and will then die.

2 To provide a barrier against leakage of the coronal seal which would allow invasion of micro-organisms into the root canal.

3 To reduce inflammation of the periapical tissues or remnants of vital pulp if time does not allow its complete removal.

4 Calcium hydroxide has a variety of uses but it is thought that the increase in pH encourages deposition of hard tissue and so promotes healing. It is also useful in the treatment of cases of chronic wet canals.

There are large numbers of canal medicaments, many of them offering wild claims of success. It is suggested the contents on the label are examined and those containing powerful concentrations of bactericides should be discarded.

Parachlorphenol. A 1% solution gives adequate bactericidal properties yet is relatively non-toxic to tissue. 35% camphorated parachlorphenol is not recommended as it damages vital tissue. The 1% solution may be made up at a local chemist or drugstore.

Metacresyl acetate (Cresatin)[1]. This is used in cases of vital pulp extirpation because of its sedative effect.

Ledermix[2]. This product is available in the form of a paste and a cement. The contents of the paste are:

Triamcinolone acetonide	1%
Demethylchlor tetracycline HCL	3%

in a water soluble cream containing triethanolamine, calcium chloride, zinc oxide, sodium sulphate and polyethylene glycol 4000.

The active ingredients are the broad spectrum antibiotic and the corticosteroid which produces an anti-inflammatory effect. Although controlled studies are lacking, the paste is used as an inter-appointment canal medicament when the patients have presented in pain.

277

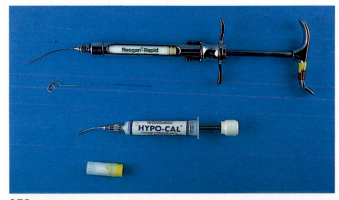

278

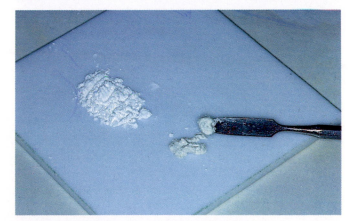

277 Calcium hydroxide. There are several commercial preparations. Two are illustrated. Reogan[3] is contained within a cartridge and is injected into the canal using a hypodermic syringe and wide bore needle. Hypocal[4] consists of a barrel containing the calcium hydroxide which is extruded by twisting a plunger.

Pure calcium hydroxide may be obtained as a powder from a local chemist or drugstore and mixed with sterile water or local anaesthetic solution (**278**). The mix should be made thick and placed in the root canal with a small carrier. The mix is then packed into the canal with pluggers or a carrier such as a Messing Gun[5].

ROOT CANAL SEALERS

A wide variety of sealers is available, suggesting that the ideal has not yet been discovered; indeed all sealers are soluble. The purpose of a sealer is to fill the minute spaces which remain between the filler and the walls of the root canal. It follows that only small quantities of sealer are required and the final thickness of sealer should be as thin as possible.

Sealers may be broadly classified according to their composition:

Eugenol   Non Eugenol   Medicated

Eugenol. Eugenol-containing cements form the group most widely accepted in teaching hospitals. Basically the group may be sub-divided into those that contain silver and those that are silver free. The inclusion of silver in the sealer recommended by Rickert in 1931 has been criticised because it stains dentine a dark grey. Note the grey margin beneath the crown (**279**).

Grossman's formula replaced silver with another radiopaque substance, barium sulphate.

Kerr Pulp Canal Sealer (1931)[1].   This contains a powder and liquid.
Constituents:

Powder: Zinc oxide   Liquid: Oil of cloves
        Silver (precipitated molecular)   Canada balsam
        Oleo resins (white resin)
        Thymol iodide

The setting time is a little longer than Tubliseal.

Tubliseal (1961)[2].   This is a two paste system which is easier to mix than a powder and liquid system. Constituents:

Base: Zinc oxide   Catalyst: Eugenol
       Oleo resins   Polymerised resin
       Bismuth trioxide   Annidalin
       Thymol iodide
       Oils and waxes

Setting time approximately 20 minutes on pad, five minutes in the canal. Other examples in this group are Procosol radiopaque silver cement, Procosol non-staining cement, Grossman's sealer and Wach's paste.

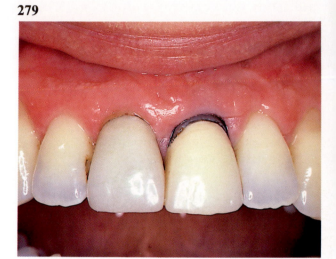

279

Non-Eugenol. These sealers do not contain Eugenol and consist of a wide variety of chemicals. Chlorapercha, a combination of chloroform and gutta percha, and a similar formulation by Nygaard-Østby, which contains Canada balsam and rosin in addition to chloropercha, have been criticised because of their shrinkage.

Diaket (1951)[3].   This consists of a fine powder and thick viscous liquid. Chemically Diaket is a polyketone. A medicated variety, Diaket A, is included in the next section. The setting time for Diaket is 8 minutes on the mixing slab and somewhat quicker in the mouth. A second bottle is provided which contains a solvent for the sealer.

AH26 (1957)[1]. This consists of a yellow powder and viscous resin liquid. AH26 is an epoxy resin base with a bisphenol diglycidyl ether liquid. The formulation has been altered recently with the removal of silver as one of the constituents. On occasion there may be a severe inflammatory response to the sealer which subsides after some weeks. The setting time is 36 to 48 hours at body temperature and at room temperature 5-7 days.

Medicated. Provided the principles of root canal preparation and filling are observed there is no justification for the use of therapeutic sealers. In fact the use of powerful chemicals such as formaldehyde which will produce necrosis and tissue fixation will prejudice the success of root canal treatment. The main attraction for the use of these materials is the claim that the time consuming classical method of root canal preparation is not required as the medicated sealer will sterilise the contents of the root canal.

The addition of heavy metal ions is potentially dangerous as these are disseminated throughout the body. The principle of adding corticosteroids to mask the chemical effects must also be challenged.

Diaket A. Chemically this sealer is similar to Diaket but it also contains the disinfectant Hexachlorophene. Diaket is one of the few medicated sealers which does not contain paraformaldehyde.

N2 (1970)[2]. Many claims have been made for this material but one of the problems of testing it has been the variation in the formulation.

N_2 refers to the so-called second nerve. For some years two different types of N_2 sealer were marketed, normal and Apical. A single N_2 sealer is now available, Universal, and the formulation has been altered with the removal of hydrocortisone, prednisolone and barium sulphate.

The corticosteroids are now added to the cement separately as hydrocortisone powder or Terra Cortril. Constituents:

Powder:		
Zinc oxide		68.51g
Lead tetroxide		12.00g
Paraformaldehyde		4.70g
Bismuth subcarbonate		2.60g
Bismuth subnitrate		3.70g
Titanium dioxide		8.40g
Phenylmercuric borate		0.09g

Liquid: Eugenol
Oleum Rosae
Oleum Lavandulae

Endomethasone[3]. The formulation of this sealer is very similar to N2. A pink antiseptic powder is mixed with eugenol. Constituents:

Powder:		
Zinc oxide		100.00g
Bismuth subnitrate		
Dexamethasone		0.01g
Hydrocortisone acetate		1.60g
Thymol iodide		25.00g
Paraformaldehyde		2.20g

Liquid: Eugenol

Spad. This material is advertised as a one-visit non-irritant radiopaque filler and sealer. It is a bakelite type resin which consists of a powder and two liquids.

Powder:		
	Phenylmercuric borate	0.16g
	Calcium hydroxide	0.94g
	Hydrocortisone acetate	2.00g
	Paraformaldehyde	4.70g
	Titanium oxide	6.30g
	Barium sulphate	13.00g
	Zinc oxide	72.90g
Liquid L—	Glycerine	13.00g
	Formaldehyde solution	87.00g
Liquid L.D.	Hydrochloric acid	20.00g
	Resorcinol	25.00g
	Glycerine	55.00g

Spad is recommended by the manufacturers for pulpotomies in both deciduous and permanent teeth and as a root-filling paste. It is suggested for the treatment of acute endodontic infections and for teeth with periapical areas. In the latter cases small quantities of Spad are introduced into the periapical areas deliberately because it is thought that the sterilising effect accelerates healing.

The manufacturer's instructions concerning root canal preparation state "Ream the canal or canals quickly to just short of the apex if possible (2-3 reamers of different sizes maximum)."

The setting time is 24 hours, during which time small quantities of formaldehyde gas are released.

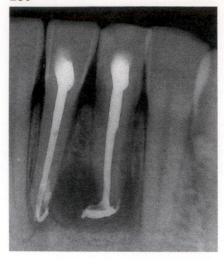

Iodoform paste (1928). This paste is absorbed by the body and any seal achieved at the time of root filling is short lived. The paste is often used without a metal or gutta percha point. The paste is introduced with a spiral root canal filler. The material is very radiopaque as may be seen from the radiograph (**280**).

Constituents:

Powder   Iodoform

Liquid   Parachlorphenol
         Camphor
         Menthol

ROOT CANAL FILLING PASTES

The main disadvantage with the available root filling materials both metal and gutta percha is that they require a sealer. The theoretical attractiveness of removing the sealer and producing a single interface between the filling material and the canal wall should be apparent. Two methods have been produced which are available.

Hydron. Hydron is a hydrophilic gel with barium sulphate added for radiopacity. The gel is Poly-2-hydroxy ethyl methacrylate. The paste is injected into the root canal system using a special device.

There is some doubt as to the stability of the polymerised material, its ability to seal the canal system, and its tissue tolerance. The material is not very radiopaque (**281**).

Lee Endofill[1]. Lee Endofill is an injectable silicone resin. It is reported to be non-irritant to tissues and stable. The paste is a distinctive pale pink colour and sets to a rubbery solid similar to gutta percha. Before setting the paste has a low viscosity allowing good adaptation. The setting time is adjustable from 10 to 60 minutes.

There have been several filling techniques suggested. A precision endodontic syringe may be used to inject directly into the canal or the material may be used with a gutta percha cone as a filler.

281

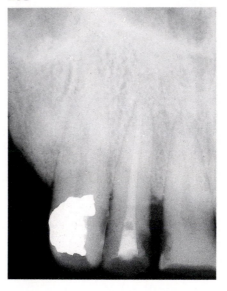

SPREADERS, PLUGGERS AND HEAT CARRIERS

All these instruments are used for the condensation of gutta percha into the root canal.

Spreaders. The instruments are used to force gutta percha laterally against the walls of the root canal and provide a space for the introduction of more cones. The instruments are tapered and have a sharp pointed end.

There are several different diameters of spreader.
The largest size that reaches to within 1 or 2 mm of the working length without binding is the correct one to use. An accessory cone of corresponding size is selected.

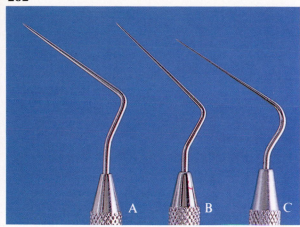

282

Three spreaders of different sizes are shown (**282**) with the largest on the left.

A   D11 — Hu Friedy[1]

B   D11T — Hu Friedy[1] (T standing for thin)

C   RC25S — Premier[2]

283

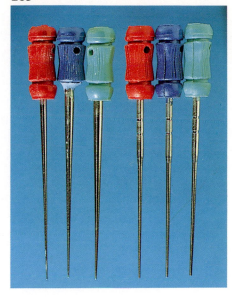

Although most spreaders and pluggers have long handles, short handled instruments are available.

Examples of colour coded finger spreaders on the left and pluggers[3] on the right are illustrated (**283**).

284 Pluggers.   A plugger is similar in design to a spreader except that the end is blunt. The main component of force is vertical rather than lateral.

A   Prima instrument[4]   The black marks denote 20 and 25 mm from the tip.

B   5/7 Plugger[5]   This is a double-ended plugger which may also be used as a heat carrier.

Kerrs produce a range of plugger sizes with 20 and 25 mm markings on the shank. The chapter on filling the root canal shows a selection of Schilder pluggers.

Heat Carriers are used to carry heat to the gutta percha already placed within the root canal. Several instruments may be used as heat carriers. A selection is shown (**285**).

A   Kerrs No. 3 Spreader[6] which is recommended by the author as a heat carrier.

B   5/7 Hu Friedy plugger.

C   PCA D4[7]. The instrument is sharp pointed and has a bulbous portion at the end of the shank which retains the heat.

A new form of battery-operated heat carrier is being introduced shortly which shows promise. This has been produced by Dr Howard Martin in conjunction with Dentsply.

284

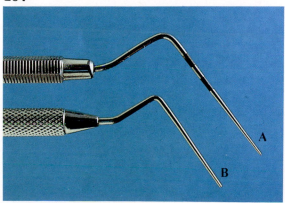

285

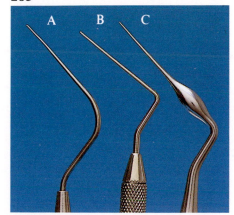

6 Rubber dam J. J. Messing

IS RUBBER DAM ESSENTIAL IN ENDODONTIC TREATMENT?

Many dentists answer this question in the negative. They consider that the use of rubber dam is academic and difficult and do not use it again after they leave dental school.

The chief benefit of rubber dam is the security it provides against inhalation or ingestion of dropped root canal instruments, especially apt to occur when patients are supine. This danger is averted by many who attach a safety chain (parachute) (286) to the handle of each instrument. This method is cumbersome and wastes time, because it necessitates the application of the chain each time the instrument is changed, and is obstructive when space is limited.

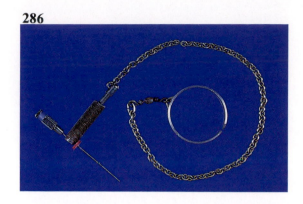

286

However, there are other valid reasons why rubber dam should be used:

(1) Irrigating fluids are prevented from entering the mouth (287).

(2) Contamination of the endodontic system by saliva is prevented, thus enabling the operator to obtain and maintain an aseptic field. This is of paramount importance when attempting the elimination of infection from the canal system.

(3) A clean, dry field is obtained.

(4) Tongue and cheek are retracted, enhancing visibility and accessibility.

(5) With rubber dam in place, the patient is unable to converse freely and use a mouthwash, thus saving time and allowing uninterrupted concentration on the treatment.

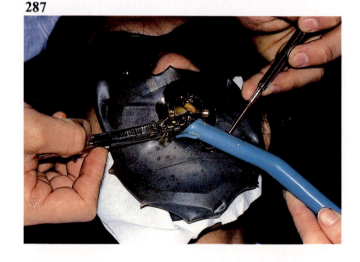

287

HOW LONG DOES IT TAKE TO APPLY RUBBER DAM?

It is rarely necessary to apply the dam over more than one tooth. However, if the tooth lacks adequate bulbosity or is likely to disintegrate under the pressure of a clamp (eg when a copper band or aluminium crown has been cemented), it may be necessary to anchor the dam at a distance from the affected tooth, with isolation of two or more teeth (288).

Where anterior teeth are severely imbricated it is advantageous to isolate a number of teeth, in order to obtain good access to the lingual surfaces. It is customary to place a clamp on a canine or premolar on either side.

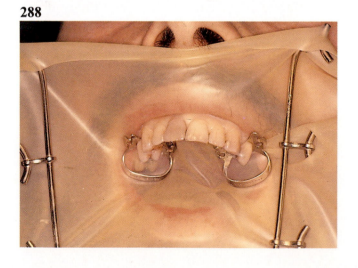

288

Provided an adequate range of clamps is available and there is a modicum of assistance provided, the time required for the application of the dam should not exceed thirty seconds for a single tooth and sixty seconds for multiple teeth. Furthermore, as a practical economy, the same sheet of rubber may be used throughout the treatment, provided it remains undamaged and is scrubbed with an antiseptic soap at the conclusion of each treatment. It is then dried, folded in a paper tissue and placed with the patient's notes in a folder.

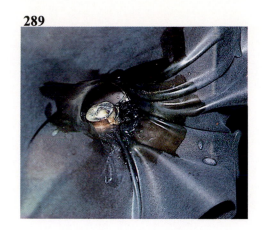
289

PREPARATION OF THE TOOTH PRIOR TO PLACEMENT OF THE RUBBER DAM

In the section on root canal preparation, the need to remove caries, leaking restorations and hyperplastic gingival tissue overlying cavity margins, has been stressed. Furthermore, badly mutilated teeth, especially where there is tooth loss cervically, need to be restored. This will prevent leakage of saliva into the pulp chamber by allowing the rubber to fit closely around the neck of the tooth.

When a posterior tooth is so broken down that it is not possible to apply a matrix band, a copper band (**289**) or stainless steel orthodontic band, or an aluminium crown form (**290**) can be cemented for the duration of the treatment. The area of the access cavity, if already opened up, should first be filled with gutta percha, which is easily softened by heat and removed to regain access to the canals. It is essential that any cemented object be free from occlusal stress, and the edges of copper or steel bands must be contoured and rounded to avoid trauma to the soft tissues.

When a band is cemented, it is advisable to avoid clamping it, at least on the day it is cemented, because the pressure of the clamp may fracture the cement.

Rough, overhanging margins of restorations can prevent fitting of the dam around the cervix of the tooth. They should be trimmed or the restorations replaced.

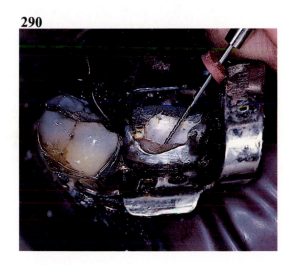
290

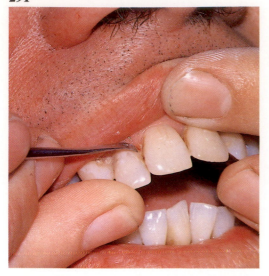

291

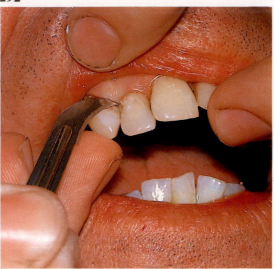

292

Composite resin and amalgam can be trimmed with a fine T.C. blank bur in the turbine handpiece. However, it is possible to plane away small amounts of sub-gingival excess amalgam with a 'chisel' scaler (G2) (**291**), or a Swann-Morton scalpel, No. 11 (**292**).

WHICH CLAMPS SHOULD BE USED?

Whenever feasible the dam should be retained solely by a simple clamp, placed on the tooth being treated (**293**). Retention of a clamp is affected by lack of adequate bulbosity of the crown, which in turn may be related to under-eruption or malposition of the tooth. In such cases, common sense and ingenuity will provide effective solutions in the majority of cases. Two vital factors influence further the retention of the clamp on the tooth. Firstly, the jaws of the clamp must be sharp so that they can grip the smooth enamel surface, and secondly the points rather than the centres of the arcs of the jaws, must contact the tooth making four point contact (**294**). Otherwise the clamp will exhibit a tendency to pivot at its mid-point and spring off the tooth.

There is a large variety of clamps available, but the author has found that the clamps shown (**295-298**) will be effective in the majority of cases.

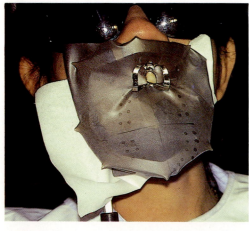

293

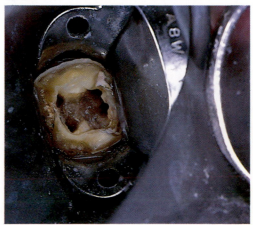

294

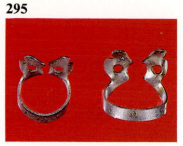

295

Ash no. 0/no. 1

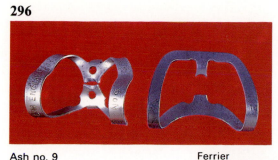

296

Ash no. 9

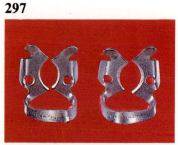

297

Ash no. 10/no. 11

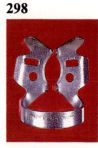

298

Ash no. 7a

The Ferrier Clamp (**299**) is especially useful for short or undercontoured teeth, and for roots which have lost the bulk of their crowns.

The use of wingless clamps (**300**) is a matter of personal choice. They are less bulky than winged clamps and thus, are better for molar treatments on patients who gag easily.

Where several teeth are isolated, it is customary to secure the dam at either end with clamps. Alternatively, the dam can be clamped at one end and secured at the other by means of a dental wedge or massage stick placed beneath the contact area (see **309**).

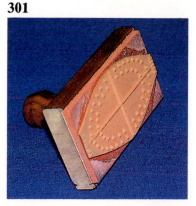

Ferrier
299

Ferrier (SSW 212)

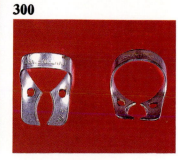

300

Wingless

THE RUBBER DAM

Rubber dam is available in a variety of widths and colours and thicknesses. Heavy duty dam is less apt to tear in use and the dark grey, black or green colours provide a contrast to the teeth, thus improving visibility. A sheet of rubber, 5-6 in. square, is placed over the mouth in such a way that the upper border just covers the tip of the nose. The hole is then punched in the appropriate area. If several teeth are to be isolated, the dam is stretched lightly over the teeth and a mark is made on the rubber over the centre of each tooth to indicate the position of each hole.

It is easier however using a rubber stamp (**301**) to mark the arches on the sheet of dam, to punch the appropriate holes which are indicated by a series of dots showing average spacing of adult and deciduous dentitions (**302**).

If each square of dam is marked in advance, the assistant may save time by punching the relevant holes at the start of the treatment. The size of hole is dictated by the size of the crown and it may be necessary to make a larger oval hole, by semi-super-imposition of two holes, when crowns are extra-large. However the minimum size of hole is more likely to prevent leakage around the neck of the tooth (**303**).

The contacts between the teeth are checked with dental floss and any rough restorations, which would prevent the passage of the dam, are reduced and smoothed with a chisel scaler, (G2), or abrasive metal strip.

It may be necessary to give a local anaesthetic or apply a topical anaesthetic cream (5% Lignocaine) if the tooth shape forces the clamp to press against the gingival crest.

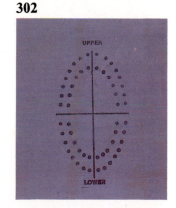

301

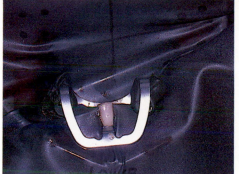

302

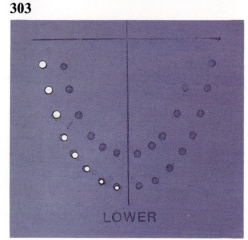

303

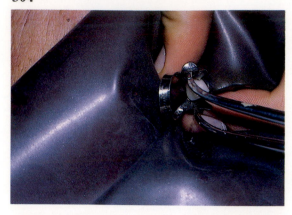

304

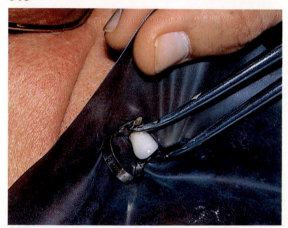

305

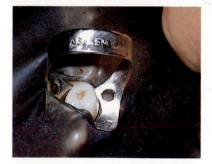

306

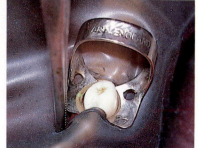

307

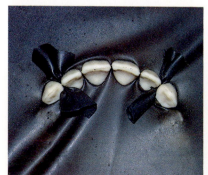

308

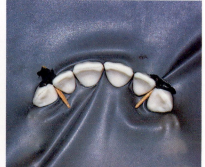

309

TECHNIQUES FOR APPLICATION OF THE DAM

1 Dam applied before the clamp. The dam is pulled over the tooth and, if indicated, over adjacent teeth prior to application of the clamp. Where contacts are excessively tight, the under-surface of the rubber may be given a light coating of cocoa butter, silicone cream or brushless shaving cream in order to facilitate its passage past a tight contact area. The dam is stretched bucco-lingually and the leading edge of each hole proximally is see-sawed through the contact and down to the cervix. When the contact is firm and broad, the passage of the inter-dental rubber may be aided by the application of pressure from dental floss, used with a see-sawing movement. The clamp should be held in the forceps until it can be seen to be stabilized and not impinging on the gingivae (**304**). With this technique it is immaterial whether or not the clamp has wings.

2 Dam and clamp applied together. The alternative technique is to attach a winged clamp to the dam (**305**), carry it into position on the tooth and release the rubber from the wings to lie around the tooth. This is best accomplished using an excavator or flat plastic instrument (Ash 156). The proximal edges are then carried through the contact areas with dental floss.

3 Clamp applied before the dam. A wingless clamp is placed on the tooth and the hole in the dam is pulled over the bow initially and then, in turn, over the jaws, and forced past the contact area with dental floss (**306, 307**).

4 Accessory methods for retaining the dam. Where teeth are under-erupted it is easier to isolate a number of teeth and either, to stabilize the dam with clamps on more bulbous teeth at some distance from the unretentive tooth, or to secure it by the insertion of wooden wedges or strips of rubber dam interproximally (**308, 309**). Wedges can be stabilized with beads of softened impression compound.

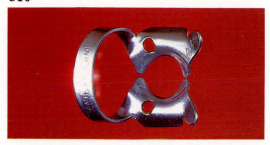

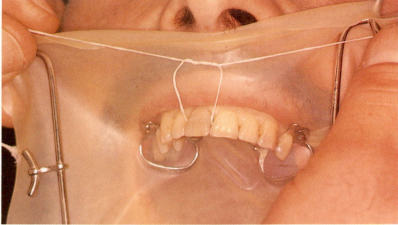

If circumstances dictate that a single clamp be applied to a tooth which lacks retentivity, a retentive clamp, as opposed to the conventional or bland clamp, should be used, eg the 'Ferrier' or (S S White 212) (see **299**) or the Ivory 14a (**310**).

When the Ivory no 9 (Butterfly) or the Ferrier Clamp is used, there is a tendency for it to rock mesiodistally. This can be prevented by stabilisation of the clamp with pieces of softened impression compound, inserted between the bows and the adjacent incisal edges and chilled under water spray (see **299**).

The dam should be inverted into the gingival sulci of unclamped teeth using a double ended, flat plastic instrument (Ash 156). This usually prevents marginal leakage but, any tendency for the dam to slip in an occlusal direction may be countered by tying a ligature of dental floss around the tooth, securing it by means of a surgeon's twist (**311**) or a clove hitch. The dam is pressed into the gingival crevice with a flat plastic instrument (Ash 156, **312**).

Before the rubber dam is retracted on the frame, a square of gauze with a central hole is placed over the mouth, thus interposed between the skin and the dam. This soaks up any saliva which tends to collect at the oral commissures and also protects the skin from the chafing effect of the rubber. Alternatively, paper tissues may be used (**313**).

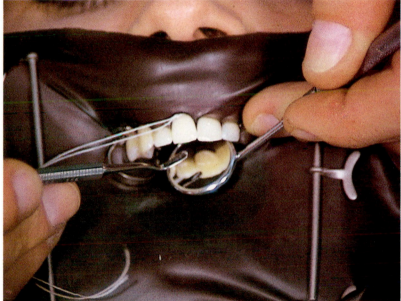

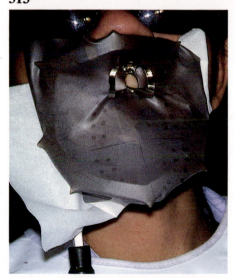

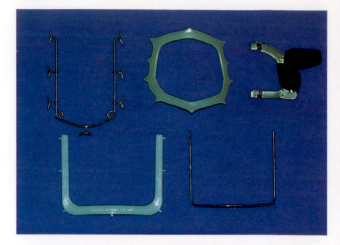

A variety of rubber dam frames are available and it is a matter of individual preference as to which is selected (**314**). The authors tend to use the Star Visiframe (s) or the Östby (Norwegian) frame (o).

The frame should be applied on the facial side of the dam because it interferes less with access by pulling the rubber towards the face.

A saliva ejector is placed under the tongue and is held by the patient so that it can be prevented from digging into the floor of the mouth.

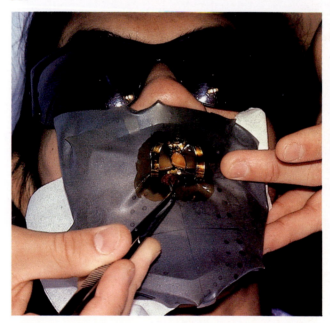

Prior to commencing treatment, the tooth, rubber dam and clamp are swabbed with a disinfectant solution, such as Povidone-Iodine or a 2% solution of chlorhexidine (**315**).

If, during the treatment, the rubber dam is torn, it should be replaced immediately. A minor leakage around the tooth can be plugged with a mix of quick setting zinc eugenolate cement.

In order to facilitate access to rubber dam instruments, it is convenient to assemble them on a tray (**316**).

a) Rubber dam punch
b) Rubber dam clamp forceps
c) Dental floss
d) Saliva ejector
e) Selection of rubber dam clamps
f) S.S.W. 212 and "butterfly" clamps
g) Gauze square
h) Östby frame
i) Fernald frame

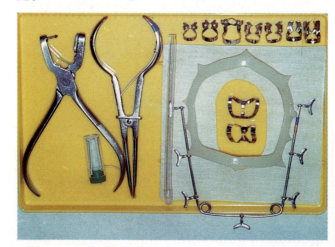

PROBLEM AREAS

Making a temporary crown. What about the crownless tooth which needs endodontic treatment and, simultaneously, restoration for the sake of appearance?

When endodontic treatment is required for a tooth which previously had a post crown or which has suffered loss of the natural crown, two problems arise. Firstly, it may be impossible to isolate the root with rubber dam. Secondly, the patient will be unhappy to face the world with an anterior space. One method recommended for restoring the crown while maintaining access to the canal, is to enlarge the coronal third of the root canal and cement a length of stainless steel orthodontic tube over which an acrylic temporary crown is constructed. The drawbacks of this technique are the limitation of size of file which can be used and the tendency to over-prepare the coronal part of the canal.

There is an alternative technique which leaves the canal free to be prepared as required.

1) Provided the mesio-distal dimension of the root is of adequate width, small diameter stainless steel retention pins are placed halfway between the canal and root surface in the mesial and distal aspects of the root, and the projecting ends are bent over to increase retention (**317, 318, 319**). Care is exercised to ensure that they do not impede access to the canal. Many authorities object to the use of self-tapping pins in pulpless teeth. They fear the risk of subsequent fracture of the root as a result of propagation of fracture lines caused by stresses in the dentine. Therefore, cemented pins may be used for retention. However, because this technique is used only as a temporary measure, the two self-tapping pins, used where indicated, should be cut off level with the dentine at the conclusion of the treatment and the crown replaced with a post-retained temporary crown.

2) Approximately 5.0 mm of the canal coronally is enlarged so that a size 70, or 80 GP cone will fit tightly to that point. Lower incisors, if wide enough for the technique, can be enlarged to size 50.

317

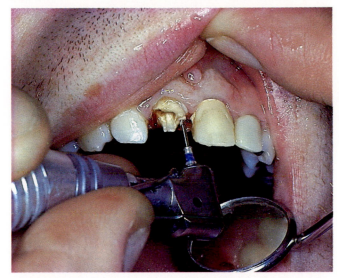

318

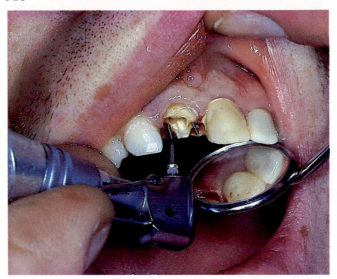

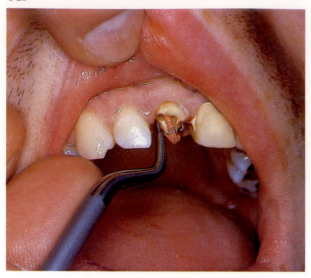

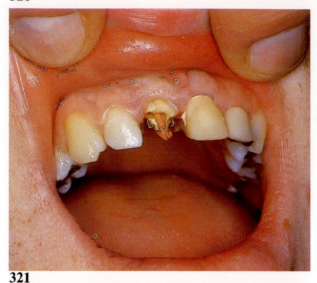

321

3) A GP cone, lubricated with petroleum jelly, is shortened and jammed home so that the coronal end lies in the area of the access cavity (**320**).

4) A polycarbonate or cellulose acetate crown form is trimmed and fitted, ensuring the adaptation of the gutta percha cone to lie in relation to the lingual fossa (**321**). Holes are pricked in the incisal angles of the crown form so that air entrapment may be avoided.

Hyperplastic gingival tissue covering the margins should be eliminated using an electro-surgical technique or scalpel (**322**).

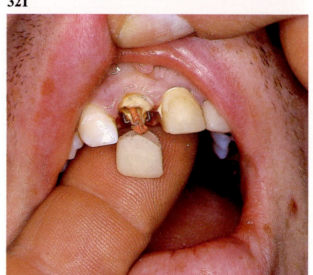

322

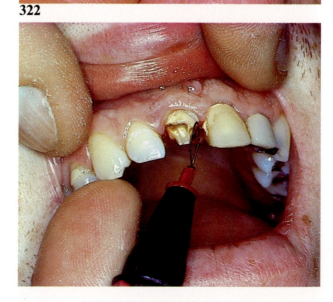

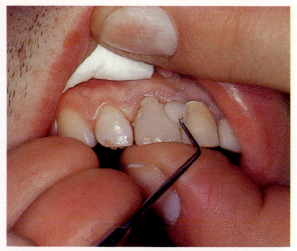

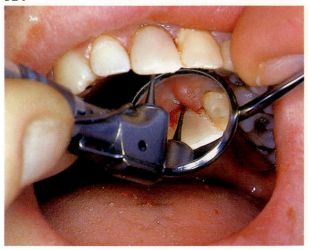

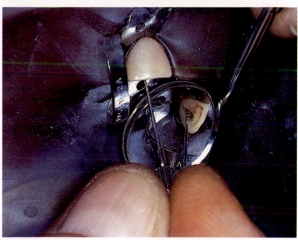

5) The crown form, filled with composite resin, is placed over the root and held firmly in position after the removal of marginal excess of composite (**323**).

6) When the resin has polymerized, the crown form, if made of cellulose acetate, is removed and any excess resin at the perimeter is ground away to ensure a flush fit at the margin (**324**). Using a small round diamond bur in line with the axis of the root, composite resin is removed to gain access to the gutta percha core which in turn is removed. The rubber dam is applied (**325, 326**). Direct access in the line of the canal is then ensured by further drilling if required (**327**).

7) The occlusion is checked in all excursions and the crown is rendered free from masticatory stress,
a) to avoid traumatogenic occlusion, and
b) to prevent stress in the dentine around the pins.

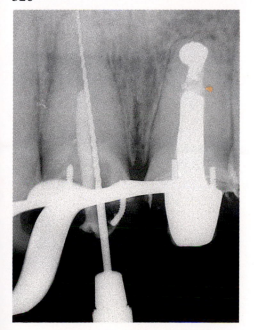

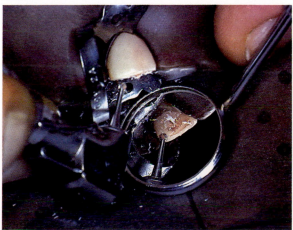

328

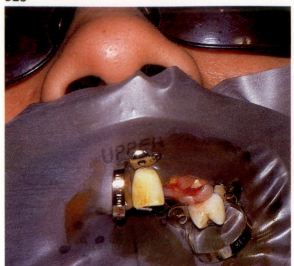

329

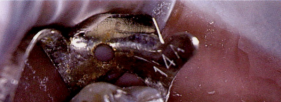
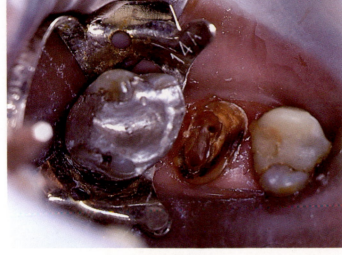

If the patient is willing to undergo endodontic treatment without replacement of the missing crown, it is acceptable to attach the dam to the neighbouring teeth and slit the dam between the holes so that the root is accessible and the dam is held firmly against the gingivae (**328, 329, 330**).

330

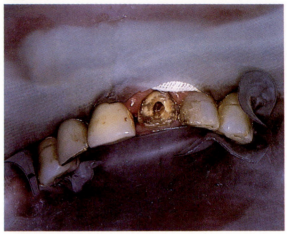

Endodontic treatment through a bridge. If there is doubt about the presence of caries beneath a crown or if the retainer is defective, it is unwise to make the access cavity through the crown. The correct policy is to remove the crown or bridge, eliminate the caries and, if necessary, make and cement a temporary crown or bridge. However if it is felt that the canals can be reached and prepared through the restoration, it is usually satisfactory to clamp the dam onto the tooth to be treated.

If this does not provide adequate isolation, a problem frequently encountered with mandibular posterior teeth, the dam is clamped at either end of the bridge or to adjacent teeth, and a slit is cut to join the holes, so that the buccal and lingual tags can be tucked under the pontic, and even sutured if necessary. This is done by punching holes in the tags, threading floss through the holes with a blunt needle and pulling the tags together with a knot, to hold them below the pontic (**331**).

Similar methods may be used for splinted teeth (**332**).

331

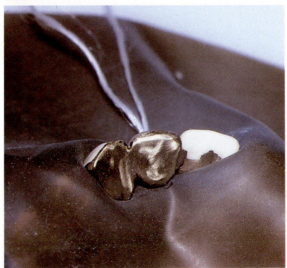

332

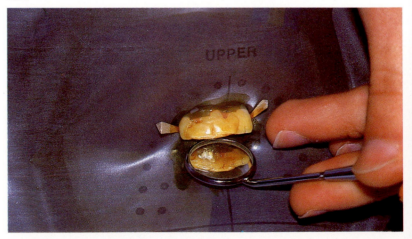

Hyperplastic gingivae in a cavity interfering with the application of the dam.   The presence of gingival overgrowth in a cervical cavity can prevent satisfactory application of rubber dam. Following the removal of caries, it is expedient to excise the unwanted soft tissue, using an electro-surgical unit, coagulate the cut vessels and dress the cavity with a reinforced zinc eugenolate cement.

When the margins of the root are submerged by gingival ingrowth, it is necessary to excise sufficient tissue to expose the margins, after which a short length of copper band, which fits tightly, is cemented onto the root.

Before the band is cemented, the coronal orifice of the canal is enlarged and a lubricated gutta percha cone is inserted, protruding a few mm. from the root. The copper band is cemented with phosphate or silicophosphate cement, and when it is hard, the cone is removed, thus providing a coronal access cavity (333). It is inadvisable to place a clamp on such a tooth, but if it is applied to a neighbouring tooth, the dam can be made to grip the copper band using, if needed, a wedge or ligature to hold it in place.

Inability to apply the rubber dam.   If for any reason the use of rubber dam is contra-indicated or impossible a pack should be placed in front of the pharynx to prevent inhalation or ingestion of dropped instruments (334). Dental floss or a safety chain is attached to each instrument. Alternatively, a reciprocating hand piece, eg Giromatic, can be used in the preparation of the canals.

333

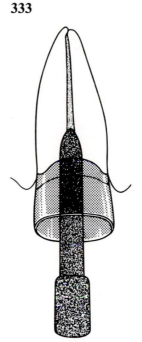

Short length of copper band cemented over root, with lubricated gutta percha cone in situ to prevent blockage of root canal.

Without the use of rubber dam, control of saliva can be a serious problem, and will demand continuous aspiration plus frequent changing of cotton rolls. A useful aid in maintaining the rolls in place is the disposable plastic cotton roll holder (335).

Endodontic treatment is difficult enough without extraneous problems such as saliva, gagging due to nauseating irrigating solutions, and the need for constant vigilance to protect the air way. Rubber dam provides alternative dimensions of access, safety and visibility (336).

334

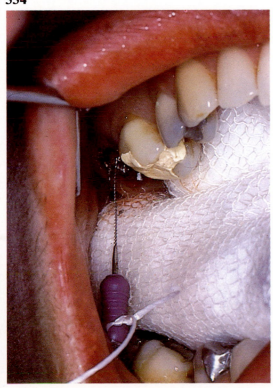

335

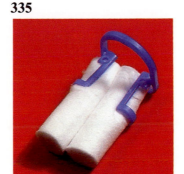

336

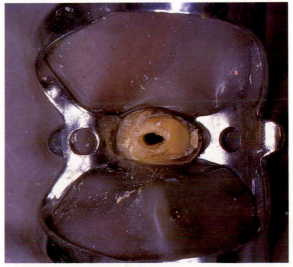

7 Treatment of the emergency patient C J Stock

The purpose of emergency treatment is to relieve the patient of pain as quickly and as simply as possible without prejudicing the long term treatment. Various types of emergency are given below with a brief description of the typical symptoms and suggested treatment.

PULPITIS

REVERSIBLE (See Chapter 3, Table 3 for a differential diagnosis of reversible and irreversible pulpitis).
Symptoms. Pain on taking hot, cold and sweet foods or drink. Lasts for several seconds. Difficult to locate.
Treatment. Remove irritant, eg faulty restoration (see **337**) and place a lining of calcium hydroxide followed by a zinc oxide cement.

IRREVERSIBLE
Symptoms. Pain initiated by heat. Lasts for several minutes to hours. Pain may be spontaneous. Difficult to locate but gradually tooth becomes tender to touch (**338**). The maxillary right first molar shows early radiographic changes around the apices of both buccal roots.
Treatment.
Anteriors and Premolars. Extirpate pulp and apply a dressing. If time allows the canal(s) should be fully prepared so that the treatment may be completed at the next visit. The access cavity is sealed. In these cases the author frequently uses a hydrocortisone/antibiotic paste (Ledermix) placed on a cotton wool pledget in the pulp chamber.
Molars. If there is sufficient time the pulp should be extirpated, the canals prepared, and the tooth dressed as above. If time is short a pulpotomy is performed as follows:

A local anaesthetic is given, rubber dam applied and the access cavity cut. The pulp is removed from the pulp chamber with a large sharp excavator. A pledget of cotton wool impregnated with Cresatin (metacresyl acetate) is placed gently, exerting no pressure on the pulp in the canal entrances, and the access cavity sealed.

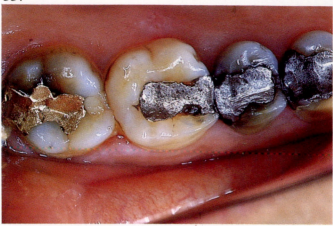

337

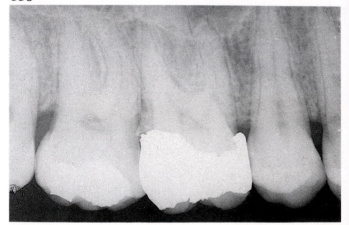

338

Difficulty may be experienced in achieving anaesthesia in a pulp which has irreversible pulpitis. Complete anaesthesia may be achieved if the following steps are taken:
1 Additional local anaesthetic palatally opposite the tooth in the maxilla and both lingually and buccally in the mandible.
2 Intra-ligamental injection mesially and distally to the affected tooth.
3 If the pulp is still sensitive an intra-pulpal local, placing the needle within the coronal portion of the pulp and injecting one or two drops of anaesthetic.

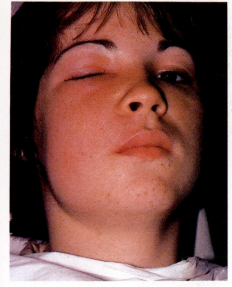
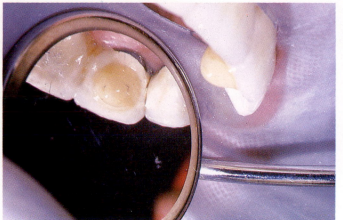
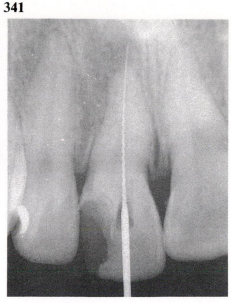

PERIAPICAL ABSCESS

Symptoms. (339) The tooth becomes mobile and exquisitely painful to both touch and heat. The tooth is slightly extruded from its socket. Cold may relieve the pain. As the swelling appears the pain decreases. The swelling is oedematous and diffuse at first but gradually localises and becomes fluctuant over several days. The most dependent part becomes reddened and starts to point. The patient may have systemic effects due to a generalised toxaemia which subsides as the abscess localises.

Treatment. As the pulp is non-vital, access may be made with an air rotor into the pulp chamber, providing a light touch is used. Local anaesthesia may be given as a block injection but no local infiltration is given because it would be painful and might spread infection. A discharge of pus and blood usually occurs (340). If this does not happen a size 15 or 20 instrument is passed through the apex deliberately (341) — the only time in root canal treatment that this step is advised — to attempt to provide drainage.

Rubber dam is applied as soon as the access to the pulp chamber is achieved. The canal is now irrigated copiously with sodium hypochlorite and the canal length measured, prepared and dried (342). A pledget of cotton wool moistened with 1% Parachlorphenol is placed in the pulp chamber and the access cavity sealed. The tooth is ground out of occlusion. The patient is reassured and analgesics are prescribed. If the patient has systemic effects antibiotics are given. The choice of antibiotic is similar to that given for conditions requiring cover. See Chapter 3. The dosage, however, is different. If Penicillin is used the dose recommended is one Amoxil sachet (3 g) followed by Amoxycillin tablets (500 mg tds) for four days starting eight hours after the Amoxyl.

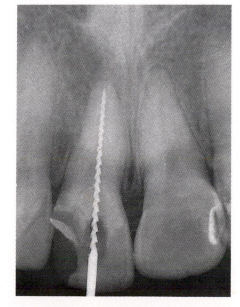

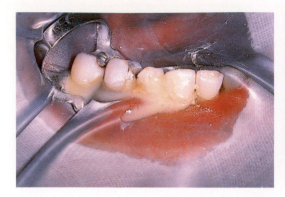
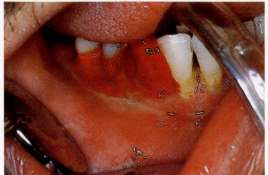
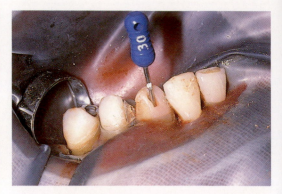

346

If the discharge from the tooth cannot be controlled by irrigation and filing, or the patient will not allow thorough cleaning of the canal(s) the tooth is left open for 24 hours. Analgesics and antibiotics are given as above. After 24 hours the canal should be prepared, medicated and sealed as described.

343, 344, 345 The patient has an acute periapical abscess of a mandibular canine. A buccal access cavity was made and there was a copious pus discharge. It was not possible to control the discharge (**344**) and the tooth was left open for 24 hours. The final picture (**345**) shows canal preparation being carried out at the second visit. The tooth was then sealed with a temporary dressing.

The best route for discharging pus is through the tooth. However, if the swelling is fluctuant it should be incised (**346**) or the pus aspirated through a syringe with a wide bore needle. The most dependent part will be reddened and pointing. The abscess is incised as follows:

1 Block anaesthesia if this is anatomically possible. If not, a local anaesthetic submucosal infiltration will be sufficient or the application of ethyl chloride spray.

2 A number 15 or 12 blade is used to penetrate the area which is about to point (**347, 348**).

3 Gentle finger pressure will encourage the discharge.

4 On rare occasions it may be necessary to introduce a piece of rubber dam cut in a 'T' shape, into the incision. The cross bar of the T is tucked into the wound and sutured so that drainage will continue. The rubber is removed after two or three days when drainage is complete.

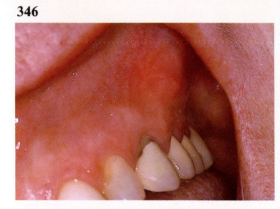

347

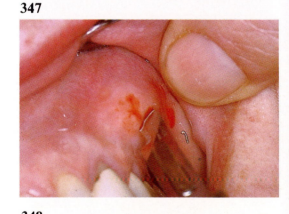

348

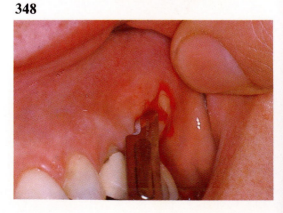

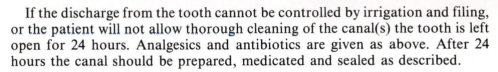

PAIN FOLLOWING ENDODONTIC TREATMENT

Pain following endodontic procedures occurs in about 15% of cases. The cause of pain is usually periodontitis.

AFTER PREPARATION

Symptoms The patient returns 24 hours later with a continuous dull ache which may become severe. The tooth is tender to touch (**349**). The teeth most susceptible are those which had a symptomless periapical area before treatment.

Possible Causes.

1 The temporary filling was high or has become so due to extrusion of the tooth from its socket.
2 The periodontal tissues were disturbed during root canal preparation either by extruded canal debris or a root canal instrument forced through the apical foramen, or lateral wall of the root.
3 Irritant or infected canal debris or vital tissue remaining in the main canal or a lateral canal.
4 Irritant canal medicament percolating through the apex.
5 Root fracture.
Treatment. Take tooth out of occlusion by grinding. If the pain is moderate or severe analgesics and antibiotics are prescribed. If over-medication is suspected remove dressing, wash out canal(s) thoroughly then redress with sterile cotton wool pledget, gutta percha and zinc oxide cement.

AFTER FILLING

Symptoms. Similar to pain following preparation but usually less severe.

Possible Causes.

1 Extruded filling material. There may be a delay in onset of pain if the sealer contained hydrocortisone (**350**). This tooth was tender for several days following completion of a root filling.

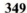

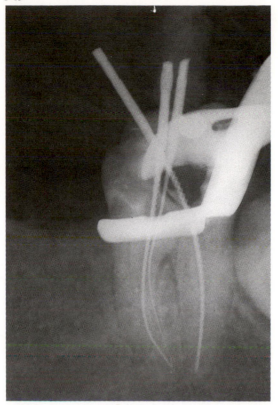

350

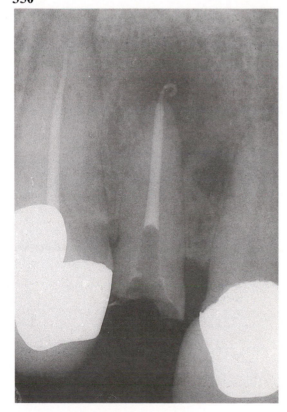

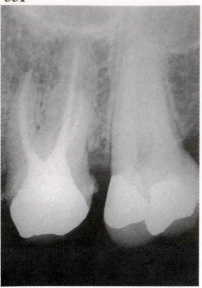

351

2 Debris or infected material extruded from the canal during filling (**351**). The patient experienced moderate pain for three days after filling the root canals. Because of the proximity of the root filling to the radiographic apices it may be conjectured that some remaining canal debris was extruded into the tissues during filling.

3 Tooth fractured during filling or a previous fracture line opened up by filling the canal(s). This molar tooth (**352**) remained tender to touch for several weeks following completion of the root filling. The radiograph shows a bucco-lingual fracture in the furcation.

4 Temporary or permanent filling material causing an occlusal interference. All excursive movements should be checked. **353** is a preoperative radiograph of a central incisor with symptoms of an early abscess. The tooth was root-filled and was then symptomless for 15 months (**354**). The patient returned with pain from the root-filled incisor described as similar to the original symptoms — a dull ache and tender to touch. Note the periodontal ligament space has almost returned to normal. There was an occlusal interference in the retruded contact position (**355**). The interference deflected the mandible forwards so that the lower incisors contacted the crown of the root-filled central incisor. The facet on the second molar is visible (**356**). When the occlusal interference was removed by grinding, the symptoms disappeared from the incisor.

352

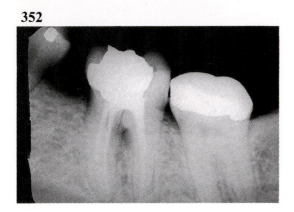

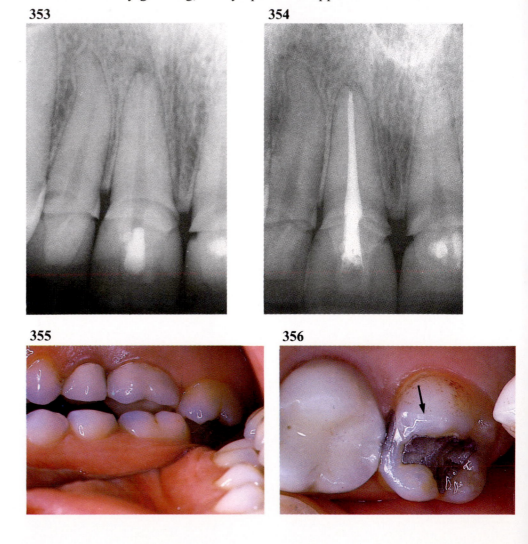

353

354

355

356

5 Pain occurring some months or years later may be due to a breakdown in the seal due to a poorly condensed root filling. A silver point root filling (357) carried out three years previously had become uncomfortable. It is unlikely that the canals are sealed, particularly the distal canal, and that toxins from the canals are leaching out into the periapical tissues.

Treatment When an assessment of the most likely cause of pain has been made the appropriate treatment is carried out.

357

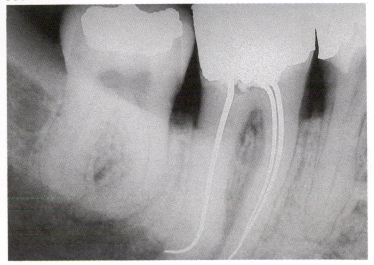

CRACKED TOOTH INVOLVING DENTINE AND PULP

Symptoms. These will vary considerably depending on the degree of involvement of the pulp. At first the patient exhibits a non-localised pulpitis which may gradually progress to periodontal pain due to pulpal involvement or mobility of the fractured segments.

358 The patient complained of reaction to hot and cold gradually becoming more severe over the previous 12 months. More recently the pain had localised and the tooth, lower right first molar, had become tender to touch. The radiograph shows a widened pdl space around the mesial root. The mesio-distal fracture line can be seen in the clinical picture (**359**). The tooth was extracted.

Treatment. If reversible pulpitis is diagnosed the pulp is protected by replacing any restoration involved with a sedative dressing and inserting a metal band (orthodontic band or copper ring) around the tooth and cementing with zinc phosphate. The tooth is also taken out of occlusion.

358

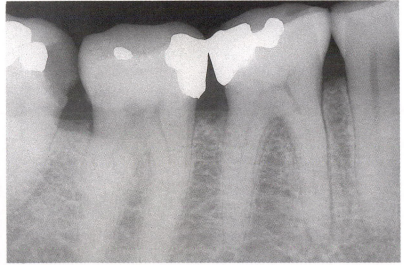

359

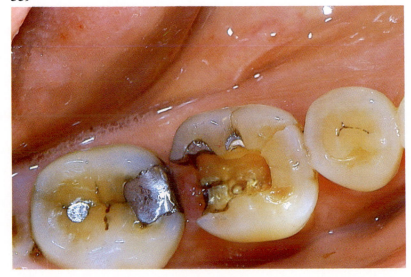

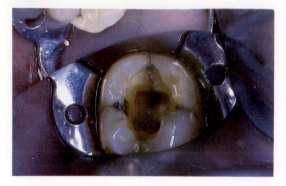

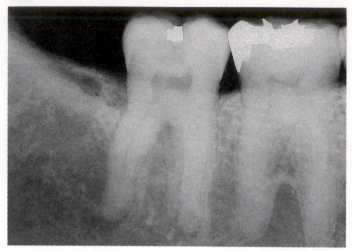

Irreversible pulpitis requires removal of all coronal restorations and extirpation of the pulp. The floor of the pulp chamber is examined and, if fractured, part or all of the tooth should be extracted. If there is a mobile fractured segment it should be removed and a decision taken on whether the tooth is restorable or not. If the tooth is savable a metal band is cemented around the tooth and the access cavity dressed (360). The patient's symptoms were diagnosed as irreversible pulpitis and the pulp removed. The fracture line is visible in the distal wall of the tooth. The fracture extended into the distal wall of the canal but did not involve the floor of the pulp chamber. The fracture is not visible on the radiograph (361) although there is a radiolucent area on the distal root around the apex and the distal surface of the root. A metal band was cemented around the tooth (362), a dressing placed and the tooth removed from occlusion. The patient's symptoms subsided and the tooth was root treated. The prognosis in these cases is poor but if the tooth is crowned it may be preserved for some years.

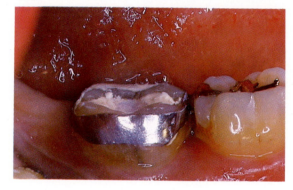

TRAUMA

The majority of accidental injuries to teeth occur in children. Prompt and correct emergency treatment is obviously of paramount importance to reduce the effects of permanent damage. Patients who have presented with fractured teeth must be carefully examined so that all the injuries are discovered and appropriate treatment given. Missing tooth fragments may be buried in the lip (363). Separate radiographs must be taken if necessary.

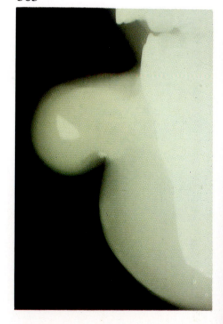

FRACTURES OF THE CROWN

Exposed Dentine. In these cases it is unlikely that the pulp will be affected. In **364** the patient had fractured his incisors, involving enamel and dentine, some 15 years previously. The teeth responded to pulp tests and the radiograph showed a normal periodontium (**365**). The risk of damage to the pulp depends on several factors — the distance from the fracture to the pulp, the time lapse between injury and treatment and the age of the patient, because a young tooth will have wide dentinal tubules. A more likely cause of pulp necrosis in a fractured tooth is impaired circulation of the pulp due to a simultaneous luxation injury. At the emergency appointment the results of vitality tests should be recorded and rechecked after two to three months and the parallel radiographs compared.

Treatment   The dentine should be protected with a liner and the tooth restored with an etch-retained composite (**366, 367**).

Exposed Pulp   The aim of treatment is to preserve a vital inflammation-free pulp which has re-established a continuous hard tissue barrier. This is achieved by pulp capping or pulpotomy and, if this is not possible, then by extirpation of the pulp and root canal treatment.

364

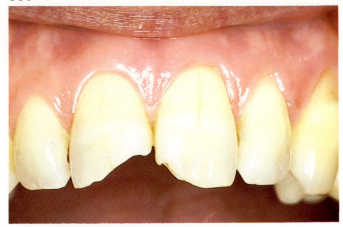

365

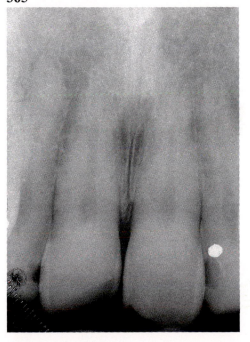

366

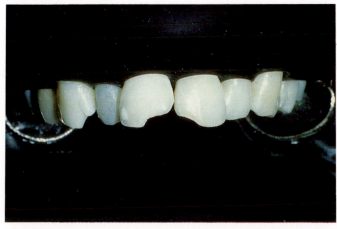

367

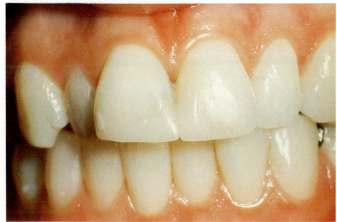

Treatment — Pulp Capping.   Pulp capping is only carried out if the exposure is very small and the treatment can be undertaken shortly after injury. The tooth is isolated with a rubber dam and the fractured surface washed with saline. When the exposure site has stopped bleeding it is covered gently with a calcium hydroxide liner and restored with a restoration which reduces micro-leakage, eg etched composite. Care is taken to ensure that calcium hydroxide is placed directly onto the pulp tissue and no blood is trapped between tissue and liner as this will impair healing.

Pulpotomy.   The treatment involves the removal of damaged and inflamed tissue to a level of clinically healthy pulp followed by a calcium hydroxide dressing. Pulpotomy is indicated in immature teeth as a temporary or in some cases permanent measure to allow complete root growth. The procedure is carried out as follows:

1 Give local anaesthesia.
2 Isolate with rubber dam and wash with a mild disinfectant eg sodium hypochlorite.
3 A high speed abrasive diamond bur is used to remove pulp down to healthy bleeding tissue, usually at the cervical level. A high speed diamond causes the least damage provided adequate cooling water spray is used. If overheating due to depth of penetration is likely then a slow speed round bur is used.
4 Wait for haemostasis and wash with saline.

5 Cover pulp stump with calcium hydroxide using no pressure and place directly onto tissue. The cavity is sealed with zinc oxide and the remainder of the crown is restored with an etch-retained composite.
6 The vitality tests are checked and parallel radiographs are taken at six months and annually until root growth is complete.

368   A pulpotomy was carried out following a fracture of the upper right central incisor. Two follow up radiographs show continued root growth (**369, 370**). Rarely two problems may arise:
1 Irritation dentine continues to be laid down resulting in almost complete sclerosis of the root canal.
2 Internal resorption.
If there is radiographic evidence of either sclerosis or internal resorption the pulp should be extirpated and the tooth root filled.

Pulpectomy.   In the majority of cases of pulpal exposure in mature teeth with fully formed roots, the pulp should be extirpated and the tooth root filled. If there is a reason why the final obturation should be delayed calcium hydroxide may be used as an intermediate root canal dressing.

368

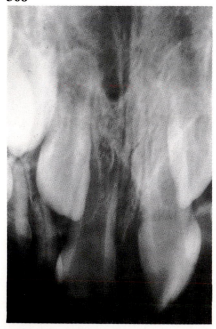

369

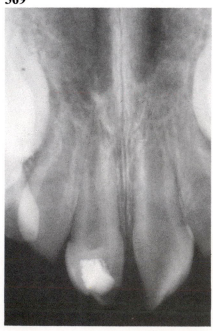

370

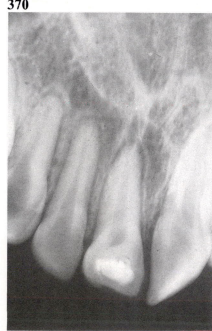

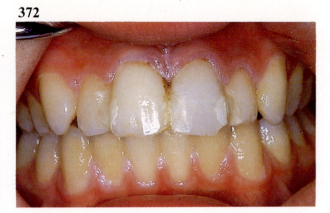

371

372

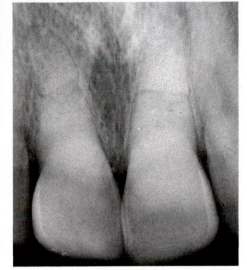

373

FRACTURES OF THE ROOT

Vital Pulp. Trauma may produce paraesthesia in the pulps of affected teeth which makes vitality tests unreliable. The loss of sensation may last for a few weeks to months.

If the fractured tooth is mobile it should be splinted. The simplest form of splinting is by acid-etching the adjacent enamel surfaces and joining the tooth to its neighbours with composite resin (see **371, 372**). The splint should remain for two to three months.

If there is displacement, this should be reduced with digital pressure before splinting.

In many cases the pulp may remain vital and no treatment is required. **373** is a radiograph of an untreated 12 year old fracture. Both incisors are vital and symptomless.

374

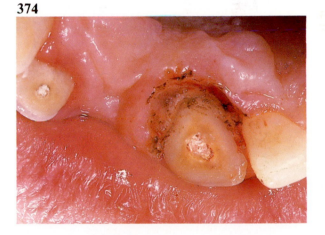

375

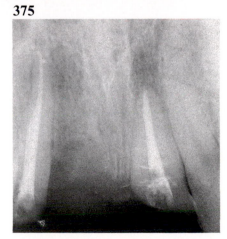

The position of the fracture in the root is important. If the fracture line involves the gingival crevice it will be subject to contamination. In these cases a temporary treatment may be used:

1 Local anaesthetic.
2 Removal of coronal fragment.
3 Remove pulp from coronal fragment (**374**).
4 Extirpate pulp, prepare and root-fill (**375**).
5 Place a post in the root canal which protrudes from the root face.
6 Fit and cement coronal fragment.

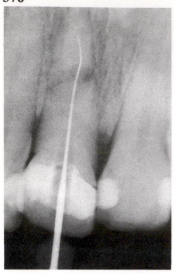
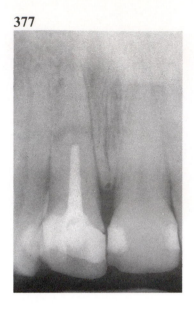
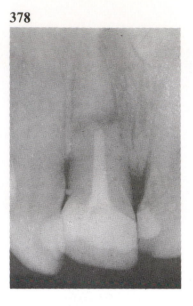

Necrotic Pulp—Root Canal treatment of coronal portion. On occasion the pulp in the coronal segment becomes necrotic but the apical portion remains vital. In these cases only the coronal portion is root-treated. If it is not possible to prepare an apical stop within the canal, calcium hydroxide is used to encourage the formation of a hard tissue barrier (376). The upper right central incisor was fractured and the pulp became necrotic in the coronal segment. There was a sinus associated with the fracture line. The diagnostic instrument was deflected by the partially displaced apical segment. The coronal portion of the root was root-filled (377). A follow up six months later showed no symptoms and no sinus (378).

Root canal treatment of both fragments is necessary if the entire pulp is necrotic. This treatment is only carried out if there has been minimal displacement of the apical fragment as it is the fracture line site which is difficult to seal.

Root canal treatment of the coronal segment and surgical removal of the apical portion. This treatment is used when the canal in the apical fragment has a necrotic pulp and is not accessible.

LUXATED AND AVULSED TEETH

In luxated teeth, if there is any evidence to suggest that the pulp is necrotic the tooth should be root-treated.

All replanted teeth should be root-treated 7-10 days following replantation. The only exception is if the tooth has a wide open apex and had been returned to its socket within minutes after luxation, as a percentage of these teeth show a vital response to pulp testing after an interval.

Any sign of internal or external resorption should be treated by root canal therapy using calcium hydroxide for a period before the canal is obturated with a final filling material. In the Author's opinion it would be advisable to use calcium hydroxide in all cases of luxation and avulsion for a period of at least six weeks prior to the root-filling material being placed.

Replantation of avulsed teeth should be accompanied by tetanus prophylaxis and antibiotic cover as inflammatory resorption is significantly related to injured pulp tissue. A lateral incisor was totally avulsed in a rugby football accident. The tooth was replanted on the field and later a splint placed. The radiograph taken ten days later shows root treatment was initiated (379). A follow up radiograph (380) nine months later showed the central incisor required root treatment. Possible replacement resorption on the lateral incisor mesial surface of the root was noted. 15 months later a follow up radiograph (381) shows advanced replacement resorption of the lateral incisor. It is apparent with hindsight that this tooth should have been treated with calcium hydroxide dressing for 6-8 weeks before root canal filling with gutta percha.

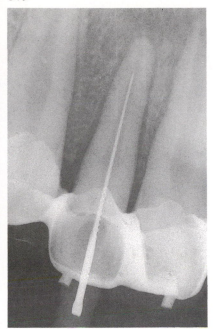

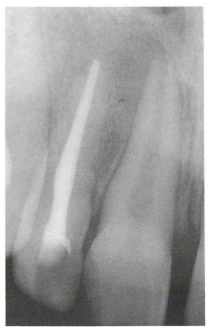

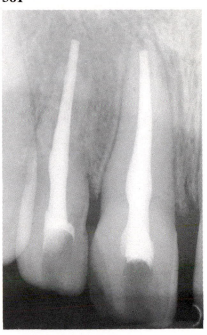

Splinting. A wide variety of methods of splinting loose teeth have been suggested. The length of time that a splint should be left in position varies according to the type of injury:

Replantation	1 week
Luxation	2-3 weeks
Luxation with alveolar fractures	3-4 weeks

Interdental wiring with etch-retained composite may be used as a splinting device. If facilities are available an alginate impression may be taken after covering the teeth with paraffin gauze dressing[1]. A model is cast and a vacuum formed splint made. Retention holes are drilled (see **382**). The splint is then cemented in position using Kalzinol or polycarboxylate cement (**383**).

382

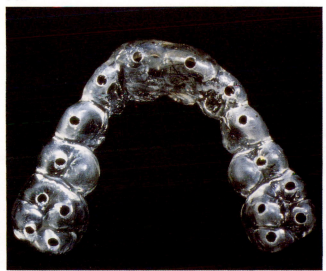

383

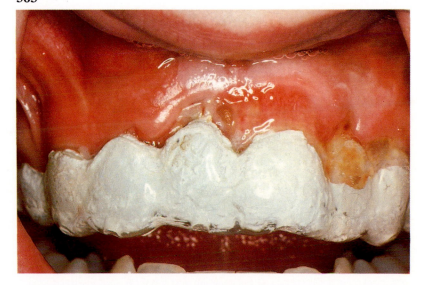

8 Access Cavities C J Stock

RULES FOR ACCESS CAVITIES

Removal of roof. The first step is to locate and remove the entire roof of the pulp chamber so that its walls are continuous with the access cavity (**384, 385**). Any pulpal remnants left in the pulp chamber will break down and cause the crown of the tooth to discolour. In addition during preparation of the canal the debris left in the pulp chamber may be pushed down the canal by instruments and cause infection.

Direct line access. The shape of the access cavity should be cut so that the coronal walls do not deflect instruments during root canal preparation (**386**). Access should be in a direct line with the apical third of the root canal.

The radiograph taken from the mesio-distal direction (**387**) shows that direct line access into incisor, canine, and mandibular premolar teeth involves the incisal edges, and in mandibular premolars the buccal cusp. So as not to compromise with the restoration of the crown of the tooth, the access cavity should be cut close to, but not involving, the incisal edge. The two photographs (**388, 389**) show a case for overdentures where the crowns of the teeth are to be removed. It is evident that direct line access is on the labial surface.

384

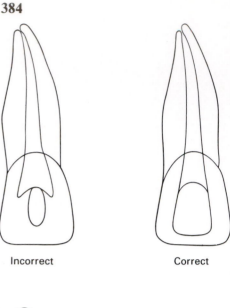

Incorrect   Correct

385

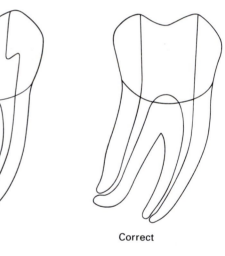

Incorrect   Correct

386

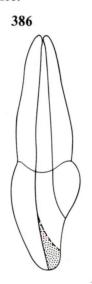 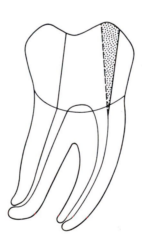 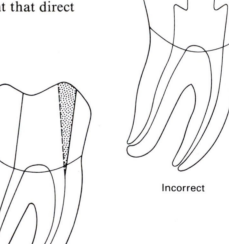

387

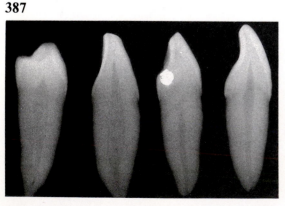

388

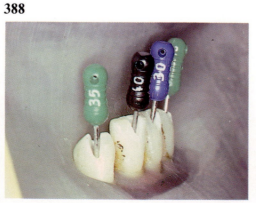

389

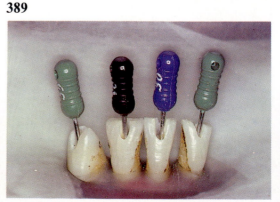

108

390

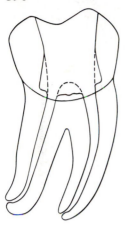

Avoid damage to floor. Particular care must be taken not to damage the floor of the pulp chamber (**390**). The photograph (**391**) shows that the floor of the pulp chamber in the molar has been flattened with a bur which makes the location of the canal orifices much more difficult. The natural floor tends to guide an instrument into the canal orifice. The floor of the pulp chamber in the mandibular molar is illustrated (**392**). Note the hump in the centre of the floor which will deflect the point of an instrument.

391

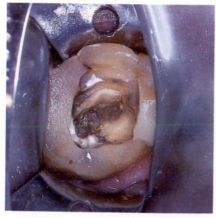

392

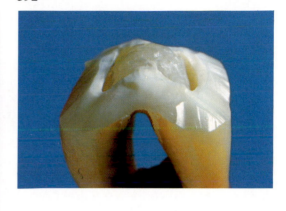

393

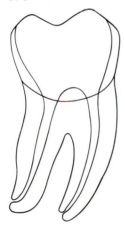

Conserve tooth substance. The access should not be made so large that the walls of the tooth will be unnecessarily weakened (**393**). The tooth must be capable of being restored.

Resistance form. The access cavity should be bevelled to prevent the coronal filling material from being depressed into the tooth and so breaking the seal.

The temporary amalgam restoration has been displaced because no bevel was made (**394**). The access cavity in the second illustration has been altered to provide resistance form for the filling (**395**).

394

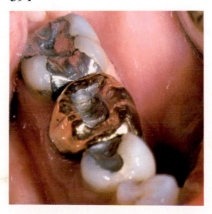

395

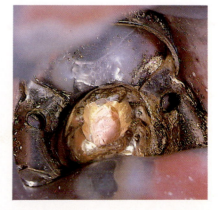

CUTTING THE ACCESS CAVITY

Cutting the access cavity may be divided into three stages —
locating the pulp chamber with a bur, secondly removing the
roof of the pulp chamber, and finally completing the shape of
the cavity.

Stage 1. A tapered tungsten 701 friction grip bur is used to
locate the pulp chamber. In anterior and premolar teeth the bur
is held in the main axis of the tooth (**396**). If the preoperative
radiograph shows a fine canal this stage is carried out before
the rubber dam is placed so that the orientation of the tooth is
not lost.

In posterior teeth the handpiece head and bur are held in
front of the preoperative radiograph which has been taken with
a paralleling technique (**397**). The depth and angle of
penetration from the occlusal surface may be estimated.

The initial penetration in posterior teeth is directed towards
the main axis of the largest canal, that is the palatal canal in the
maxillary teeth and the distal canal in the mandibular teeth
(**398**). The pulp chamber will be at its widest in this area.

Stage 2. A No. 6 round bur in a slow handpiece is used to
remove the pulp cornua and remainder of the roof of the pulp
chamber. The bur is placed in the pulp chamber and a cutting
action used only on the withdrawal stroke so that the roof is
lifted off the chamber (**399**).

Stage 3. The access cavity shape is completed using a non-end
cutting, tapered, diamond friction grip bur (**400**). It is
important to ensure that the walls of the pulp chamber are
continuous with the walls of the access cavity and that the
cavity is bevelled to provide resistance form for the temporary
restoration (**401**).

396

397

398

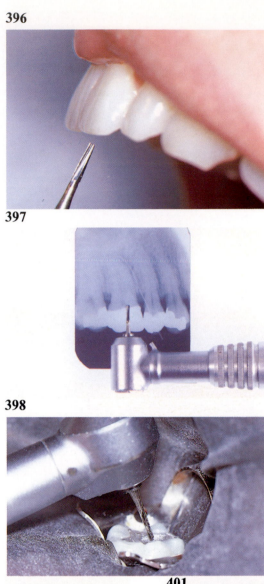

399

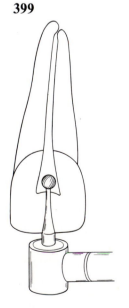

400

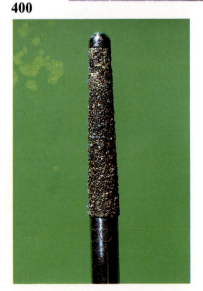

401

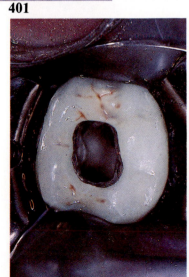

FINAL SHAPE OF ACCESS CAVITY

Diagrams and extracted teeth have been used to illustrate the shape of access cavities. The final size of the cavity will be dictated not only by the rules outlined on pages 108, 109 but by the size of the pulp chamber. In the younger patient the access will tend to be larger and in the older patient it will be smaller. It should be mentioned that the cavities illustrated are classical in outline. In practice many restorations will be removed to prevent contamination of the root canal.

MAXILLA

Central and lateral incisors. To achieve direct line access to all parts of the canal the cavity will encroach almost onto the incisal edge (**402, 403**). The cingulum should be preserved as far as possible as this portion of the tooth is important in providing retention for a jacket crown.

Canine. The cavity is similar to that of the incisors except that the palatal cut involves more of the cingulum (**404, 405**). This will allow instrumentation of the bulge in the palatal wall which lies above the cingulum. The buccal extent of the cavity should be almost to the incisal edge.

First and Second Premolars. The oval outline is similar for both premolar teeth. The buccal and palatal extensions end approximately in the middle of the cuspal slopes (**406, 407**). The width of the cavity will be about one third of the mesio-distal width of the occlusal surface.

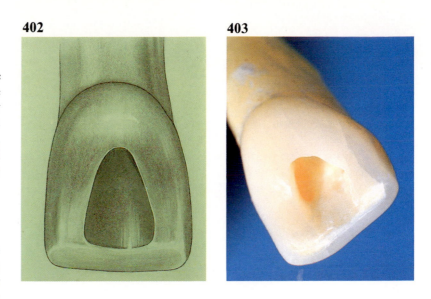

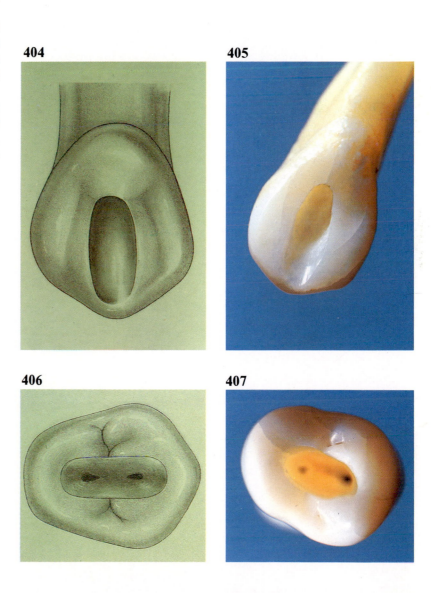

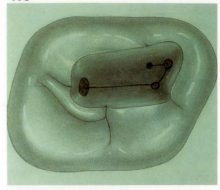

First molar. The shape is rhomboidal rather than triangular and lies nearer the mesial aspect of the tooth (**408, 409**). The mesio-buccal extension of the cavity cuts into the mesio-buccal cusp. Most of the palatal cusp is preserved due to the direction of the palatal canal. The palatal wall of the cavity is broader than illustrated in many textbooks as this follows the shape of the pulp chamber.

Second molar. The outline (**410**) is similar to the first molar except that it is flattened mesio-distally in keeping with the pulp chamber and the occlusal surface of the tooth.

MANDIBLE

Central and Lateral Incisors. Direct line access would be through the incisal edge (**411, 412**) and this coupled with the high incidence of two canals means that the access cavity must be wide bucco-lingually and up to the incisal edge. If the tooth is to be crowned following root treatment then the incisal edge may be involved. Note that the cavity is relatively narrow mesio-distally.

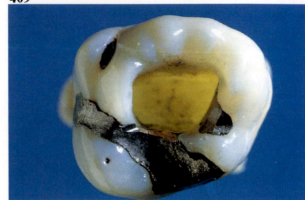

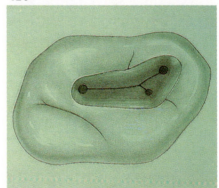

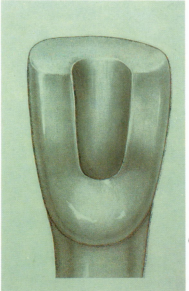

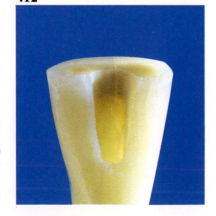

Canine. Same as Central and Lateral Incisors. The incidence of two canals in mandibular canines is lower than centrals and laterals but still significant (**413, 414**).

Premolars. The buccal cusp tip lies over the central axis of the tooth so the oval-shaped cavity should lie as far buccally as possible encroaching towards the tip of the buccal cusp (**415, 416**). If the tooth is to be cusp-covered following root treatment the access may involve the buccal cusp tip.

First molar. The access is rhomboidal in shape lying in the mesial part of the occlusal surface with the bucco-mesial corner of the cavity involving the mesio-buccal cusp. The distal aspect of the access must be wide enough to allow for the high incidence of two canals in the distal root or one broad canal (**417, 418**).

Second molar. The position of the access cavity is similar to the first molar (**419**). The distal aspect of the cavity is narrower due to the low incidence of two canals in the distal root. The overall shape is triangular rather than rhomboidal.

413

414

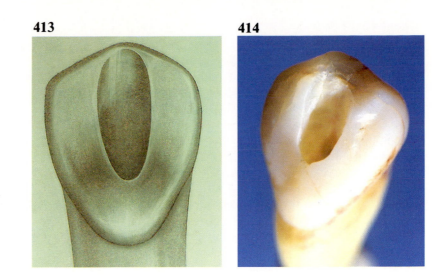

415

416

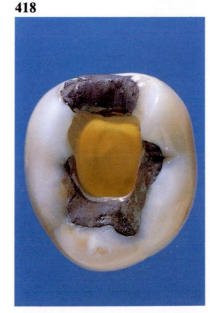

417

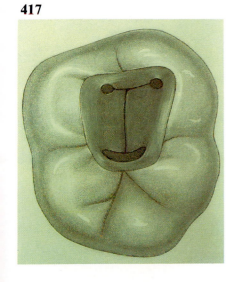

418

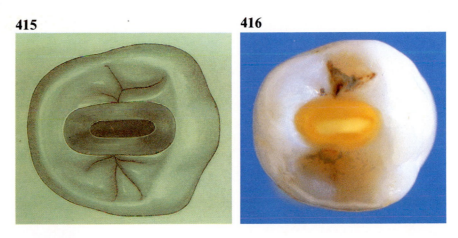

419

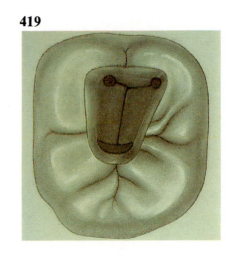

LOCATION OF CANAL ORIFICES

Sometimes it is difficult to locate a canal orifice in the floor of the pulp chamber, particularly in posteriors. A thorough knowledge of the number of canals likely to be present and their location is essential. A good preoperative radiograph or, on occasion, two radiographs taken from different angles, is useful. The radiograph showing the mandibular incisors (420) appears quite straightforward until a second radiograph is taken from a different angle which shows the incisors have two canals (421).

Some methods used to locate canals are as follows:

1 Access should be made to allow a good view of the whole of the floor of the pulp chamber (422). It may be necessary on occasion to remove a cusp, for example the mesio-buccal cusp of a maxillary molar to allow access into the canal so that it can be prepared. The pulp chamber should be cleaned thoroughly with sodium hypochlorite solution. The two illustrations show that the floor of the pulp chamber is usually darker than the walls (423), and the canal orifices tend to be situated at the corners of the floor (424).

2 A DG 16 canal explorer is used to feel along the floor of the chamber at the expected site of the canal orifice (425).

3 Binocular loops[1] are useful providing a good view of the floor of the chamber (426). Magnification is x 2. The loops may be fitted to any pair of spectacles.

420

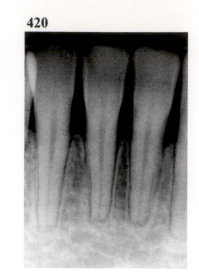

421

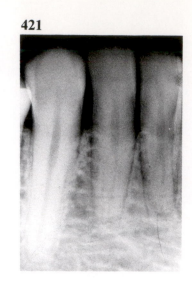

422

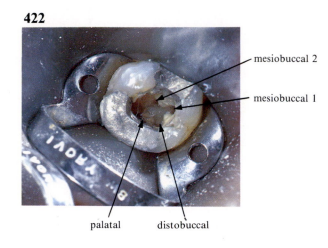

mesiobuccal 2

mesiobuccal 1

palatal   distobuccal

423

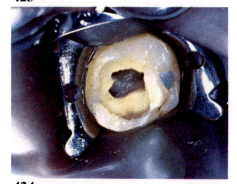

424

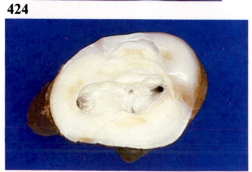

425

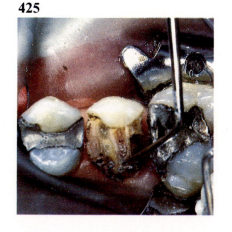

426

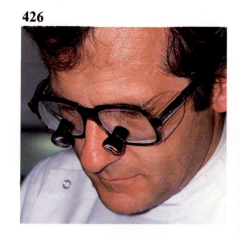

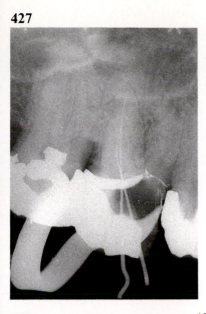

427

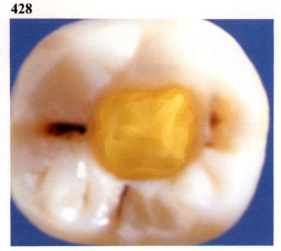

428

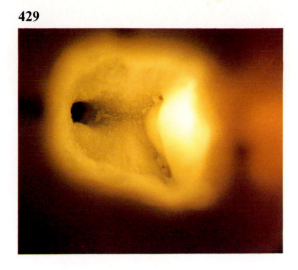

429

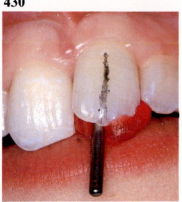

430

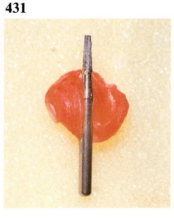

431

4   In posteriors one canal may be located but it is not possible to decide which one. An instrument is placed in the canal and a radiograph taken (**427**). Identification is made by using the buccal object rule. (See page 146).

5   Transilluminating the tooth using a fibre optic light may show the position of the canal orifices (**428**). The light is placed at gingival level. A better result is obtained if ambient light is reduced by deflecting the dental operating light (**429**).

6   Dyes such as iodine may be used which show the canal orifice as a darker area. This technique is used rarely.

7   As a last resort a bur may be used. A hole 2.0 mm in depth is cut where the canal orifice is expected and parallel to the long axis of the tooth. If the canal is not located then the bur should be removed from the handpiece placed in the bur hole and retained with soft wax (**430, 431**). A pencil line is drawn on the buccal surface of the tooth and a radiograph taken (**432**). A two dimensional picture will be obtained helping to provide correct alignment of the bur. Further penetration into the root may be carried out (**433**).

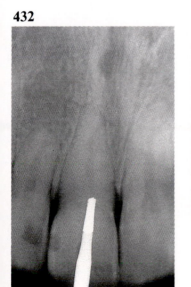

432

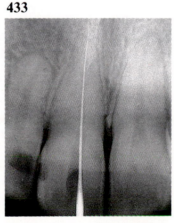

433

434

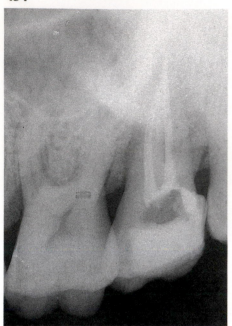

If a canal cannot be located the remainder of the root canal system is prepared and filled. **434** shows an upper left 7 which was abscessed and periodontally involved. The disto-buccal canal could not be located but the remainder of the canal system was filled, prior to periodontal treatment.

COMMON FAULTS WITH ACCESS CAVITIES

Too Small. When the access cavity is too small instruments will be deflected by the coronal tissue and it will not be possible to remove all the contents of the canal (**435, 436**).
Incomplete Removal of Roof. Pulp cornua project into the roof of the chamber and so may be exposed during access cavity preparation (**437**). It is common in premolar and molar teeth to see that although the canals have been instrumented the roof of the pulp chamber is still largely intact (**438**). The floor of the pulp chamber is darker.

436

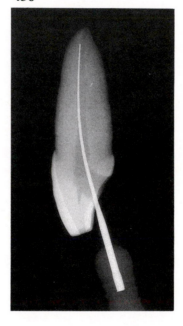

435

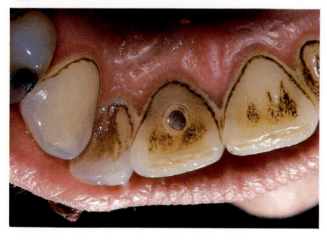

438

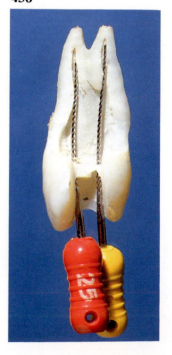

437

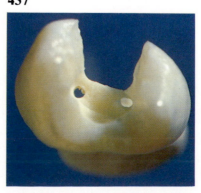

439

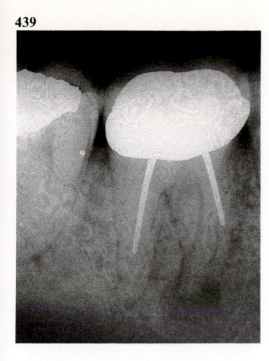

440

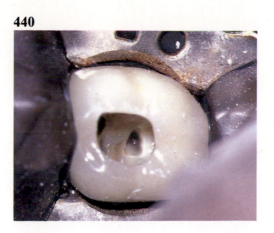

441

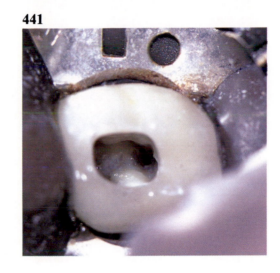

(**439**) The radiograph shows a root filling that was failing. Access was made and the silver points extracted from the canals (**440**). The roof of the pulp chamber was then removed (**441**).

442

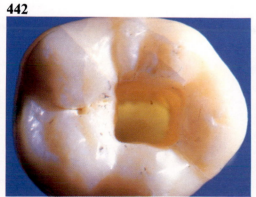

443

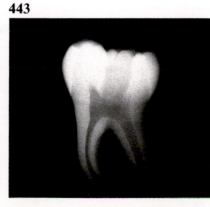

Wrong Place. Making the initial access in the wrong place will ultimately mean destruction of a large amount of tooth substance when the correction is made. The access into the mandibular molar is too far to the distal (**442, 443**).

444

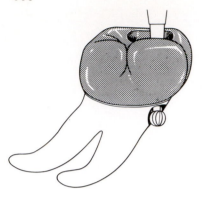 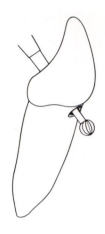

Perforation Through Crown or Root. This may occur in anterior teeth when the initial penetration of the bur is not in the long axis of the root. In posterior teeth there is a particular danger when a tilted tooth has been uprighted by crowning (**444**). The preoperative radiograph should always be examined before access is attempted.

445

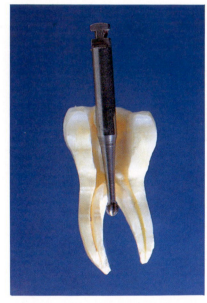

446

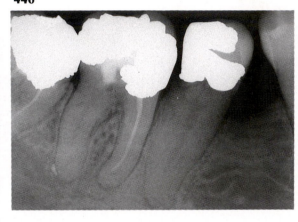

447

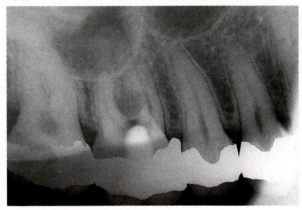

Perforation into Furcation. Too deep penetration with a bur in multirooted teeth can result in perforating the floor of the pulp chamber between the roots (**445**). Two cases are shown, one in a mandibular molar (**446**) and one in a maxillary molar (**447**) where this has occurred. Note the bone loss particularly in the maxilla.

448

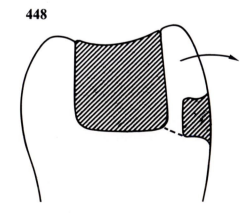

Weakened Cusps. When the access cavity has been cut the remaining tooth substance should be examined (**448**). If it has been weakened it should be reduced or a metal band must be cemented around the tooth.

9 Root Canal Anatomy C J Stock

A thorough knowledge of root canal anatomy is essential for successful endodontics (**449**). Before treatment is started a preoperative radiograph must be taken. If there is any doubt about the number of roots or the root canal configuration a second radiograph should be taken from a different angle. The size, shape, and position of the pulp chamber and root canal should be studied. If the canal becomes indistinct at a point in the root it usually indicates that the canal has bifurcated. This can be seen in the examples of the two mandibular premolars (**450, 451**).

449

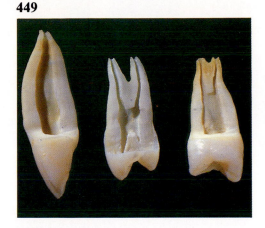

AVERAGE LENGTH OF TEETH (mm)		
	Maxillary	Mandibular
Central Incisor	22.5	20.7
Lateral Incisor	22.0	21.1
Canine	26.5	25.6
First Premolar	20.6	21.6
Second Premolar	21.5	22.3
First Molar	20.8	21.0
Second Molar	20.0	19.8
(Adapted from Black)		

450   **451**

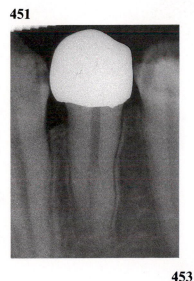

A knowledge of the average length of teeth will help determine the depth of insertion of the initial instrument into the canal (See table above).

The diameter of the root canal decreases towards the apical portion, reaching its narrowest point 1.0–1.5 mm from the apex of the root (**452**). The canal then widens out to the apical foramen. The shape of the narrowest portion may be round, oval or serrated. The direction of the canal at the apical foramen is usually at an angle to the main canal. The apical foramen is found anywhere between 0 and 3 mm from the apex of the root. The radiograph demonstrates the widening of the apical foramen (**453**).

453

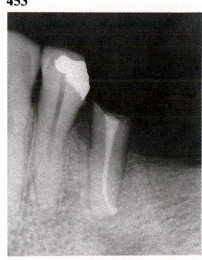

452

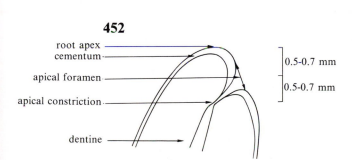

root apex
cementum
apical foramen
apical constriction
dentine

0.5–0.7 mm
0.5–0.7 mm

454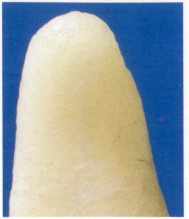

455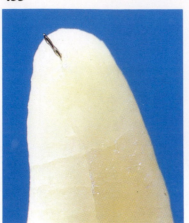

456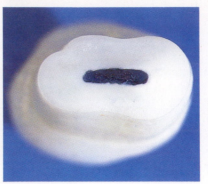

457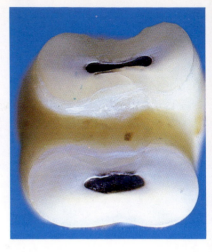

458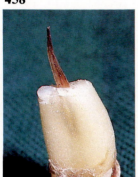

The photographs of the root end from different viewpoints (**454, 455**) show how, on a radiograph, the instrument tip would appear to be at the apex when in fact it has perforated. A root filling should terminate 1.0-2.0 mm from the radiographic apex.

The shape of a root canal is irregular and varies in each tooth and in each mouth. As a general rule the outline of the canal (**456**) follows the outline of the root surface. Many roots are flattened mesio-distally, and so their canals are broad, bucco-lingually and narrow, mesio-distally (**457**). There is a tendency for these canals to become separated into two distinct canals. Some canals contain finlike grooves in their walls (**458, 459**).

PERCENTAGE OF TEETH WHICH MAY CONTAIN TWO CANALS IN ONE ROOT

	Mandible	Maxilla
Central and Lateral Incisors	40	RARE
Canine	18	RARE
First Premolar	23	84*
Second Premolar	6	40
First Molar		
Mesial Root	87	Mesio buccal root 1st and 2nd molars 60
Distal Root	30	
Second Molar		
Mesial Root	87	
Distal Root	5	

*62% have two separate roots.

Many teeth contain two, or very occasionally, three canals in one root. The table gives the approximate percentage incidence based on studies by various workers.

459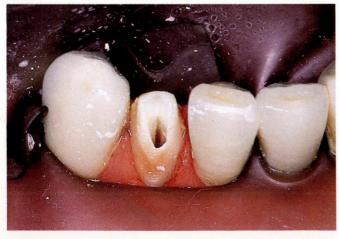

There is a considerable variation in the configuration of root canals that may be found in one root. Frank Weine (1982) lists 4 different types which may be found

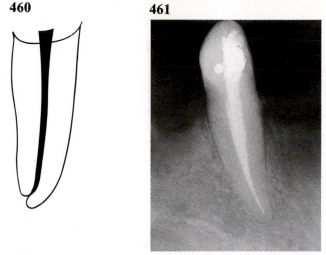

Type 1 Single canal from pulp chamber to apex (**460, 461**).

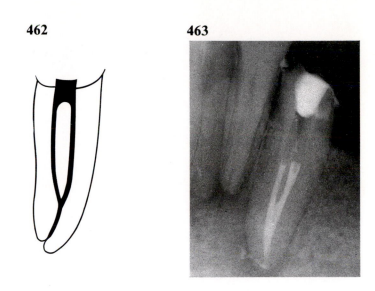

Type 2 Two separate canals leaving the pulp chamber but merging short of the apex to form only one canal (**462, 463**).

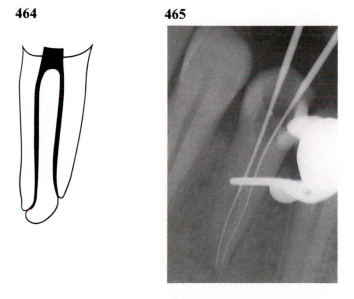

Type 3 Two separate canals leaving the pulp chamber and exiting from the root in separate apical foramina (**464, 465**).

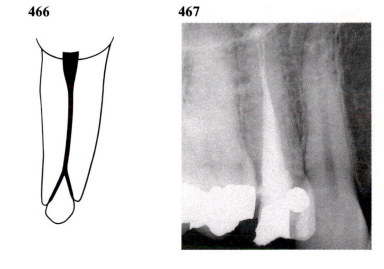

Type 4. One canal leaving the pulp chamber but dividing short of the apex into two separate canals with separate apical foramina (**466, 467**).

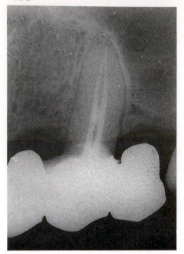

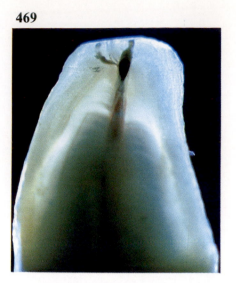

Other configurations do occur, but less commonly. When two distinct canals are present in one root there may be a considerable number of anastomoses (**468**).

Apical delta, lateral and furcation canals. Several branches may occur from the main canal in the apical 1.0-2.0 mm, forming the apical delta (**469**).

Lateral canals occur in approximately 50 per cent of all permanent teeth. These canals leave the main canal at right angles, and although some may be blind-ending sacs the majority communicate with the root surface (**470**). These lateral canals may occur anywhere along the length of the root and will vary in size from a few microns to as wide as the main canal (**471**).

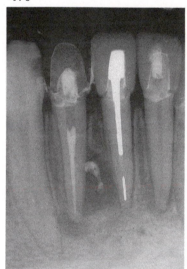

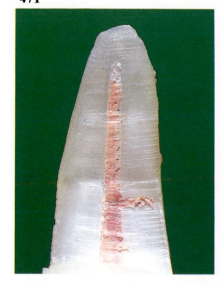

472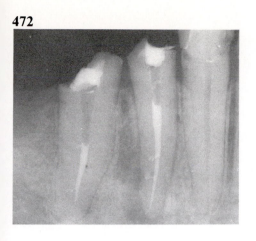

473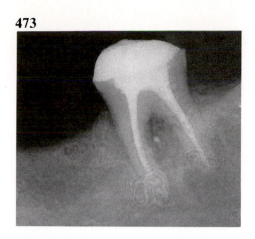

The relevance of lateral canals in endodontics is as channels of communication between the main canal and the periodontal tissues. Toxins from the pulp space may affect the periodontium or conversely toxins from a periodontal pocket may affect the pulp (**472, 473, 474**).

474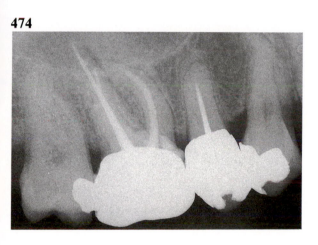

475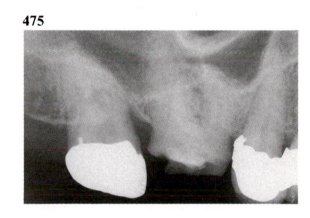

The root canal system gradually reduces in size due to the deposition of secondary or irritation dentine. Note the apparent lack of canals in the molars in the radiograph (**475**). Irritation to the pulp will hasten this process due to caries, trauma, excessive wear or operative procedures. The older patient will require a smaller access cavity than the younger patient. No canal becomes completely sclerosed, hard tissue is laid down by the pulp which obliterates the pulp chamber then the coronal portion of the canal. As deposition of the secondary dentine continues, the pulp becomes more fibrous and less vascular. Occasionally, it is no longer able to support itself and so dies, leaving the apical portion of the root canal patent.

476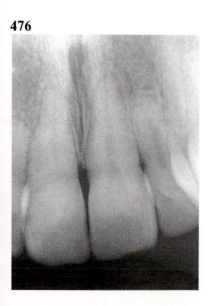

477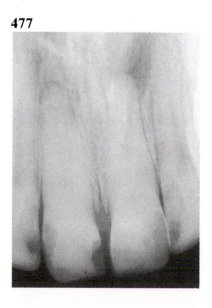

The right central (**476**) received a blow three years previously. The canal is much smaller than the left central.
477 History of trauma some years previously shows almost total obliteration of the canals in both incisors. The teeth do not respond to pulp testing. The left incisor has a radiolucent area associated with the apex.

478

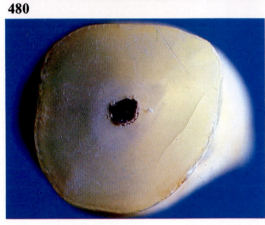

478 Central and Lateral Incisors. The teeth are labially inclined. The root of the central incisor tends to be straight, the lateral incisor frequently has a distal curve in the apical portion of the root (**479**). The shape of the cross section of the canal is oval in both teeth but tends to become round in the apical third (**480**).

479

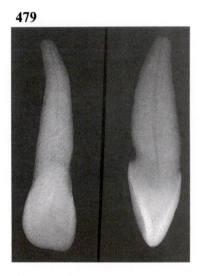

Lateral incisor

480

481 Canine. The tooth is labially inclined. The root tends to be straight or have a distal curve near the apex. The apical few millimetres of root may be tapered and thin allowing only small sized instruments during preparation before there is a danger of perforation. The canal in the middle third is broad labio-palatally forming a bulge. Towards the apex the canal becomes round in cross section (**482**).

481

482

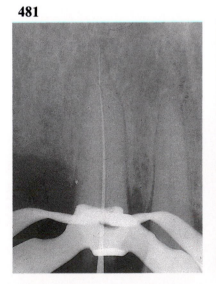

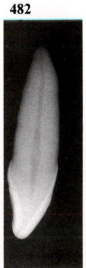

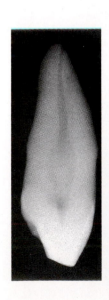

483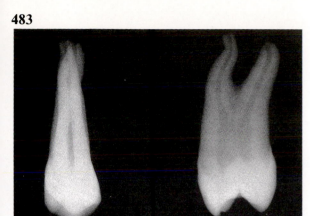

484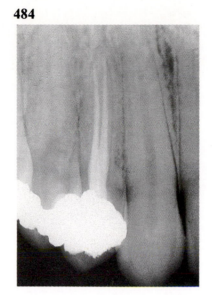

485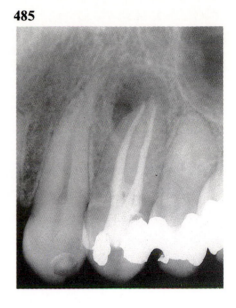

483 First Premolar. 62% have two roots, the remainder have one (**484, 485**), and on rare occasions three. The majority of teeth have two canals (85%). The floor of the pulp chamber extends well into the roots and is wide bucco-palatally.

486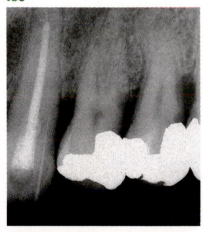

Three rooted premolars are difficult to detect preoperatively. Close examination of the radiograph (**486**) will show the presence of two separate buccal roots. The second case (**487**) shows three canal orifices, two buccally and one palatally and a radiograph of the completed root filling (**488**).

487

488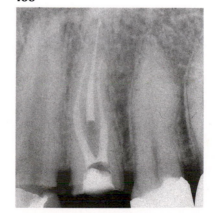

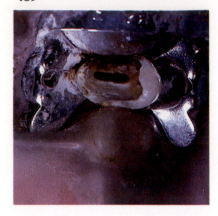 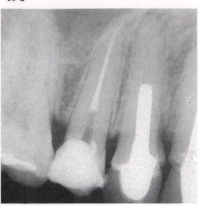 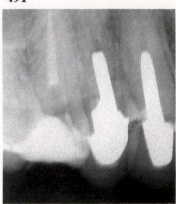

489   **Second Premolar.**   The single root usually contains one canal which is broad bucco-palatally. Two canals occur in 25% and two separate roots in 15%. **490** and **491** show two views of a root-treated second premolar. The extent of the canal bucco-palatally is only evident in the second oblique view.

492   **493**   **494**

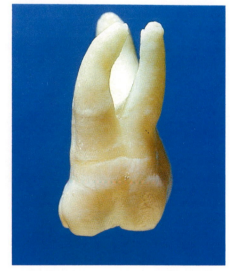 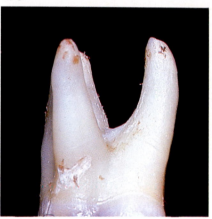 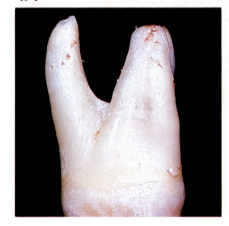

Distal view   Mesial view

492   **First Molar.**   The first molar normally has three roots, two buccal and one palatal. The disto-buccal root tends to be straight and round in cross section (**493**). The canal opening onto the floor of the pulp chamber is not related to a cusp but lies centrally.

    The mesio-buccal root is curved towards the distal and is broad bucco-lingually (**494**). It normally has a groove on both the mesial and distal aspect.

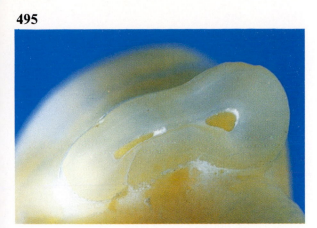

495

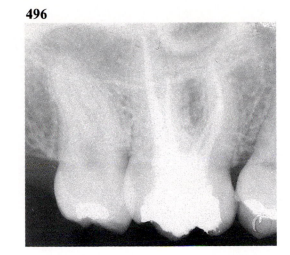

496

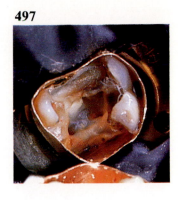

497

The sectioned molar (**495**) shows two canals in the mesio-buccal root and this occurs in 60% of cases (**496**). If the mesio-buccal root has only one canal it will be broad bucco-lingually but narrow mesio-distally.

497 The opening of the mesio-buccal canal onto the floor of the pulp chamber is beneath the mesio-buccal cusp. The main mesio-buccal canal is the most buccally situated and is the larger of the two.

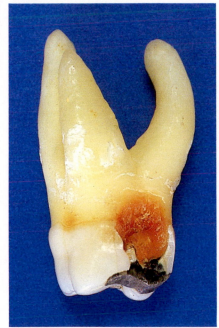

498

The palatal canal curves towards the buccal which cannot be seen clinically from a radiograph (**498**). The canal is oval in a mesio-distal direction. The canal opens onto the floor of the pulp chamber under the mesio-palatal cusp.

Second Molar. The second molar is similar to the first molar. The pulp chamber is flattened mesio-distally reflecting the shape of the crown (**499**). The roots tend to The incidence of a second canal in the mesio-buccal root is lower than in the first molar.

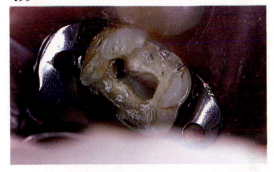

499

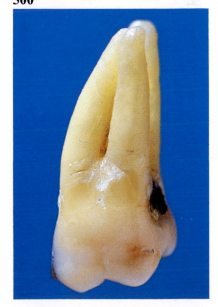

500

501

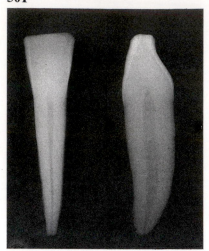

502

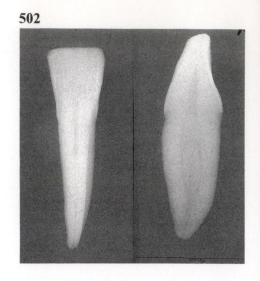

CANAL ANATOMY OF MANDIBULAR TEETH

Central and Lateral Incisors. 40% of these teeth contain two canals. Configuration is Type 1 60% (**501**), Type 2 35% (**502**) and Type 3 5%. After the molar teeth the incisors are the most difficult to root treat because of the complex canal anatomy.

503

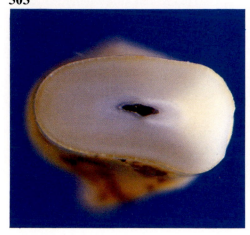

When there is one canal it is broad bucco-lingually (**503**) and narrow mesio-distally. **504** shows a cross section containing 2 canals which are rounder in shape.

504

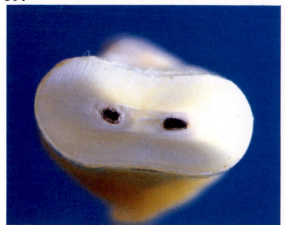

Shallow grooves run vertically in the root on the mesial and distal surfaces (**505**) decreasing the root width and increasing the likelihood of a lateral perforation during canal enlargement beyond size 70.

505

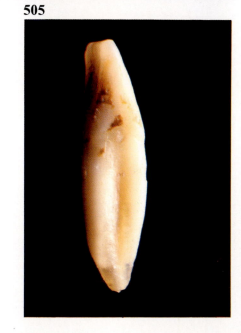

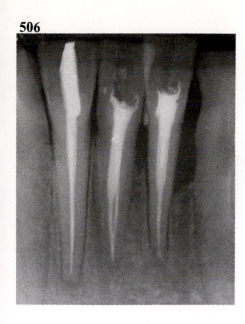

506

The incisor root canals tend to be ovoid throughout their length. **506**, showing three incisors root-filled, illustrates a Type 1 configuration in the lateral and left central. The right central shows a Type 2 canal system. Note the bone loss associated with the left central and the lateral canal.

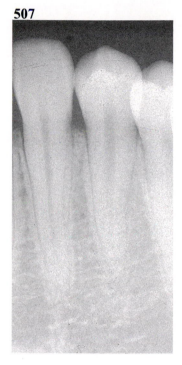

507

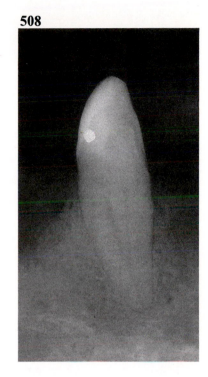

508

507 Canine. The canine is single rooted but in rare cases two roots may be present. Teeth with one root may have canal configurations Type 1, Type 2 or Type 3. The canine is the longest tooth in the mandible but its length is also the most variable. The incidence of two canals is 18% (**508**).

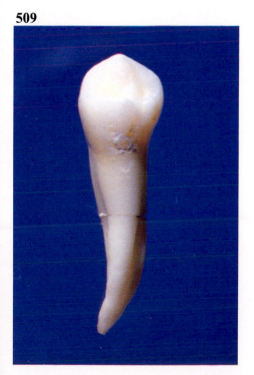

509

509 First Premolar. Usually one canal is present but 27% of first premolar teeth contain two canals at some point along their length, on rare occasions three are present. The canal configuration is mainly Type 4. When a second canal is present it will be situated lingually. The canal is wide bucco-lingually (**510**).

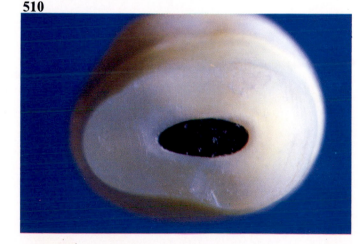

510

511

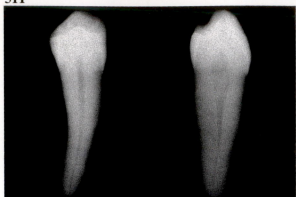

512

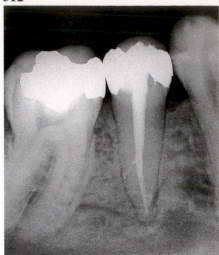

511 Second Premolar. The second premolar has fewer variations than the first premolar. The canal is wide bucco-lingually and Type 1 is the most common configuration. There is frequently a distal curve in the apical portion of the root. There is a clinical impression of a high incidence of lateral canals (**512**).

513

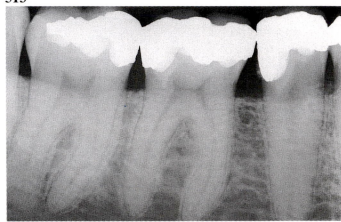

First Molar. The tooth usually has two separate roots. The mesial root (**513**) has two distinct canals in 87% but half of these merge to have a common apical foramen. The direction of the mesial canals from the pulp chamber is mesial, then a gradual curve to the distal. The mesio-buccal canal is more curved than the mesio-lingual. Both canals also curve towards the midline of the root. There are frequent communications between the mesial canals along their length (**514**). If the canals are separate there are often grooves in the midline wall (**515**). In cross section the canals lie nearer the distal aspect of the root increasing the possibility of perforation during preparation.

514

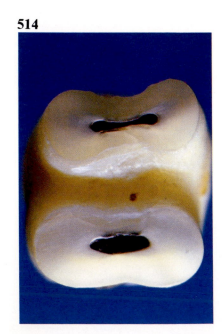

515

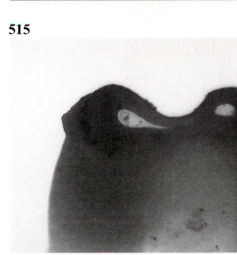

516

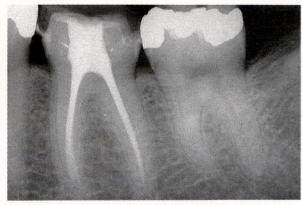

517

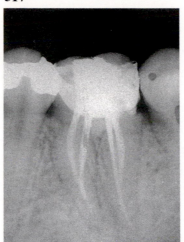

518

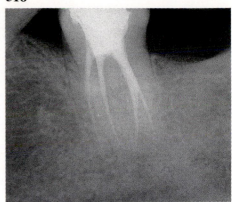

The distal root contains a canal configuration Type 1 (**516**) 70%, or Type 2 (**517**), 3 or 4 (**518**) 30%. When one canal is present it is broad bucco-lingually (**519**).

519

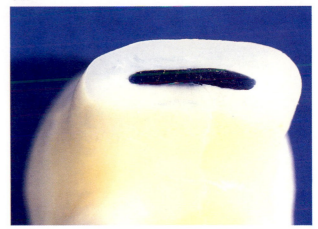

The mesio-buccal canal opening is beneath the mesio-buccal cusp while the mesio-lingual canal is nearer the midline. The distal canal opening lies centrally slightly behind the middle bucco-lingual fissure. **520** and **521** show the floor of the pulp chamber and the canal entrances in a three- and four-canalled first molar.

520

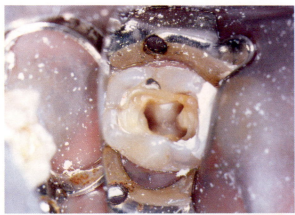

521

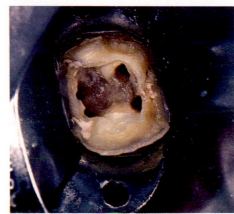

522

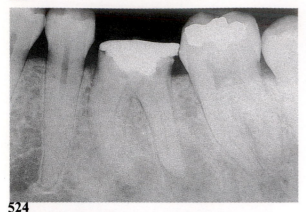

523

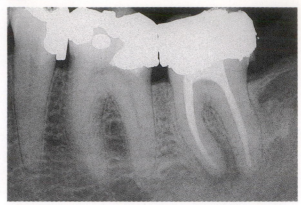

524

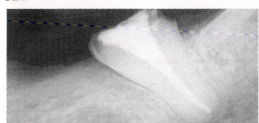

Second Molar. This is similar to the first molar except for a lower incidence of two canals in the distal root. The roots tend to be closer together (**522, 523**). The mesial root usually contains two canals, but occasionally one is present. In these cases the canal will be broad bucco-lingually. Rarely, there is one root and one canal (**524**). Occasionally a C-shaped canal occurs (**525**) when the distal canal extends mesially to include the mesio-buccal (**526**) and, more rarely, the mesio-lingual canal as well. These C-shaped canals are difficult to fill and are not visible on the preoperative radiograph.

525

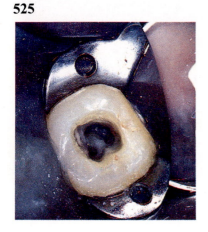

526

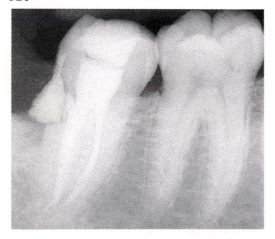

10 Preparation of the Tooth C J Stock

Before embarking on the root canal preparation any restoration(s) in the tooth should be examined and the state of the periodontal tissues assessed. Planning at this stage may prevent problems arising during and after the root treatment. Preparing the tooth should take into consideration:

REMOVAL OF FILLINGS

Any carious, leaking or suspect restorations must be removed. The amalgam illustrated is obviously leaking and should be removed (**527**).

PERIODONTAL CONDITION

The presence of any gingival inflammation or periodontal pocketing should be assessed (**528**).

In posteriors the furcation should be probed to see if there is any involvement. In this case the probe may be passed into the furcation area of the second molar in a mouth which has poor oral hygiene (**529, 530**).

The reasons why the periodontal condition should be examined before root canal treatment is started are to:

A. Give the patient oral hygiene instruction, particularly around the tooth in question, so that the gingival condition will be healthy before the final restoration is placed. On removal of the old crown in this case (**531**), gingival irritation is evident around the distal aspect of the tooth.

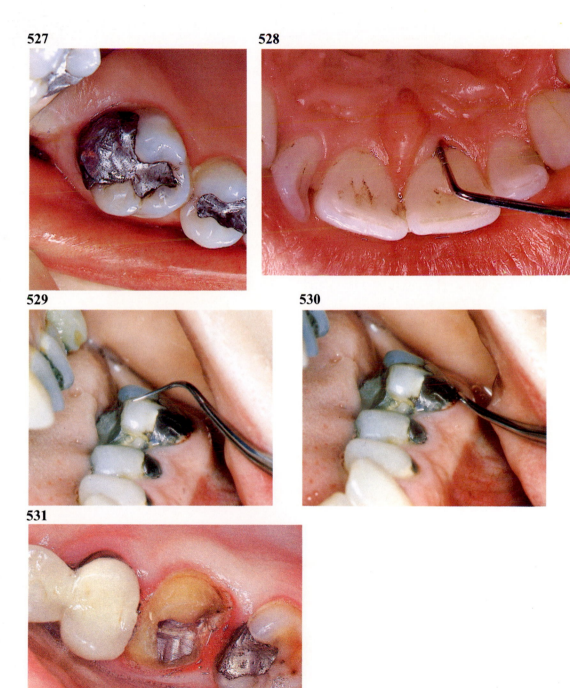

527

528

529

530

531

B. Make it possible for the patient to clean effectively by smoothing or replacing restorations which have ledges. The ledge shown on the radiograph on the mesial aspect of the crown must be reduced or the crown removed (**532**).

532

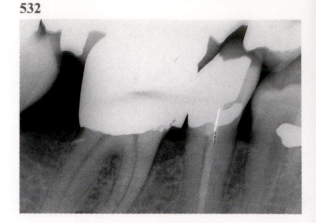

534

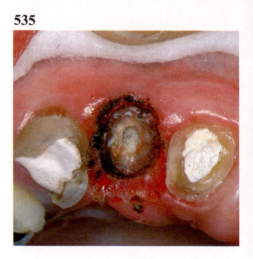

533

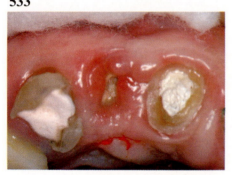

535

C. Assess if a crown lengthening procedure is needed to allow placement of the clamp. The case illustrated (**533-537**) shows a proliferation of gingival tissue around the root face of a lateral incisor. Electro-surgery was used to remove the tissue so that the clamp could be placed. **534** shows the electro-surgical tip used.

536

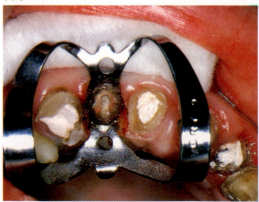

537

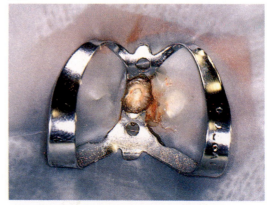

WEAKENED CUSPS

Removal of restorations may leave weakened unsupported cusps and these should be reduced. Failure to do this can result in fracture of the cusp wall or a vertical fracture involving the crown and root.

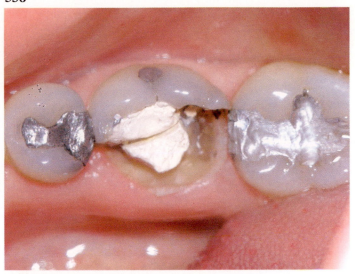

538

538 In this case the patient returned several days after the canals had been prepared with a fractured crown. The lingual wall had been weakened and as a result fractured. If the lingual wall had been reduced at the first visit it would have been better able to withstand masticatory stress.

539, 540 Root canal treatment had been started in this tooth, but the walls had not been reduced. The result was a vertical fracture through the crown and root. The tooth had to be extracted.

539

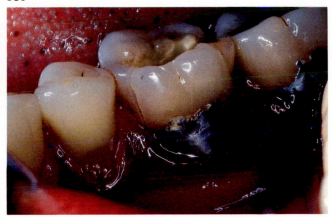

540

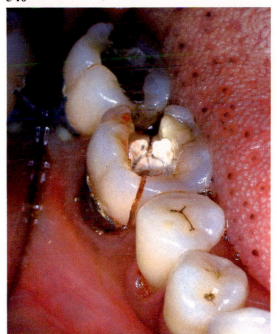

METAL BANDS

Metal bands, or crown forms, which may be used are shown in **541**.
- A Copper Ring[1]
- B Orthodontic band[2]
- C Aluminium Crown form[3]
- D Isoform temporary crown[4]

A suitably contoured metal band should be cemented around the tooth with zinc phosphate cement in the following cases:

1. When the loss of tooth substance makes it difficult to isolate with rubber dam. **538** will require a cemented band before the treatment can be considered, so that the tooth may be isolated.

541

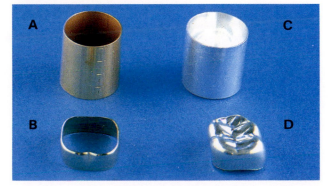

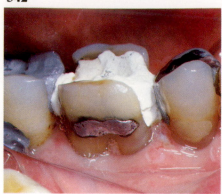

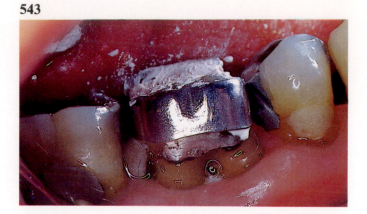

2. There is a danger of the tooth fracturing during treatment in molars and premolars. The molar shown (542, 543) with weakened walls and a buccal restoration is an obvious candidate for a metal band.

3. The tooth already has an incomplete fracture which must be prevented from spreading.

544

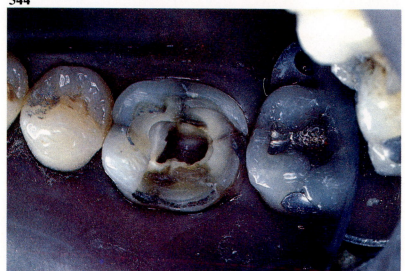

544 shows a first mandibular molar which has a fracture line in both the distal and buccal walls of the crown. The tooth must be banded before root canal treatment and the tooth taken out of occlusion. The prognosis is still poor but by banding these teeth and later crowning it may be possible to preserve them for some years.

A band is fitted as follows. The band is selected and trimmed with scissors to fit around the tooth (545). Care should be taken to smooth the cut edges with a stone (546) and fit the band so that it does not damage the soft tissues.

545

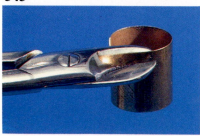

546

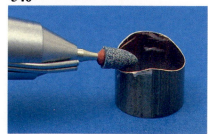

547

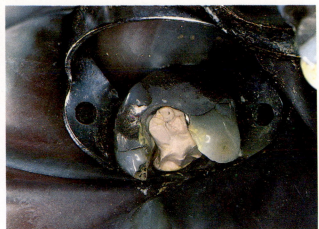

548

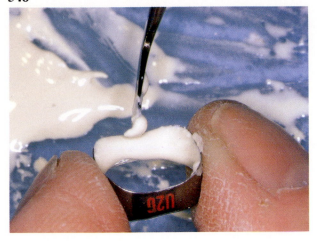

549

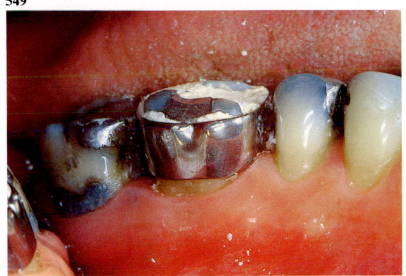

Stick gutta percha is softened and placed over the roof of the pulp chamber (**547**). Zinc phosphate cement is placed inside the band (**548**) and around the tooth, and the band seated (**549**).

The remaining cement is then thickened by the addition of more powder and pushed into the cavity to cover the gutta percha (**549**). The band should not be clamped at that visit as it could be displaced. **550** shows a copper ring which had not been smoothed and a traumatic ulcer (arrowed) may be seen (**551**). The copper ring has been smoothed.

550

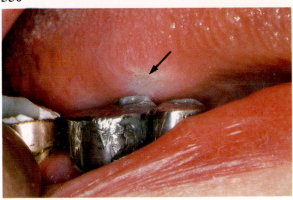

551

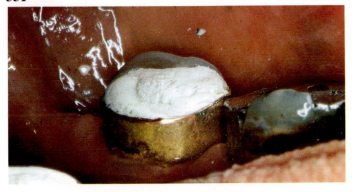

552

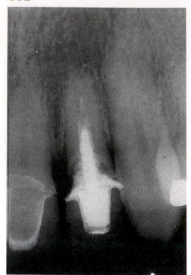

553

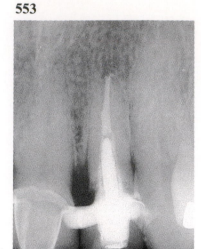

554

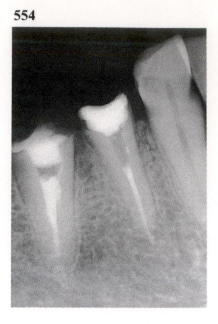

555

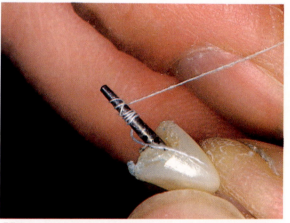

556

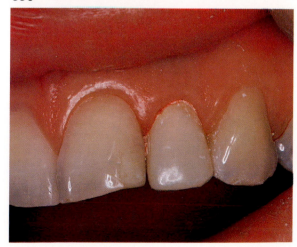

POST CROWNS

It is difficult to produce an adequate seal to protect the periapical tissue in between appointments during root canal treatment of post crowned teeth.

There are four ways in which this problem may be tackled:

1. Carry out the root canal treatment in one visit as was done here (**552, 553**). This involved removing the old post, preparing and filling the root canal and providing new post space so that the temporary post and crown could be fitted.

2. The patient may agree not to have a temporary crown between visits. The canal is prepared, dressed and the coronal portion sealed (**554**).

3. Prepare and seal the root canal coronally, then fit an acrylic tooth into the space by acid etching it with composite to the adjacent teeth.

4. If it is necessary to place a temporary post and crown, a better fit can be obtained by winding a strand of gauze around the temporary post (**555**) and sealing with a temporary cement such as Tempbond[1] (**556**).

CROWNS

Cutting an access cavity through an existing full crown will endanger its retention by weakening the core material or dentine. The crown should first be examined for caries, decementation or marginal deficiencies, the periodontal condition should also be checked. Radiograph (**557**) shows a crown that should be removed as it has deficient margins.

The second molar on the radiograph (**558**) should be root-treated through the crown providing it does not need replacing. In cases where the crown requires renewal, it should be removed before starting the root treatment because access into the pulp chamber and canal system will be made easier as the two cases below demonstrate (**559, 560**). If the crown can be replaced temporarily a good inter-appointment seal can be obtained.

557

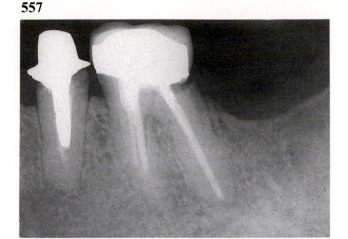

558

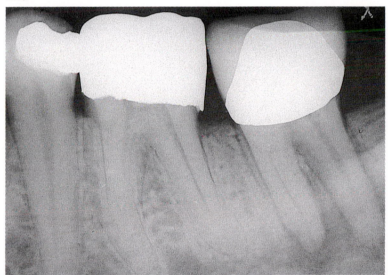

559

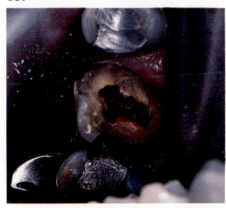

560

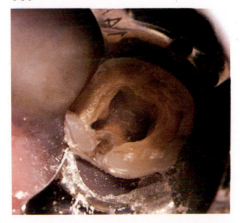

BRIDGES

When a bridge abutment requires root treatment the bridge should always be checked to see if it has been decemented. A Briault probe is hooked under the pontic, near the retainer, and pressure applied to remove the bridge. If bubbles are noted around the retainer margins this indicates decementation. In this case the bridge has to be removed (**561, 562**).

The posterior bridge shown in the radiograph (**563**) has marginal leakage under the mesial aspect of the retainer on the first molar. The bridge will have to be removed.

There is a danger of decementation of a bridge retainer if root treatment has been carried out through the bridge. If it is necessary to carry out root treatment without removing the bridge great care must be taken, using the preoperative radiographs as a guide, to remove the minimum of tooth substance or core material during access cavity preparation (**564, 565**).

561

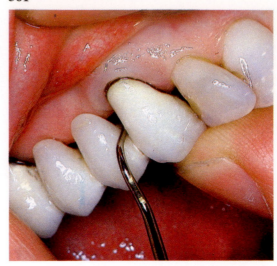

562

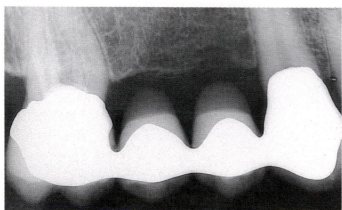

563

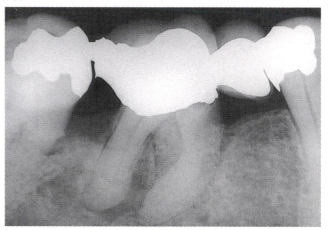

564

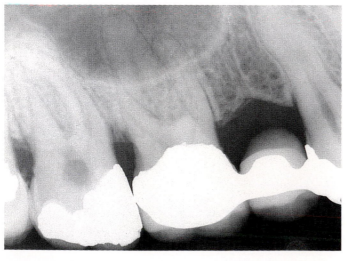

565

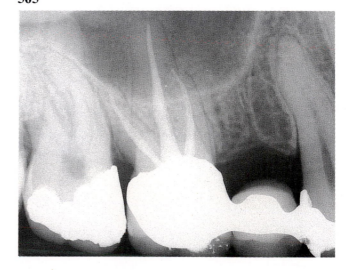

11 Preparation of the root canal C J Stock

OBJECTIVE

The objectives of root canal preparation are to:
1. Remove all organic debris from the root canal system.
2. Eliminate bacteria from the root canal.
3. Shape the canal so that it can be obturated with a root filling material.

PROBLEMS WITH LARGER SIZED INSTRUMENTS

As the size of root canal instruments increases their flexibility decreases. The larger sizes are stiff and problems arise when they are used to prepare the root canal. These problems are:
1. The apical portion of many roots is narrow, so that if large instruments are used they could lead to perforation (567, 568).
2. The majority of teeth have curved roots, particularly in the apical one third. The curvature in the root is negotiable with small instruments but larger instruments tend to straighten the canal out by cutting dentine from the outer wall of the curve at the apical end of the canal (569). This is referred to as apical flaring or zipping. The photograph (570) shows three plastic blocks[1] each one containing a curved canal.

(a) The unprepared canal. The circular shape at the end of the canal represents an apical area.
(b) The canal has been straightened by the larger instrument and an apical flare or zip has been produced.
(c) The zipping effect is close to the end of the canal and has enlarged the apical foramen. The canal would now be difficult or impossible to obturate so that an hermetic seal is produced.

Dentine is removed from all parts of the canal walls so that the original shape is maintained and a tapered preparation produced with the narrowest part at the apical end (566).

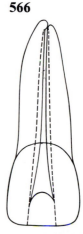

566

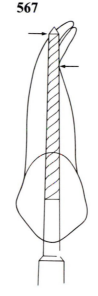

567

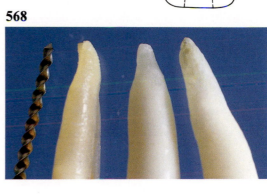

568

3. Forcing stiffer instruments into the canal may produce ledging and eventually perforate the wall of the root (571). Radiographs (572-574) demonstrate a case of poor canal preparation which has been corrected:

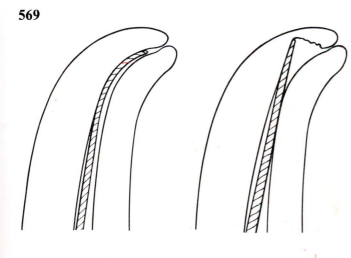

569

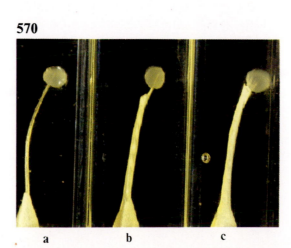

570

a   b   c

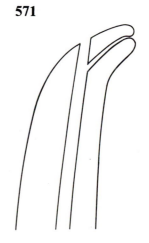

571

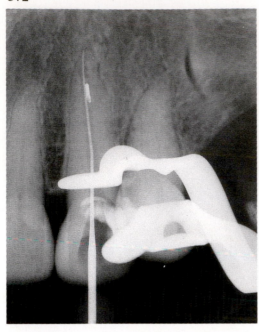

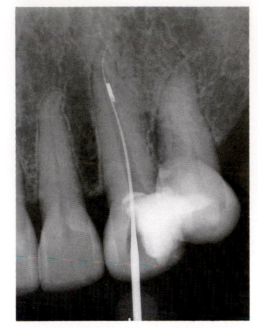

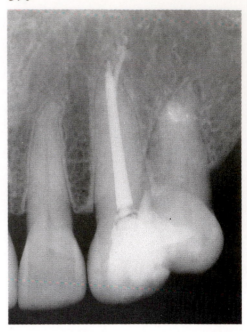

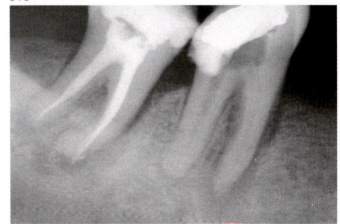

572 The canine has been prepared by forcing large instruments into the canal which has perforated. The root apex may be seen curving distally beyond the perforation.

573 A small flexible instrument has negotiated the canal to the apex.

574 The root canal is finally obturated.

575 Another case shows a molar root filling with an area associated with a mesial root. The canal(s) in the mesial root has not been prepared correctly and there has been a perforation. The apical portion of the canal has not been instrumented or filled.

4. The vigorous use of successively larger instruments at the full working length may force debris through the apical foramen into the periapical tissues. Figure **576** shows a canal that has been instrumented extruding a column of debris. It is not surprising that after-pain can occur following root canal preparation.

To overcome these problems the method of root canal preparation advocated is the step back technique.

576

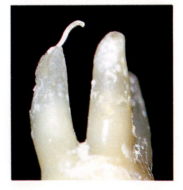

REMOVAL OF PULP TISSUE

The first step in preparing the root canal is to remove any vital pulp tissue. The largest barbed broach which will fit loosely in the canal is selected. Barbed broaches should be used in the straight part of the canal only (577).

NEGOTIATION OF CANAL

Placement of the first cutting instrument into the canal is important and should be done with care and minimal force. The diagram (578) shows that a straight instrument will tend to bind on the wall of the canal rather than follow the curve. In fine canals a curve is placed in the apical 2-3 mm of the instrument. A small reciprocating movement will allow the instrument tip to seek its way into the canal and follow the curvature. The choice of size of instrument will be dictated by the size of the canal. An 06, 08 or 10 will be necessary in a fine canal. The curve in the instrument is placed by inserting the tip into a sterile cotton wool roll (579) and bending the shank as shown. Note that the curve is gradual and not a sharp bend (580).

Problems may be encountered in negotiating and widening fine tortuous canals. Copious amounts of irrigation are used but additional help may be required. EDTA (ethylenediamine tetra-acetic acid) which is a chelating agent, softens the dentine making it easier to remove. The most convenient form is a paste such as RC Prep[1] which contains 15% EDTA, and 10% Urea peroxide which acts as a lubricant in addition to its chelating properties.

It is inadvisable to use EDTA to help complete negotiation of a canal as the softening effect on the dentine may encourage the tip of the instrument to start its own canal. In these cases Glyoxide (a mouth wash), Hibiscrub[2] or K.Y. jelly may be used as lubricants.

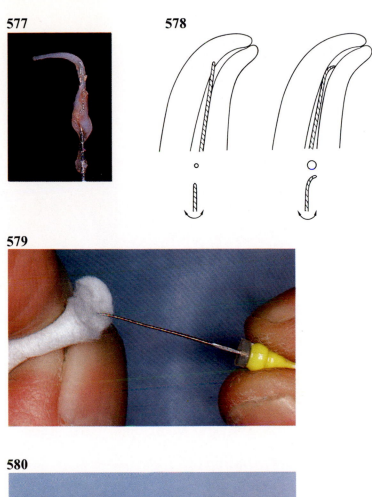

577

578

579

580

581

2.0 mm

working length

ESTABLISHING CANAL LENGTH

A rough estimate is made from the preoperative radiograph and a knowledge of the average lengths of teeth. The instrument is inserted 1-2 mm short of this length and a radiograph taken. The correct working length is 1 mm short of the radiographic apex. From the radiograph the correct working length may be determined by estimating the distance between the tip of the instrument and the apex. In the diagram (581) the diagnostic instrument is 2 mm short of the "radiographic" apex so the working length will be 1 mm more than the measured length. If the

143

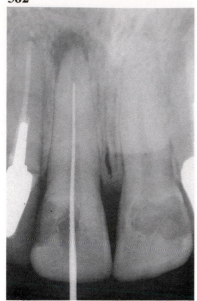

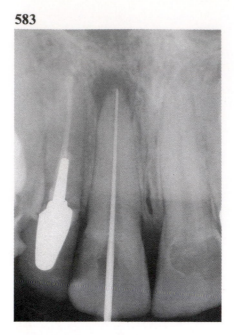

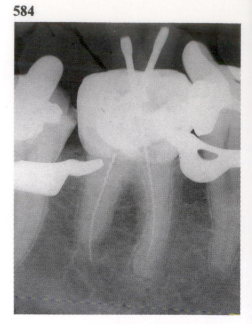

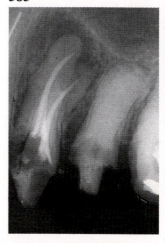

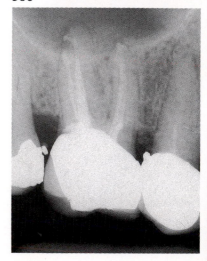

diagnostic length is wrong by 3 mm or more the instrument should be adjusted and another radiograph taken. In the case shown (582) a second radiograph was necessary. The working length may be calculated by reducing the measured length by 0.5 mm (583) from the second radiograph.

Electronic Measuring Instrument. Two of these devices have been mentioned briefly in the chapter on instruments and materials. The principle on which these devices is based is sound and in clinical practice they have been found to be accurate in the location of the apical foramen. The advantages of using an electronic device for measuring are:

1. It is difficult to locate the radiographic apex on some teeth, particularly posteriors. In **584** the position of the apex of the distal root on the radiograph is uncertain.

2. The apical foramen may be located up to 3 mm from the radiographic apex. Two examples show the main apical foramen opening onto the surface of the root some distance from the radiographic apex (**585, 586**).

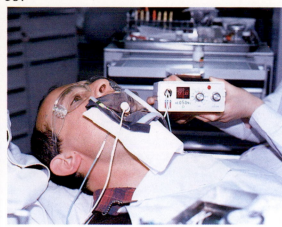

587 The Neosono D in use.

By locating the foramen short of the apex the electronic device will prevent perforation, which could occur if only the radiographic length was used.

3.   A considerable reduction in the number of radiographs necessary may be made. This is particularly useful in cases of pregnancy or if the patient does not wish to have radiographs taken.

4.   It is quicker and simpler to measure the length electronically than it is to take and develop a radiograph.

However, with all these devices there are some disadvantages. These are:

1.   A period of learning is required to understand when the readings are reliable.

2.   Occasionally the reading is definite, appears accurate, but may be incorrect by several millimetres.

The devices are a most useful addition to the armamentarium but do not replace radiography. Some guidelines concerning their use are given below (**587, 588, 589**):

(a)   Always use with rubber dam as any fluid seepage will make the readings unreliable.

(b)   The more recent devices will measure in a damp canal but the pulp chamber and canal entrance should be dried with a pledget of cotton wool.

(c)   When the access cavity is cut through a metal restoration, care must be taken to prevent the instrument contacting the restoration and producing a false reading.

(d)   In vital teeth take the reading as soon as the pulp is exposed. A partially extirpated and bleeding pulp would not give a correct reading.

(e)   If the canal contains blood necrotic tissue or any dissociating ions it should be dried with paper points before a reading is taken.

(f)   Sodium hypochlorite if used must be dried from the canal before measuring.

(g)   The devices may be used to locate a perforation and its site in the wall of the canal. This is done by inserting a small instrument with a curve at the tip and gently exploring the canal walls.

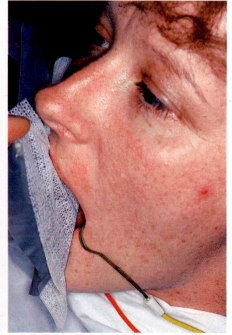

588 The hook may be placed over any part of the lip.

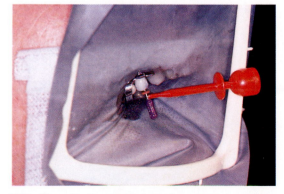

589 The clip is attached to the reamer or file, which is then advanced into the canal.

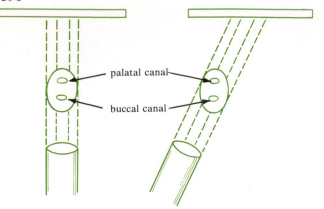

590

palatal canal

buccal canal

BUCCAL OBJECT RULE

When there is more than one canal it is necessary to identify each one on the radiograph. The buccal object rule states that if the radiograph is taken from the mesial the buccal canal will appear as the most distal one on the radiograph (**590**). When taking radiographs to measure working length of all premolars and molars, the X-Ray cone should be placed mesially and directed distally. The radiograph (**591**) of a first premolar has been taken with the X-Ray cone placed mesially. The distal diagnostic instrument on the radiograph arrowed is in the buccal canal. On the radiograph of the second molar (**592**), the middle diagnostic instrument which appears straight lies in the mesio-buccal canal.

THE STEP BACK TECHNIQUE

The principles of the step back technique should be used for the preparation of all root canals. There are three stages:

Stage One.   Establishing Apical Stop.

Once the working length has been measured filing the canal may be started. The aim of filing is to remove all the irregularities from the walls of the canal and leave them smooth and cone shaped. The file is introduced gently to the correct length using a small contra-rotating movement. A planing action is used, pressing against the full length of the wall and gradually moving clockwise around the circumference of the canal (**593**). Filing repeatedly in one area will produce a groove. Canals which are wide bucco-lingually may have finlike grooves in the walls. Buccal and lingual filing will open up these grooves, remove the organic debris and make it possible to obliterate them with a filling material.

591

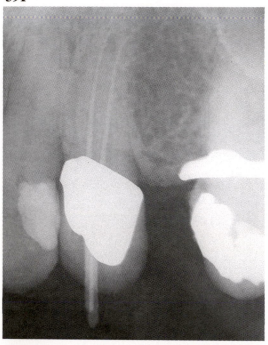

592

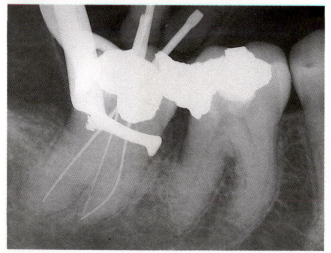

593

over-filing in any area will produce a groove

groove removed by filing

file

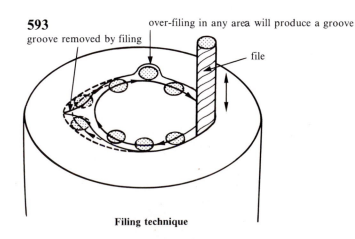

Filing technique

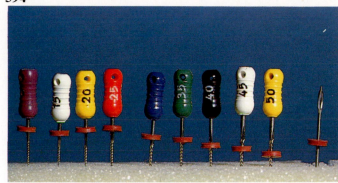

595

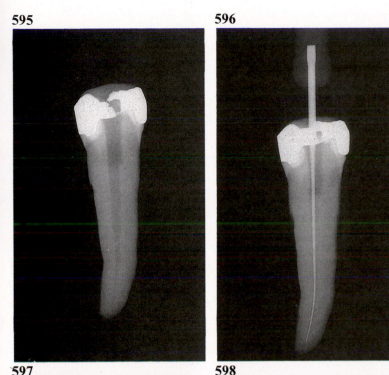

596

597

598

All instruments inserted into the canal should be marked at the correct length with a rubber stop or marking paste. To produce an apical stop accurate filing and measuring is necessary. In the photograph (**594**) the 10, 15, 20 and 25 sizes have been marked at the correct length.

The step back technique is demonstrated on the extracted mandibular premolar (**595**). If the canal had been curved then a similar curve would have been placed near the tip of the instrument.

596 The canal is fine so the size 10 is first introduced into the canal to the full working length and filing commenced.

597 A size 15 is then used.

598 When this feels loose at the working length the size 10 is reintroduced to remove any accumulated debris. The process is termed recapitulation. After each increase in size of instrument the previous size is inserted into the canal to prevent the canal from becoming blocked. This procedure is unnecessary in larger canals.

The sequence of files in this case was 10 - 15 - 10 - 20 - 15 - 25 - 20.

599 The first stage is now completed with the formation of an apical stop.

599

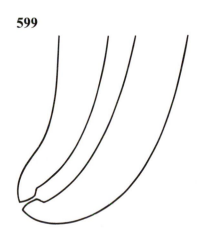

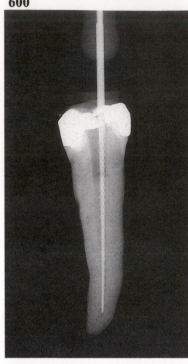

600

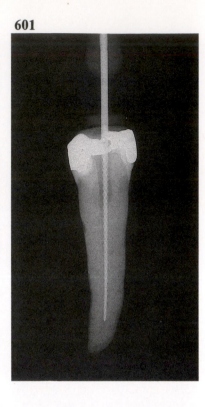

601

Stage Two. Stepping Back.

Each larger instrument is inserted 1 mm less into the canal. Recapitulation is carried out between each increase in instrument size by inserting the largest instrument size used in Stage One (in this case 25) to the full working length.

600 A size 30 is placed 1 mm short of the working length and the canal filed. The size 25 is then used briefly to ensure patency of the canal to the full working length.

601 Size 35 — 2 mm short.

602 Size 40 — 3 mm short.

603 Size 45 — 4 mm short.

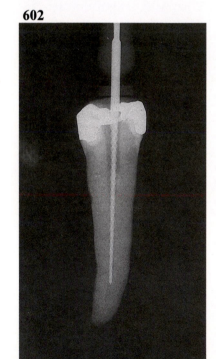

602

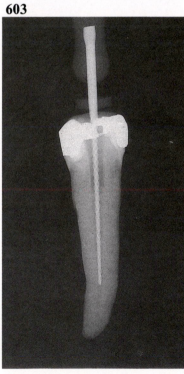

603

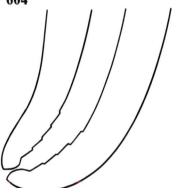

604

604 The diagram shows the flared shape of the canal. In practice the steps in the canal wall are minimal.

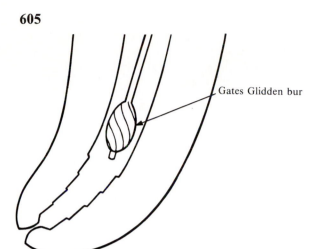

605

Gates Glidden bur

606
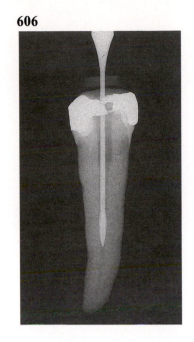

607
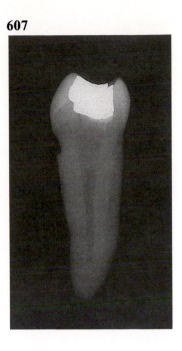

Stage Three. Completion of Preparation.

A suitable sized Gates Glidden bur is used to complete the coronal taper (**605**). The bur is inserted into the straight part of the canal (**606**) and a cutting action made only on the withdrawal stroke. Any small ledges are removed by filing with the last instrument used at the full working length.

The final radiograph (**607**) taken from the mesio-distal aspect shows the gradual taper produced in the coronal part of the canal.

It is not possible to stipulate the largest instrument used in stage one to produce the apical stop due to the variation in canal anatomy. Generally in a fine curved canal the size will be 25 and in a larger straighter canal a minimum of size 40.

ANTICURVATURE FILING

There is a risk in the preparation of curved canals that the inner aspect of the curve may be perforated. **608** shows a case where the mesio-buccal root of an upper left first molar was perforated. Some extrusion of sealer can be seen on the distal aspect of the root. The tooth was extracted and the extent of the perforation is visible (**609**).

Abou-Rass (1980) has described the inner aspect of the curved root as the danger zone and recommended anti-curvature filing. This involves filing, during the preparation of the root canal, away from the danger zone. A technique verified by research (Lim 1987) recommends a circumferential filing technique filing the buccal, mesial and lingual or palatal walls of the root canal in the ratio of 3:1 with the furcal wall.

608
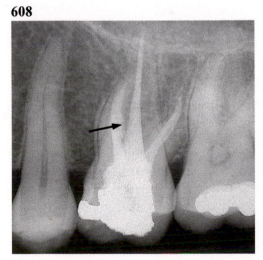

609
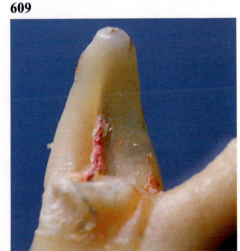

IRRIGATION

During preparation of the root canal copious amounts of irrigant should be used. The solution is injected without force into the pulp chamber (**610**). Sodium hypochlorite 1-2% is the currently accepted irrigant. When the preparation is complete the canals should be dried with paper points.

MEDICATION

The medicament of choice is placed on a cotton wool pledget in the pulp chamber (**611**). If the medicament is a liquid the pledget should be dipped into it, then squeezed dry in a sterile cotton wool roll. (See Chapter 5 on basic instruments and materials for types of medicament).

TEMPORARY SEAL

Dry or medicated cotton wool is placed in the pulp chamber and covered with softened stick gutta percha. A final seal is then placed (**612**). A variety of temporary filling materials may be used: Chemfil, Intermediate Restorative material (IRM), Cavit or amalgam.

610

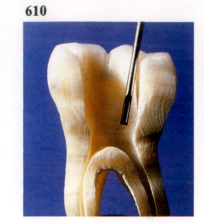

611

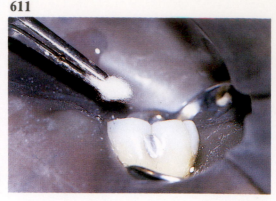

612

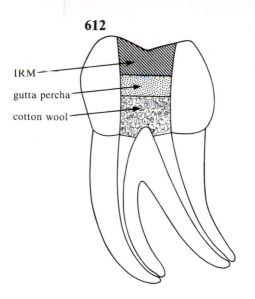

The author has found IRM, an acrylic-reinforced Zinc oxide, a good long term temporary filling material due to its hardness and resistance to wear.

If the layer of gutta percha is not inserted into the access cavity, fragments of the temporary seal may fall into the canals and block them. An example of amalgam falling into the distal canal is shown (**613, 614**).

613

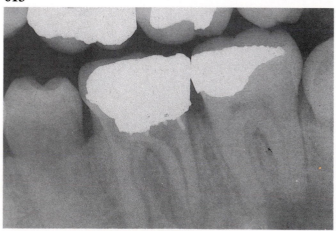

614

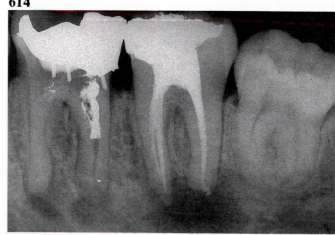

CHECKING THE OCCLUSION

615 A high temporary filling is the commonest cause of pain following root canal preparation. The tooth should be checked in all excursive movements to ensure the filling is not high.

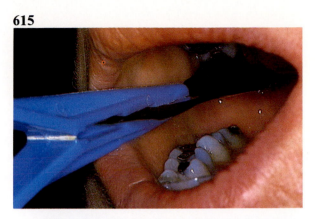

SUBSONIC AND ULTRASONIC TECHNIQUES

Handpieces have been introduced which are designed to transmit either subsonic or ultrasonic vibratory movements to root canal files. At the time of going to press there is relatively little published research concerning the subsonic devices. Early reports are conflicting but these devices may well have a useful place in the preparation of root canals.

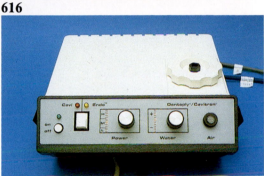

ULTRASONIC ROOT CANAL PREPARATION

The use of ultrasound in the preparation of the root canal has been developed largely by Martin and Cunningham. Several ultrasonic scaler units are now available with an endodontic function (**616**). **617** shows the head of the handpiece with a diamond file. Instruments are changed using an Allen key. (**618**).

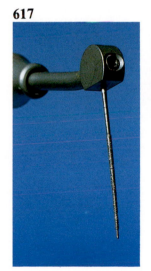

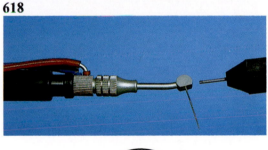

Ultrasound consists of acoustic waves which have a frequency higher than can be perceived by the human ear. A root canal instrument placed in the handpiece will oscillate at 25,000 cycles per second and have a displacement in the region of 23 microns at the tip. The units contain an irrigation system operated by a foot switch; the irrigant recommended is sodium hypochlorite at a strength of 2.5 per cent weight by volume. The irrigant under pressure passes through the handpiece and down the shank of the instrument into the root canal.

There are several studies claiming that preparation techniques using ultrasound will remove more debris from the root canal walls than conventional hand instrumentation. Acoustic streaming (**619**), which is a severe turbulence of the irrigant produced by the vibrating shank of the instrument within the canals is thought to be responsible for the increased cleaning ability. The diagram **619** shows the sound waves passing down the shank of the instrument and the arrows represent the eddies set up in the irrigant. The acoustic streaming effect allows a fast and efficient replacement of the sodium hypochlorite. Some fragmentation of the debris in the root canal also occurs, together with a small rise in temperature of the irrigation fluid which increases the speed of dissolution of the organic debris.

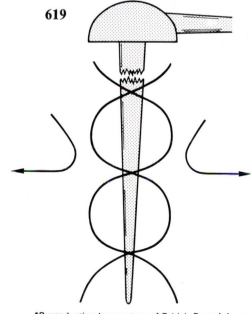

*Reproduction by courtesy of British Dental Journal.

Figures **620** (left and right) illustrate the ramifications found in the apical portions of teeth. Both root canals have been prepared by hand filing (left) and ultrasonic filing (right); sodium hypochlorite was used as the irrigant in both teeth. Debris remains in the fins of the hand filed tooth while the ultrasonically prepared tooth is clear. In this way areas of the root canal wall will be cleaned which cannot be reached by an instrument (Cunningham 1982). Sodium hypochlorite will partially dissolve the organic matter and the remainder, together with other canal debris, is easily flushed out of the canal by the operator. Sound waves will also rupture cell membranes so that the bactericidal effect of sodium hypochlorite is enhanced.

The instruments used are K files and diamond coated files (**621**). Each type is manufactured in 3 sizes. ISO sizes 15, 20 and 25 for the K file and 25, 35 and 45 for the diamond files (the diamond file size 25 is slightly larger than the ISO size). It has been demonstrated that both types of instruments have a greater cutting efficiency when used with ultrasound compared to hand operated (Martin 1980). The technique of filing using ultrasound differs from the conventional method. Two movements are used, a light circumferential filing stroke remembering that the file will cut on both insertion and withdrawal; and a circular motion maintaining the file at the same depth.

The technique used for preparation has been described in a booklet (Caulk Dentsply 1984) but the author uses a slight modification (see Table 1). In curved canals the K files should be precurved before use and the diamond files restricted to the straight part of the canal. In the author's experience the only problem with preparing root canals with ultra sound is the lack of 'feel' of cutting dentine; this presents a very real danger of stripping and perforating the inner aspect of the curve so that an anticurvature filing technique is essential.

The use of sodium hypochlorite as the irrigant of choice is causing some concern and research into a suitable alternative continues.

There are two disadvantages with sodium hypochlorite. Firstly, it is corrosive to most metals so the cost of the ultrasonic units is high; secondly, patients will not tolerate leakage of the irrigant into their mouths so that rubber dam is essential with this system. It is arguable that this second point might be an advantage as it promotes the use of rubber dam, so helping to raise the standard of endodontics.

The benefits of ultrasonic preparation appear to offer a more efficient and faster method of cleaning and shaping root canals. Provided further research substantiates these early claims, endosonics will become an important aspect in root canal treatment.

620 (left)

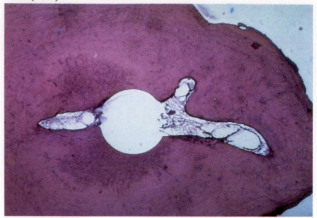

620 (right)

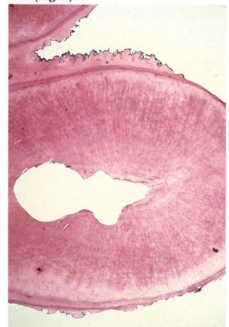

621

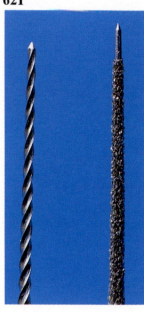

Table 1   Endosonic canal preparation

FINE CANALS	LARGER CANALS
Determine canal length	Determine canal length
Hand file to size 15	
Endosonic file size 15	
Endosonic file size 25	Endosonic file size 25
Small Gates Glidden	Gates Glidden
Endosonic diamond size 25	Endosonic diamond file 25 (35)
Provide stop with 25 hand file	Provide stop with hand file

Each instrument should be used until it feels loose in the canal before the larger size is tried.

12 Filling the Root Canal C J Stock

OBJECTIVE

The root canal system should be obturated to prevent any exchange between the canal and the periodontal ligament. Contamination of the root canal may occur due to microleakage of the coronal restoration or periodontal disease uncovering a lateral canal (**622**). Pulp tissue remnants and/or micro organisms will be present even after the most thorough mechanical and chemical preparation and these must be sealed within the root canal. Any ingress of tissue fluids will provide a culture medium for the micro organisms and allow diffusion of toxic products into the periodontal tissues.

ROOT FILLING MATERIALS

The materials available for filling root canals may be divided into fillers and sealers. All sealers are absorbable, so the minimum amount should be exposed to the periapical tissues. **623** shows a case of extrusion into the periapical tissues of a sealer.

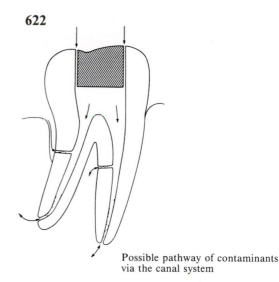

622

Possible pathway of contaminants via the canal system

624 The radiograph taken two months later shows the sealer has been resorbed. The solid or semi-solid filler should take up the bulk of the canal space, fitting as well as possible near the main apical foramen, and condensing the sealer into the remaining small gaps along the walls of the root canal.

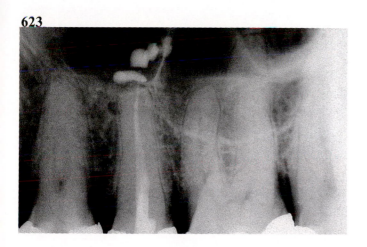

623

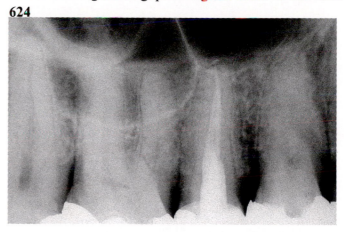

624

FILLERS
Gutta percha has been used as a root filling material for over 110 years. Two types of gutta percha point are produced: the standardised point, or cone, which conforms to the International Standards Organisation (ISO) and the non-standardised or accessory point. The latter is presented in a variety of sizes, such as extra fine, fine or medium, but vary according to the manufacturer. The difference between the two types is apparent from figure **625**, the non-standardised point being much more tapered.

Despite the introduction of numerous other root canal filling materials, GP is the most widely used filler. It is well tolerated by tissue and is compressible within the root canal.

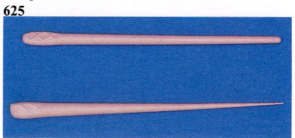

625

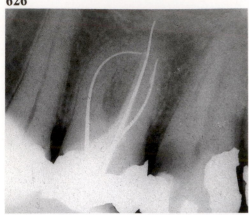

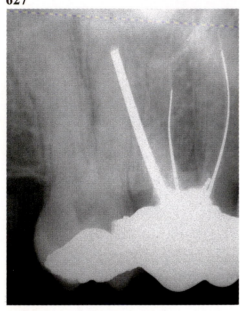

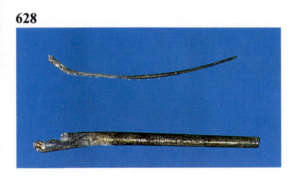

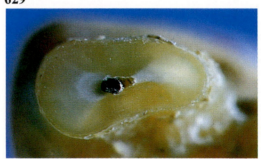

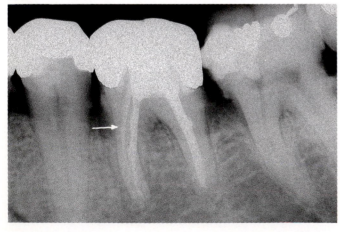

Silver. **626** The radiograph was taken 36 years after the tooth had been root filled. The tooth was functional, symptomless and there was no sinus present. Despite the considerable success of silver points since their introduction some 50 years ago, there is now evidence that they may cause late failures. The disadvantages of silver points are:

i) silver corrodes in the presence of tissue fluids within the root canal and the corrosion products are cytotoxic. The silver points which have been removed from the first molar show black corrosion products (**627, 628**).

ii) silver points provide a poor fit as they are round in cross section whereas root canals are usually oval or irregularly shaped. The very root canals where one would choose to use a silver point because of difficult access, such as the mesio-buccal canal in maxillary molars (**629**) or mesial canals of mandibular molars, are the least suitable for silver points, owing to their irregular shape.

iii) silver is non-compressible and so cannot be adapted to the shape of the canal.

Titanium. Messing (1980) suggested the use of titanium points. These are more rigid than silver points, do not corrode, and are well tolerated by tissue. However, like silver points, they are non-compressible and rely on the sealer to obturate the canal.

630 shows a molar with the mesio-lingual canal (arrowed) filled with a titanium point. The remaining canals have been filled with gutta percha. Note the internal resorption.

Plastic. Plastic points have been suggested as a root filling material but suffer from the same disadvantages as titanium. They also tend to be brittle and so have little place as a root filling material.

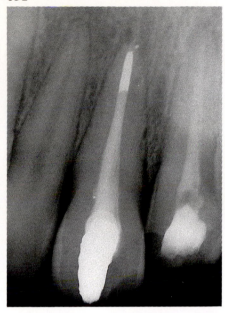

Amalgam. This material satisfies most of the requirements for the ideal root filling material, being well tolerated, non-absorbable and capable of forming a good seal.

631 The central incisor has a sectional amalgam. The remaining canal space has been obturated with laterally condensed gutta percha.

The two main disadvantages are that it is difficult or impossible to remove and requires the root canal to be prepared to at least size 40 to the full working length for correct placement and condensation. In addition some research has cast doubt on the ability of amalgam to produce a seal. This may be due to the technique used rather than the material itself.

ROOT FILLING TECHNIQUES

When to Fill. The root filling is completed when the tooth is symptomless and the canal dry or capable of being dried with one or two paper points.

Number of Visits. The accepted technique has been two visits, the first to prepare and shape the root canal and the second to obturate the canal space. There is now a trend to complete the root treatment in one visit but this is only recommended in certain circumstances. The operator requires experience to select one visit cases, but a rough guide is given below.

One visit	Two or more visits
The tooth should be symptomless	Tooth is tender to percussion
The pulp vital or partially vital	Symptomless but with apical area
Pulpless, but with no apical area	Wet canals, difficult to dry
Sinus present	Periapical tissues disturbed during root canal preparation
Straightforward uninfected re-treatment	

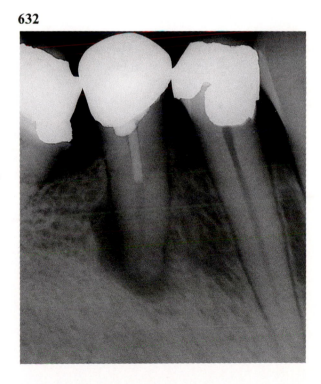

632 This is a tooth with a symptomless area. In the author's opinion such teeth, if root treated in one visit, are likely to cause the patient to return within 48 hours with an acute episode of pain.

633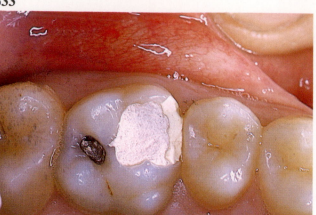

634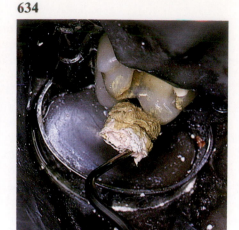

635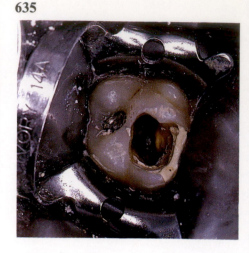

Pre-root filling Procedures. Whatever the technique for root filling chosen, certain preliminary steps are taken:

1. The patient is questioned about any symptoms since the previous visit. If the tooth is still painful the canal(s) should be re-prepared and dressed.
2. Local anaesthesia is given if required.
3. Rubber dam is applied.
4. The temporary root filling (**633**) is removed with an air rotor down to the GP, which is then teased out with a Briault probe (**634**). The cotton wool underneath is then removed, revealing the floor of the pulp chamber (**635**).
5. A paper point is inserted into each canal to check for moisture. If there is any pus or bleeding, the canal must be re-prepared and a dressing applied.
6. The largest instrument used to prepare the canal to the full working length should be inserted to check the patency of the canal and the presence of an apical stop at the correct length.

Techniques available

Sectional.

Single cone.

Multiple cone:

> Cold lateral condensation
> Warm lateral condensation
> Hot vertical condensation
> Custom made.

GP with solvents.

Thermal compaction.

Injection moulded thermo plasticised.

Pastes alone.

Sectional. This method is reserved for teeth which will be restored with a post crown immediately following root treatment. Silver, titanium, gutta percha or amalgam may be used as filling materials. The length of the apical filling should be as long as possible, yet still allowing sufficient length of post space to retain the post crown. The disadvantages of the technique are that no allowances are made for a lateral canal in the middle or coronal third of the root and it is difficult to produce a hermetic seal with any of the materials.

636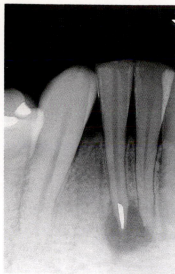

637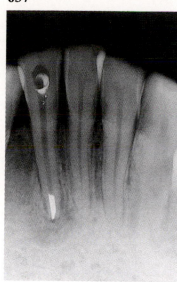

Two examples of sectional root fillings are illustrated.
Case 1 A mandibular incisor (**636**) with an area was root-treated using a sectional amalgam. The case is shown two years later. Healing appears to be complete (**637**).

638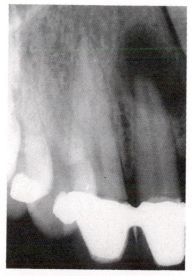

Case 2 A maxillary incisor with a radiolucent area (**638**) was root-filled using a sectional silver point (**639**). Follow-up radiographs were taken four years later (**640**) when it could be seen that healing was taking place, but a small area still persisted. In the final radiograph (**641**), two years afterwards, it is clear that the silver point had become dislodged because it did not fit.

639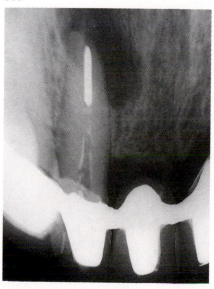

640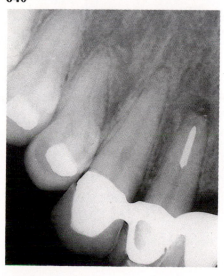

641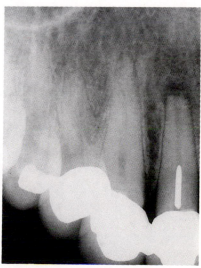

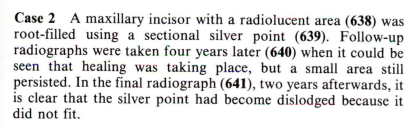

642

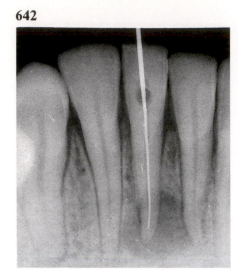

643

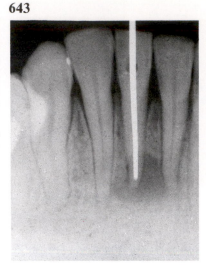

644

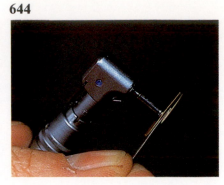

Sectional Silver or Titanium Technique
The length of the canal is measured. **642** shows the diagnostic instrument in position. The canal is prepared round in the apical few millimetres with a reamer or file using the reaming action. A similar sized point is selected and fitted into the root canal to the correct working length. The point should fit so that there is resistance to withdrawal or tug back. The length is checked by taking a radiograph (**643**). If the point is slightly too large it may be reduced in size by placing between two sandpaper discs, rough sides facing each other, in a slow handpiece (**644**).

645

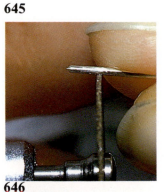

646

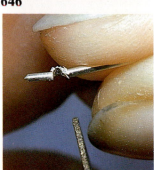

647

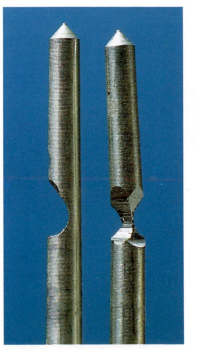

648

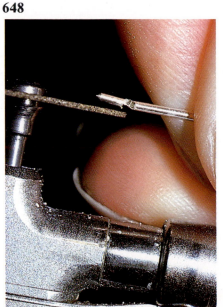

649

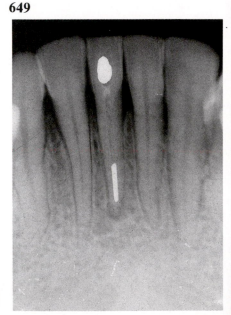

645, 646, 647 The apical 3-5 mm of point is then half sectioned with a carborundum disc or air rotor bur.

648 Any protruding rough edges must be removed, as shown, with a disc.

The point is coated with the sealer of choice and inserted to the working length, using a firm pressure to keep the point fully sealed. The shank is rotated and withdrawn, leaving the sectioned tip in position (**649**).

Messing precision apical silver or titanium points
Sectioning metal points, as described in the previous section, can present difficulties. The point may break off in the wrong position in the canal or not at all. To overcome this, apical silver or titanium tips[1] are produced. The tips are available in 3 mm and 5 mm lengths and 12 ISO sizes. The tips contain a screw thread projection, which engages in the end of the shaft (**650, 651**). A handle may be fitted over the shaft and adjusted to the correct working length of the canal, with the tip attached. The point must fit at the full working length with tug back. The length is verified with a radiograph. The tip is coated with sealer and inserted into the canal to the correct working length. Maintaining apical pressure, the handle is rotated anti-clockwise to unscrew the tip. The shaft is then withdrawn, leaving the tip in situ.

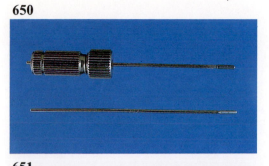

650

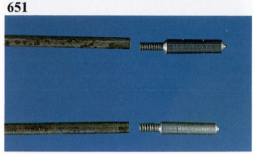

651

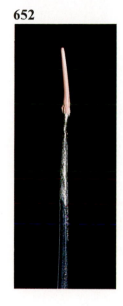

652

Gutta percha
The technique is similar to silver and titanium sections. A GP point is fitted to the correct length and then 3-4 mm cut from the tip. A wire or hot root canal plugger of smaller diameter than the GP point is heated and attached to the cut end of the tip (**652**). A mark is made on the metal shank at the correct length and the tip coated with sealer. The tip and plugger are inserted into the canal to the working length and twisted to disengage the plugger from the tip. This is a poor method of attempting to seal the apical third of the canal, as it is not possible to condense the tip adequately.

Amalgam
An amalgam apical seal has several advantages over the other sectional techniques: no sealer is required, it is well tolerated by tissue should small portions be extruded, and it does not rely on the shape of the root canal being round. The main disadvantages are firstly that it cannot be removed easily and, secondly, that the apical few millimetres have to be prepared to a size sufficiently large to allow the introduction of the amalgam carrier. The smallest size of amalgam carrier which can be manufactured is the Dimashkieh carrier. This is a flexible, spring loaded amalgam carrier, with an outer diameter of 45, 60 or 80, corresponding to the ISO sizes. The three Dimashkieh carriers are shown on the left (**653**) with their corresponding condensers on the right. The canal is prepared, dried and the correct carrier size selected. The carrier is loaded by pressing the tip into freshly mixed amalgam (**654**). The working length is marked on the shank and the carrier inserted to the full length, withdrawn 1 mm, then the amalgam is ejected by depressing the head of the handle (**655, 656**). The carrier should never be used to condense the amalgam.

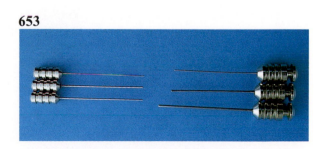

653

654

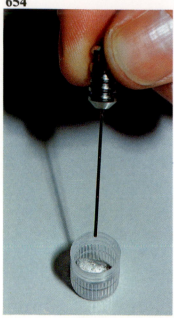

655

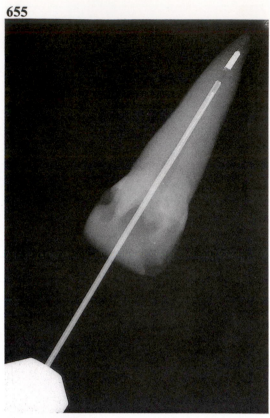

656

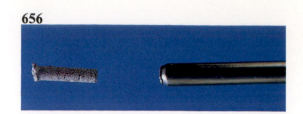

The carrier is withdrawn and the amalgam condensed, using the matching condenser supplied. The amount of amalgam in the apical portion of the canal is calculated by the length of the mark from the incisal edge (**657, 658**). Several increments are required to fill 3 mm of the apical portion of the canal. The radiograph (**659**) shows an amalgam root filling and the remainder of the root canal has been filled with laterally condensed gutta percha. It is simple to remove sufficient GP to allow post space with either a Gates Glidden drill or a heated instrument.

657

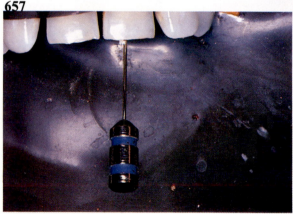

659

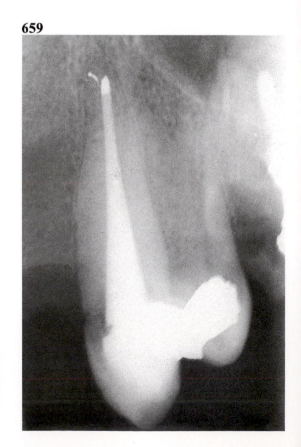

658

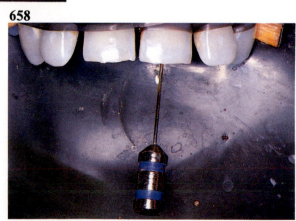

Single Cone and Sealer. A GP point, silver point or titanium point may be used with a suitable sealer; whichever point or sealer is selected, it is fitted to the full working length. The point should have tug back or resistance to removal. If the gutta percha point is too loose, a portion is cut from the tip with sharp scissors and the end re-tried. Once this is achieved, the point is coated with sealer and introduced gently into the canal to the full length.

Metal tips may be made to fit by the method described under 'Sectional Silver or Titanium Technique'. Haemostat forceps may be used to grip the point at the correct working length so that the point may be reinserted to the correct length with ease. The single cone method is quick and easy to use but, on the other hand, it does not obliterate the canal. At best the apical 2-3 mm will be filled but the remainder of the canal is unlikely to be round, so there will be large gaps, only partially filled with sealer. On rare occasions, it may be necessary to use a titanium point when a canal cannot be widened sufficiently, due to difficult access or extreme curvature. For example the mesio-buccal canal in the maxillary first molar (**660**).

Cold Lateral Condensation. The object of lateral condensation is to obliterate the entire canal system with gutta percha and sealer.

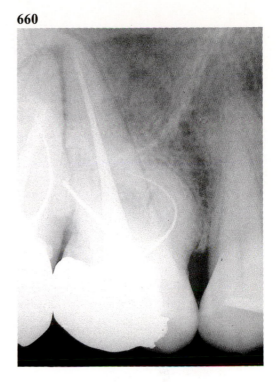

660

Instruments required:

Gutta percha, standardised cones

Gutta percha, non-standardised cones (accessory points):
    Extra fine
    Fine
    Medium

Sealer of choice

Endo locking tweezers, one for each canal

Spreaders: more than one size may be necessary.

Technique
The pre-root filling procedures are first carried out as described on page 156. A spreader is selected and introduced into the canal to ensure that it will reach to within 1 or 2 mm of the full working length. If this is not possible, the canal has been incompletely prepared and should be widened. A spreader is in the correct position in the canal (**661**).

A standardised gutta percha point or master cone is chosen normally one size bigger than the largest instrument used to reach the full working length. A master cone is fitted 0.5-1 mm short of the working length in each canal (**662**). If the GP point is too large a smaller one is selected. If the point is a loose fit, a small portion may be cut from the tip (**663**).

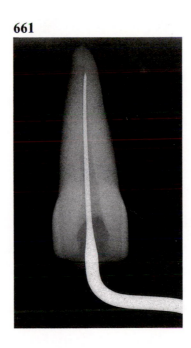

661

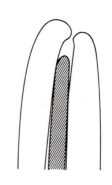

662

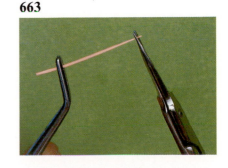

663

This is necessary as, during condensation, it will be moved up to the apical stop and so produce a better fit and also reduce the risk of an overfill. A radiograph should be taken to check the position of the master cone(s) (664) at this stage or half way through condensation, in which case a better indication of the final result will be given.

664

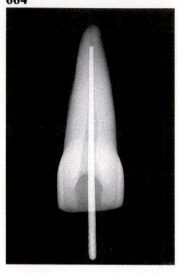

665

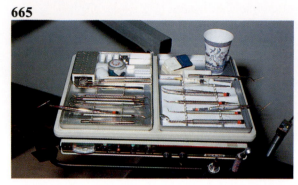

666

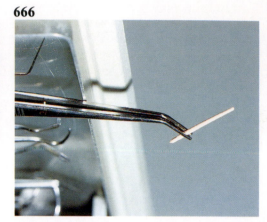

667

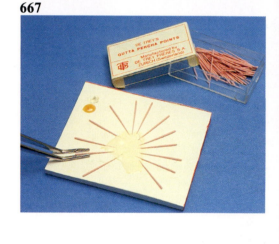

After fitting, the cone(s) are removed, using endo locking tweezers, and placed on the bracket table still clipped to the points at their correct level (665, 666). The sealer is now mixed and accessory points of the appropriate size placed on the mixing pad (667). The master cones are coated with sealer and inserted into their respective canals. It is easier to fill the most difficult canals first and then complete the larger, more accessible ones. The order in molars would be mesio-buccal, disto-buccal and palatal in the maxilla, and mesio-buccal, mesio-lingual and distal in the mandible.

The spreader is pushed gently into the canal (668), displacing the master cone to one side. The spreader is removed and an accessory cone coated with sealer is inserted into the hole (669) made by the spreader.

668

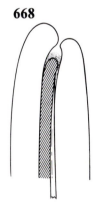

669

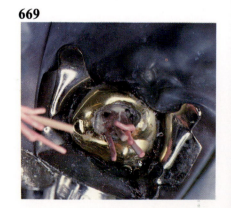

670

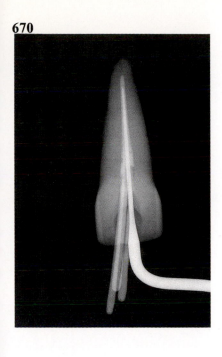

This is repeated. More pressure may be used now on the spreader (**670**) as the master cone has been wedged into place and should not pull out. The spreader is rotated while fully seated to free it from the GP and removed after a short pause to prevent the GP from springing back and closing the space. After several points have been placed, and at least one in the other canals which have coated master cones in place, it is difficult to see the entrance to the canal. A heated plastic instrument is used to cut off the excess GP down to the canal opening on the floor of the pulp chamber (**671**).

671

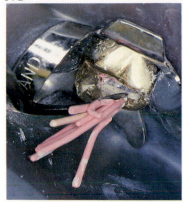

672

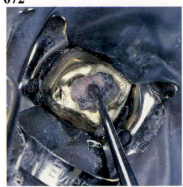

673

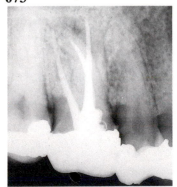

674

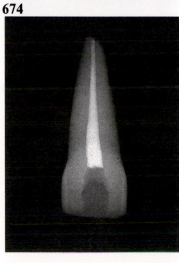

The canals are filled in this way until it is not possible to place another accessory cone further than 2-3 mm into the root canal. The excess GP is then removed with a heated plastic instrument and additional sealer placed on the floor of the pulp chamber. Pink stick GP is now warmed and placed in the pulp chamber. This is condensed firmly onto the floor to seal any furcation canals (**672**). A final long cone radiograph is taken as a check and a record (**673**). The finished radiograph of the central incisor shows a well condensed root filling (**674**). The diagram shows the master cone has moved up to the apical stop (**675**) and that some accessory cones have reached to within 1 or 2 mm of this point.

675

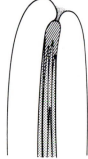

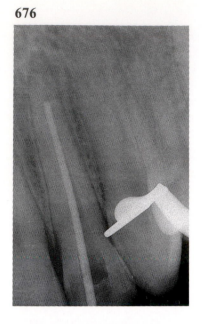

676

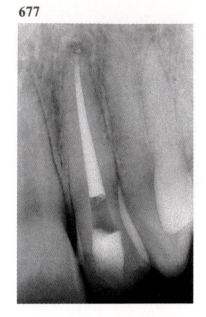

677

A suitable temporary dressing is placed in the access cavity over a pledget of cotton wool; IRM or amalgam is preferred. The filling is checked to ensure it is not interfering with the occlusion. The radiographs of the master cone fitted and the filling on completion show how far the cone has been pushed into the apical end of the canal (676, 677). It is obvious that this technique will produce a reasonable fit of the gutta percha tip as it will have conformed to the shape of the canal.

Warm Lateral Condensation. This technique has evolved as a compromise between cold lateral and hot vertical condensation. The same instruments are required as for cold lateral condensation but, in addition, a heat carrier is used to warm the gutta percha within the root canal. The softened GP may then be laterally condensed more readily into the irregularities of the root canal wall. The carrier is inserted into the canal before the start of the procedure to note the depth where the instrument engages the walls of the canal. If the instrument is placed short of this depth vertical fracture of the root due to a wedging force will be prevented.

A new device has been introduced recently which is a battery operated heated plugger. This facilitates the application of heat to the gutta percha within the canal and is simple to use.

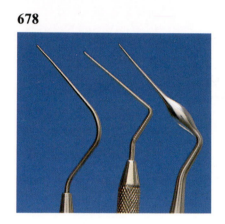

678

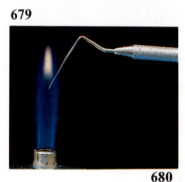

679

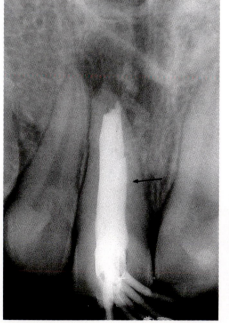

680

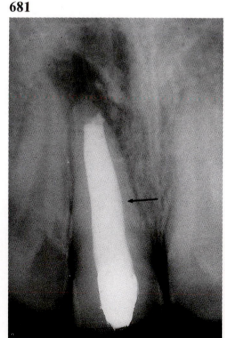

681

The technique is similar to cold lateral condensation. A master cone is fitted, sealer applied and several initial accessory points inserted. A heat carrier, (three types are shown (678), see page 83 for details), is then warmed in a flame (679) and pushed into the mass of GP within the canal. The carrier must be continually moved, using both vertical and rotational movement to prevent the shank of the instrument from sticking to the GP and dislodging it. The carrier is then removed and a cold lateral spreader inserted, followed by an accessory point. The process is repeated until the canal is filled. In the example shown (680) the canal was filled as well as possible using cold lateral condensation. Warm lateral condensation was then carried out (681). Notice the density of the gutta percha filling has been increased. See in particular the mesial canal wall (arrowed).

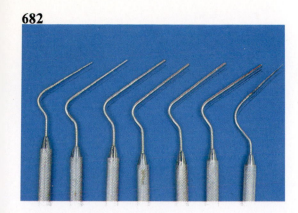

Hot Vertical Condensation. Schilder (1983) introduced this method some 25 years ago. The technique involves heat softening and condensing gutta percha until the root canal system is filled with a homogenous mass. The preparation of the root canal is carried out in a similar way to the serial or step back technique already described. The differences are:

1. Reamers and files are used alternately.

2. The working length is taken to the radiographic apex or to a point a fraction of a millimetre short.

A set of pluggers is required (682) with depth markings on the shank at 5 mm intervals. A heat carrier is also needed.

Two to four pluggers are used and these should be pre-tried in the canal. To produce maximum effect the end of the plugger must cover as large an area of gutta percha as possible, yet not impinge on the canal walls and risk their fracture. **683** shows three pluggers pre-fitted. The depth of penetration is noted on each plugger using the rings on the shank.

The master cone chosen is a non-standardised gutta percha point with the tip cut off to produce a tug back fit apically. The cone is fitted 0.5-1 mm from the radiographic apex.

The walls of the canal are lightly coated with sealer and the master cone also lightly coated is fitted. The excess GP extending into the access cavity is removed with a spoon excavator. A radiographic check is made at this stage. The apical part of the canal is now obturated using the following steps in sequence (**684**):

1. The appropriate plugger is used to condense the gutta percha.

2. The heat carrier is heated to cherry red and pressed into the gutta percha within the canal.

When the apical portion has been well condensed in this way, the final stage of completing the obturation of the middle and coronal thirds is carried out, termed back packing. The first two steps above are used in addition to a third. The sequence of operation is shown in the diagram.

3. An increment of gutta percha 3-4 mm in length is placed in the canal. These increments are cut from gutta percha cones and are approximately the width of the canal.

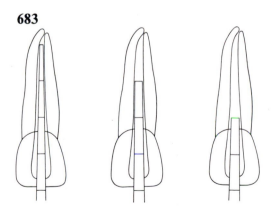

683

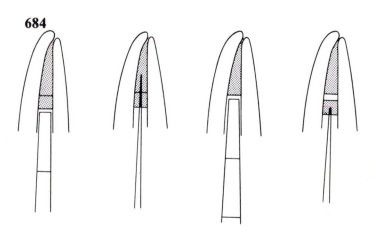

684

The larger pluggers are used at the correct levels as the canal is gradually filled with gutta percha.

685, 686 Show root canals filled using the vertical condensation technique. Note the accessory canal in the premolar which has been filled probably with gutta percha. A 'puff' of gutta percha has been extruded through the apical foramen.

685

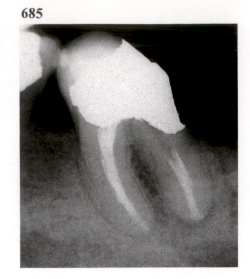

686

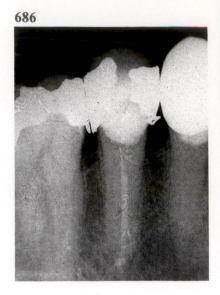

687

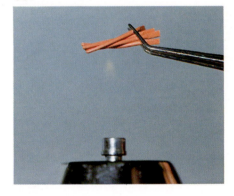

688

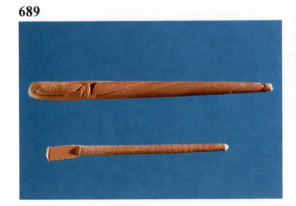

689

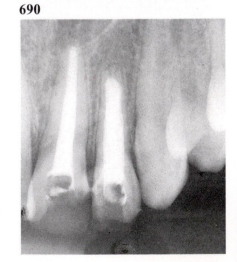

690

Custom Made Point. This technique is used only when the root canal is larger than the biggest standardised GP point. Several large cones are softened in a flame (**687**) and then rolled into a cone shape between two glass slabs (**688**). The GP should be softened sufficiently to allow a uniform mass to be formed without seams or voids. When the new cone approximates to the size of the root canal, it is chilled in water and tried. If the new cone is loose, a portion is removed from the tip; if too large, it is re-heated and rolled again between the glass slabs to a smaller diameter. The cone should be made to fit 1-2 mm from the radiographic apex. The cone is now used as the master cone and the cold or warm lateral condensation technique used to complete the root filling. The photograph (**689**) shows a custom made point and underneath a size 140 standardised GP point. The lateral incisor (**690**) has been filled with a custom made point and lateral condensation.

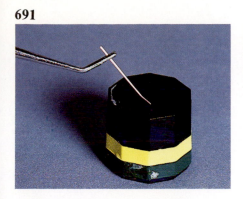

691

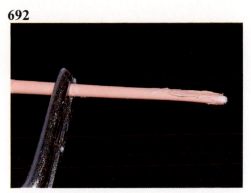

692

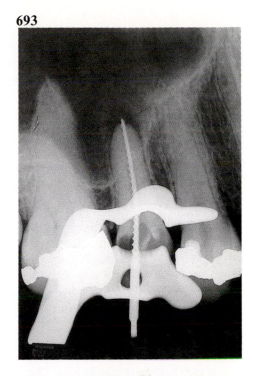

693

Gutta Percha with Solvents

Chloroform Dip

This method is useful when either there is an open apex or the apical portion of the canal is irregular in shape. The master gutta percha point is fitted as described for cold lateral condensation. The apical 2 mm of the point is then immersed into a dish of chloroform (**691**) for 3-4 seconds, removed and replaced with a firm pressure into the canal and left for several seconds. To prevent the softened point from sticking to the walls of the canal it is advisable to wet the canal with irrigant. The point is then withdrawn and allowed to dry on the bracket table for 2-3 minutes (**692**). The softened outer layers of the point take an impression of the apical portion of the canal. The drying allows the chloro percha to contract out of the mouth so that, when it is replaced and coated with sealer, a satisfactory seal may be obtained. Accessory points are now inserted, using the cold or warm lateral condensation technique already described.

693, 694 The second premolar had an open apex and has been root-filled using the chloroform dip.
695 Shows a follow-up seven months later. The area has almost resolved.

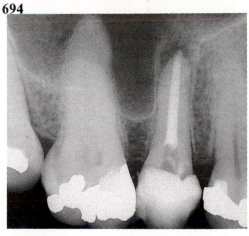

694

Chloro percha, Kloroperka, Eucapercha

Various solvents have been used but notably chloroform and oil of eucalyptus. The solvents are used to soften gutta percha and so allow its condensation into the irregular canal spaces. The main disadvantages are that the solvents evaporate, resulting in considerable shrinkage of the root filling material and also they are tissue irritants.

In the Chloro percha technique, several large standardised gutta percha points are dissolved in chloroform, producing a sticky mass, similar in consistency to zinc oxide sealer. A master gutta percha point is fitted as for the lateral condensation technique and the chloro percha used as sealer. The root filling is completed with accessory points and cold lateral condensation.

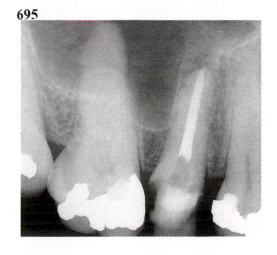

695

Kloroperka N Ø is the proprietary name and is a powder which, when dissolved in chloroform, produces a sealer similar to Chloro percha.

Eucapercha is produced by dissolving gutta percha in oil of eucalyptus. The GP is less soluble than in chloroform and the method is rarely used.

Thermal Compaction. This technique was introduced in 1978 by Dr J. McSpadden. It consists of a compactor, which is an engine operated instrument resembling a Hedstroem file but with the blades directed towards the tip.

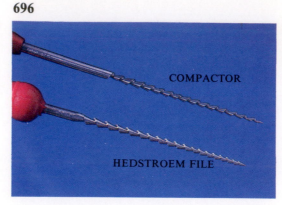

696

COMPACTOR

HEDSTROEM FILE

A McSpadden Compactor (**696** top) is compared with a Hedstroem file (**696** bottom). The instrument operates on the reverse turning screw. The conventional handpiece should have high torque and be capable of 8-10,000 rpm. The gutta percha is plasticised and forced 1 mm ahead and lateral to the compactor shaft.

The root canal preparation is carried out as already described using the step back technique.

The first step in the technique for filling the canal is to fit a master cone 1.5 mm short of the working length. The sealer is applied to the GP point. The compactor selected should be the same size as the largest file used within 1-1.5 mm of the apical stop. This is checked in the canal before the GP point is fitted and the length marked on the shank of the compactor or the nearest ring on the shaft to the correct length is noted. The compactor is inserted until a slight resistance is felt and then rotated at maximum speed. After one second, the compactor is advanced apically in one fluid movement to the predetermined depth. The compactor is then withdrawn slowly, still operating at full speed. A backing out force will be noticed, produced by the GP being forced ahead of the instrument. The compactor must not be withdrawn quickly or voids will occur. A second larger compactor may be required to condense the flared coronal portion of the canal. The whole condensation method takes only a few seconds. The extracted mandibular premolar was filled using the McSpadden compactor (**697**) and the tooth sectioned. There has been no extrusion despite the open apex.

The problems associated with this method are that the high rotational speeds involved tend to result in many fractured instruments and, in addition, a considerable amount of heat is generated very quickly. The instrument should not be kept rotating in the canal for more than a few seconds to prevent the build up of heat. The block shown (**698**) has a pre-formed canal and accessory canal. Immediately after filling with a compactor the gutta percha appeared well condensed but after several minutes the gutta percha had cooled and contracted away from the walls.

697

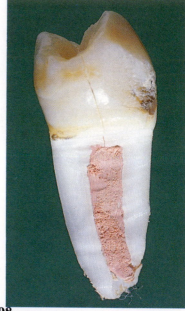

698

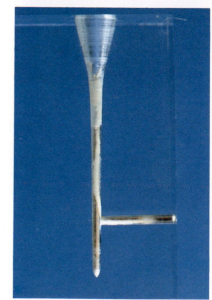

699

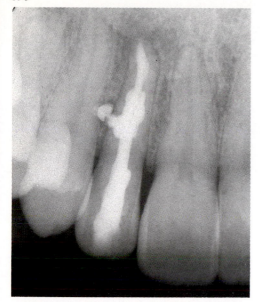

700

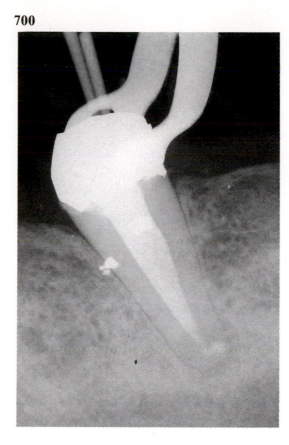

701

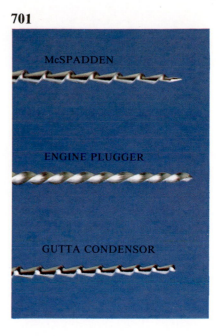

The technique has shown considerable promise, particularly in cases where other techniques would be difficult, such as internal resorption areas within the root (**699**). It has no particular advantage in fine, severely curved canals. In fact it is not recommended to introduce the compactor around curves, due to the risk of breakage.

The technique may be adapted (Tagger et al 1984) slightly as follows:

The master cone is fitted and the lateral condensation commenced with the introduction of several accessory cones until the apical 3-4 mm are filled. The compactor is then used to complete the obturation of the middle and coronal thirds of the canal. The advantage is that the middle and coronal thirds of the canal are filled quickly.

700 A second mandibular molar with one large canal has been filled using thermal compaction and lateral condensation.

Recently two other compactors have been introduced (**701**).
Top McSpadden[1].
Middle Engine Plugger[2]. This instrument is a K file design with a reverse twist.

Bottom Gutta Condensor[3]. This is similar to the McSpadden except that it is blunt-tipped and the flute depth has been reduced.

Injection moulded thermo plasticised. Two devices are now available which preheat gutta percha so that it may be injected directly into the root canal. The techniques are quite difficult to master and both devices require root canal sealer to produce an apical seal. Although the technique has advantages in some cases, such as internal resorption, it is considered to be merely another addition to the armamentarium, and has not made an advance of any significance in endodontics.

Pastes Alone. Pastes alone cannot fill the root canal spaces. The resorbable pastes, such as Kri, have no place in adult endodontics, as they are removed by the body leaving the canal as a hollow tube. It is generally accepted that pastes alone cannot satisfy the aims in endodontics. Several one-visit techniques have been put forward by manufacturers' advertising pastes. They recommend that the canal need not be cleaned and prepared and that chemical sterilisation of the canal contents is sufficient.

13 Calcium Hydroxide J. J. Messing

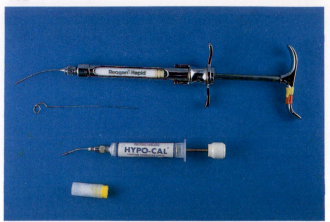

In recent years, calcium hydroxide has become one of the most useful and accepted medicaments in endodontics. It is used in the stimulation of calcific barrier formation by the pulp, at the site of an exposure, or to effect apical closure in an immature, avital tooth. It is used also as a pulpotomy dressing, a dressing in infected canals and root perforations, and a long-term expedient when root treatment must be delayed.

Calcium hydroxide possesses a powerful bactericidal action due to its high pH(12.2). In some way, not yet fully understood, using either the calcium ions or the hydroxyl ions appears to activate healing and the laying down of calcified tissue.

PULP CAPPING

Many medicaments have been tried as pulp capping agents, such as zinc eugenolate cement, corticosteroid/antibiotic cement, glycerrhetinic acid, iso-butyl cyanoacrylate and a suspension of calcium hydroxide in carboxy-methyl cellulose (eg Hypo-Cal[1] or Reogan-Rapid[2]), (**702**), or in the form of a setting cement, (eg Dycal[3], Procal[4], Life[5]).

Pulp capping in deciduous teeth is rarely successful and tends to fail also in teeth which previously have given rise to symptoms. As a useful rule of thumb, pulps should not be capped, a) if there is a history of acute or chronic pulpitis, b) the pulp is exposed in a mass of caries, c) where there has been gross contamination of the exposed pulp, d) when the pulp has been badly traumatised, eg, after a bur or probe has been thrust into the pulp, and e) where the exposure is larger than appoximately 1.0 mm in diameter.

In short, the technique should be restricted to teeth with minimal traumatic exposures, which have not been contaminated, and which respond in a normal manner to vitality tests.

Indirect pulp capping. Following removal of deep caries a layer of soft, demineralised dentine can be left over the pulp, rather than expose it. Virtual sterilisation of this layer can occur beneath a dressing of calcium hydroxide or zinc eugenolate cement. The success rate for indirect capping is greater than for direct capping. Zinc eugenolate provides a better cavity seal than calcium hydroxide, but the latter hardens the demineralised dentine and increases its radiopacity, because it stimulates remineralisation by the pulp. In consequence a calcium hydroxide base will be best protected by a zinc eugenolate lining under the coronal restoration.

Direct pulp capping. If a pulp exposure is capped after symptoms have developed, there is approximately 50 per cent less chance that the pulp will heal than in a symptom-free exposure. Success depends on the suppression of inflammatory response in the pulp and the destruction of all bacteria which have gained access to the pulp. Experiments on germ-free animals demonstrated the ability of the pulp to heal after exposure. Use of corticosteroid/antibiotic preparations will, in general, reduce the acute inflammation to the chronic pulpitis and in a small percentage of cases, provided irreversible changes have not occurred, subsequent capping with calcium hydroxide will enable the pulp to produce a dentine barrier, but results are unpredictable and pulps tend ultimately to die. Thus, it is evident that capping an infected pulp is futile. Any such treatment should be regarded as palliative and be followed ultimately by pulpectomy.

THE TECHNIQUE FOR INDIRECT PULP CAPPING

In order to avoid the risk of exposing the pulp, it is preferable to leave some softened dentine over the pulp, even when it is stained. However, all softened dentine and caries must be removed from the lateral walls and amelo-dentinal junction, with the aid of small excavators and burs. Caries on the pulpal and axial walls is best removed with large sharp excavators, sweeping the blade towards the walls with gentle strokes.

Before attending to the deep caries and subjacent demineralised dentine overlying the pulp, the rubber dam should be applied to avoid contamination by saliva.

The vitality of the pulp is established and a history is taken, in order to rule out the possibility of irreversible pathological changes.

Furthermore, a control radiograph and vitality tests, repeated at six monthly intervals over the succeeding three years, will demonstrate any alteration in the status of the pulp.

A fast setting calcium hydroxide cement, such as Dycal[1] or Life[2], may be applied to the dentine to a depth of 0.25-0.5 mm. Although, in a cavity of average depth, a restoration can be placed directly over the hydroxide base, close proximity to the pulp demands an additional zinc eugenolate or phosphate base, so that thermal shock under a metallic restoration may be avoided, when the depth of the dressing is inadequate. Despite evidence that calcium hydroxide cements, such as Dycal, can withstand pressures exerted when amalgam is condensed, there is a risk of displacing a thick layer or transmitting pressure to the pulp.

There is a wealth of clinical and experimental evidence to show that subsequent sclerosis of demineralised dentine occurs below a lining of calcium hydroxide cement. Hence there is no need to delay the placement of a permanent restoration in a previously symptom-free tooth.

Where there is a history of pain elicited by thermal or osmotic stimuli, it is advisable to place a provisional restoration over the hydroxide cement and await the cessation of symptoms before restoring the tooth. When doubt exists about the feasibility of pulp capping, it is safer to carry out a pulpectomy or pulpotomy.

THE TECHNIQUE FOR DIRECT PULP CAPPING

1. Apply the rubber dam.
2. Irrigate the cavity with sterile isotonic saline until haemorrhage has been controlled.
3. Dry the cavity with a sterile cotton pledget and cover the exposure with a suspension of calcium hydroxide in methyl cellulose, covered in turn with a fast setting zinc eugenolate base. Satisfactory results have been reported also using Dycal for capping exposures.
4. When the zinc eugenolate base has hardened, place a definitive restoration over a liner of Copalite varnish or, in anterior teeth, bevel and etch the enamel margins for a composite resin. These measures will do much to prevent micro-leakage and thus minimise the risk of contamination of the pulp, at least until a bridge of dentine has been formed, healing the exposure.

It has been demonstrated that the calcium ions in the calcium hydroxide are not present in the dentine bridge. It is considered that the high pH and antibacterial action of calcium hydroxide are the chief factors influencing the calciogenic response in the pulp.

When doubt exists about the degree of trauma to or contamination of the pulp, a corticosteroid/antibiotic dressing can be placed on the exposure for a few days after which it is replaced by Dycal or a similar product. The calmative and antibacterial effects of the dressing increase the chance of a favourable pulpal response in the short term, although subsequent radiographic and vitality tests — and developing hyper-reactivity to thermal change — demonstrate pulpitis in the majority of cases.

TREATMENT OF A DEEP CARIOUS LESION IN AN IMMATURE PERMANENT TOOTH

Closure of the apical foramen to the mature dimension is completed approximately 18-36 months after eruption of the tooth. Where there is a deep carious lesion over a vital, symptomless pulp, it is essential that the integrity of the pulp be maintained, whenever possible, by indirect capping or, if there is a small, uncontaminated exposure of traumatic origin, by direct capping. In either case an extended period of surveillance is necessary to show either continued apical development or degeneration of the pulp. In the event that the exposure is large or is surrounded by carious dentine, pulpotomy becomes the treatment of choice.

Pulpotomy is also indicated in permanent, immature, fractured incisors and canines in which the trauma involved the pulp less than 24 hours before.

PULPOTOMY

Pulpotomy is the excision of the coronal pulp, and dressing the amputation stump with a medicament. So far, the most effective drug is calcium hydroxide, because it can maintain the vitality of the pulp and stimulate the formation of calcific repair tissue. Pulpotomy is performed most often on immature permanent teeth with vital exposed pulps, although it can be used for the preservation of radicular pulp in mature posterior teeth, in which the complexity of the root canals contra-indicates total pulpectomy.

When treatment is successful, it is followed by formation of a reparative dentine bridge beneath the dressing, while the formation of the root is completed, thus closing the apex, narrowing the canal and maintaining the vitality of the pulp. The dentine bridge, although relatively impermeable, tends to have multiple defects, hence care must be exercised to prevent contamination through micro-leakage around restorations.

Most authorities advise, when apical closure is complete, that the pulp should be extirpated and replaced by a root filling. This is recommended because a percentage of teeth undergo internal resorption or progressive, accelerated dystrophic calcification of the pulp following pulpotomy. Nevertheless, pulpectomy can be delayed provided that regular radiographic and vitality checks are carried out. Careful comparison of the root apex with neighbouring teeth will give an indication of the progress of apical development, and comparison of the width of the pulp canal with neighbouring teeth will rule out dystrophic calcification.

Partial pulpotomy, in which solely the area of damaged or infected pulp in the vicinity of the exposure is excised, has been recommended. However, informed opinion is weighted on the side of removal of the whole coronal pulp.

THE TECHNIQUE FOR PULPOTOMY

1. Remove all caries and apply the rubber dam. (If this proves to be difficult in a nervous patient, cotton rolls may be used.)
2. Irrigate the cavity thoroughly with isotonic saline.
3. Dry the cavity and excise the roof of the pulp chamber by delineating its lateral extent with a small fissure bur until it can be prised away and the pulpal membrane demonstrated. The coronal pulp is then excised, using either a sharp spoon excavator (discoid or cleoid) or a slowly rotating round bur. In a single rooted tooth the line of excision should be coincident with the cervix, and in a multi-rooted tooth, with the floor of the pulp chamber.

4. Haemorrhage can be controlled by exerting gentle pressure on cotton pledgets, damped with saline. When haemorrhage has ceased, the pulp chamber is filled with a non-setting suspension of calcium hydroxide in methyl cellulose (eg Hypo-Cal[1], Pulpdent[2], Calcipulpe[3]). This dressing is covered with a 1-2 mm layer of EBA/zinc eugenolate cement which is pressed home, using minimum pressure, with a moistened cotton ball. The calcium hydroxide must be placed directly in contact with the surface of the pulp, thus elimination of blood clots is mandatory.
5. When the cement has hardened, the walls of the cavity are painted with Copal/Ether varnish and the cavity is restored with an appropriate material (**703**).

703

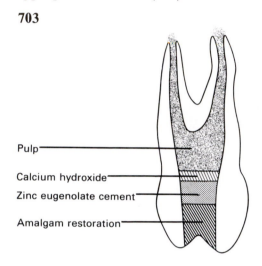

Pulp
Calcium hydroxide
Zinc eugenolate cement
Amalgam restoration

6. A control radiograph and electrical vitality test are recorded as a baseline for further checks after six months, one year and thenceforward annually. (After about 6 weeks the dentine bridge has formed, as a general rule.)
7. Once apical growth is complete, total pulpectomy and root filling should be performed so that the risk of internal resorption can be prevented.

THE USE OF CALCIUM HYDROXIDE AS A DRESSING IN INFECTED ROOT CANALS

Teeth with large periapical lesions which formerly might have been treated by apicectomy or extraction, respond well to careful bio-mechanical preparation of the canals and dressing with calcium hydroxide. Although healing can occur in response to other medicaments, calcium hydroxide controls periapical inflammation and arrests apical root resorption, due to its anti-bacterial action and the high pH which activates alkaline phosphatase.

Calcium hydroxide paste can be introduced into the canal on a spiral filler (**704**). In order to prevent an acute exacerbation of symptoms, the dressing should be inserted at the second visit. The first visit is used to prepare the canal and dress it with a bland anti-bacterial drug or an anti-inflammatory preparation, such as Septomixine[1]. If, at a subsequent visit, there is still evidence of periapical inflammation, further dressings of calcium hydroxide should be placed, as required, at intervals of two or three weeks until symptoms have abated, at which time a root filling can be inserted.

Chronic periapical osteitis associated with apical resorption will respond to long-term therapy with calcium hydroxide. The dressing is placed in the prepared canal and reviewed at intervals of three or four months until periapical healing is complete. At that stage an apical calcific barrier is usually present and prevents extrusion of the filling into the bone (see **714-716**). Such a dressing should be sealed in by means of an amalgam, composite resin or silicophosphate restoration. Temporary restorative materials are not sufficiently durable to last for an extended period.

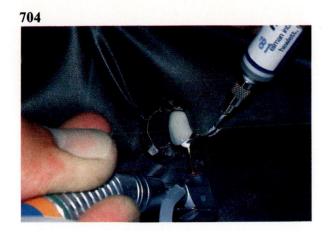

THE EFFECT OF CALCIUM HYDROXIDE ON EXTERNAL RESORPTION FOLLOWING REPLANTATION OF AN AVULSED TOOTH

When a tooth has been avulsed it should be returned to its socket as soon as possible, and kept moist until that can be accomplished. If possible the patient should be asked, after gently rinsing the tooth, to place it in the buccal sulcus, thus keeping it warm, preventing drying out and trauma to the periodontal ligament. Alternatively, after gentle lavage, the tooth can be replaced in its socket, or wrapped in a wet handkerchief and held thus in the mouth with the handkerchief protruding, or it can be stored in milk. Milk is thought to be a better storage medium than saliva because it has an osmotic pressure closer to that of blood than the hypotonic saliva. When the patient informs the dentist about the avulsion, he should be told to attend the surgery as soon as possible. If the tooth is out of the socket for more than thirty minutes, the chance that the periodontal fibres will remain viable is diminished. If the tooth has been picked up from the ground, and especially from soil, an anti-tetanus injection is mandatory. Also it is advisable to administer a systemic antibiotic for four days.

All blood clot should be removed from the socket by forced irrigation with copious quantities of isotonic saline. The socket must never be curetted to avoid damage to Sharpey's fibres still attached to the alveolus.

If the root apex is immature, there is a chance that the pulp may become re-vascularised. Thus no root treatment should be considered for about six weeks, but, should there be signs that the pulp has become necrotic in the interim, root treatment should be started immediately.

At one time, it was customary to resect the apex and fill the canal prior to replantation. It has been found that this leads to increased and more rapid replacement resorption.

A dressing of calcium hydroxide placed in the canal one week after replantation, permits the anti-bacterial action and high pH 'to exert their effects following resorption of cementum, when the calcium and hydroxyl ions permeate the dentinal tubules. On reaching the bone they stimulate the action of alkaline phosphatase to form new bone, while they discourage the acid phosphatase-based resorption of dentine, which tends to occur after about 14 days following replantation.

There is experimental evidence to show that the presence of periodontal ligament on the root of a replanted tooth inhibits osteogenesis. Thus, if it is lost, ankylosis is apt to occur after replantation, as a result of osteoclastic activity within the granulation tissue of the healing socket. However, the presence of calcium hydroxide in the root canal and consequent presence of calcium and hydroxyl ions in the dentinal tubules, exerts an inhibitory influence on the osteoclasts, thus reducing the risk of resorption and ankylosis.

After the tooth has been replanted and anti-tetanus and antibiotic injections given, it will probably need to be splinted. This can be effected, in most cases, by etching the enamel and joining the tooth to its neighbours with composite resin. A stronger splint, which does not interfere with the occlusion, can be made by bonding composite resin to the labial surfaces of the replanted tooth and two teeth on either side, and embedding a length of orthodontic ligature wire (0.5 mm) in the resin, in close proximity to the enamel. The wire is pre-bent to conform to the surface contours (**705**). This permits physiological tooth movement and thus minimises the risk of ankylosis. The splint should remain in place for one week only and the occlusion should be checked carefully to ensure the absence of premature contacts. It is advisable that the etching of enamel and fixing of the splint be done under rubber dam.

705

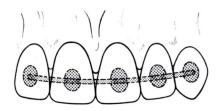

Splinting is essential in the early stages of reattachment, because excessive occlusal stress leads to an increase in replacement resorption. After approximately three weeks the tooth should exhibit a normal degree of mobility.

Thus, about seven days after replantation, to allow the patient time to get over the shock and soreness, the canal should be prepared and dressed with an hydroxide/cellulose suspension. This dressing should be left, well sealed and undisturbed for about 6 weeks, being replaced at intervals of 2-3 months for one year or longer. This long-term dressing has been shown to help in the prevention of external resorption. However, if the tooth had already been root filled, and external resorption develops, the root filling should be removed and replaced with an hydroxide dressing for about six months. Thus the resorption has a good chance of becoming arrested. The dressing can then be replaced at six monthly intervals until the bony perimeter appears to be stabilised, at which time a definitive root filling can be inserted.

Replacement resorption following replantation occurs in a large number of cases, reflecting the degree of trauma to the surface of the root or the length of time that had elapsed before the tooth was returned to its socket. In common with many other clinicians, the author has found that calcium hydroxide will not prevent resorption under such adverse conditions.

706

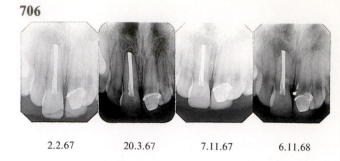

| 2.2.67 | 20.3.67 | 7.11.67 | 6.11.68 |

706 The patient was a 16-year-old male Caucasian. The maxillary right central incisor was avulsed by a blow. The tooth was brought to the surgery thirty minutes later. After resection of the apex, the canal was filled from the apical end. Progressive resorption of the root is apparent and the final radiograph shows marked loss of radicular dentine, although the tooth is still firm 17 years later (**707**).

707

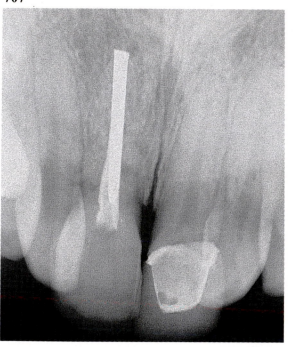

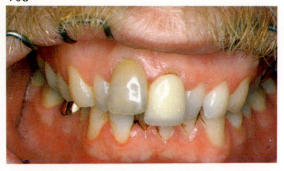

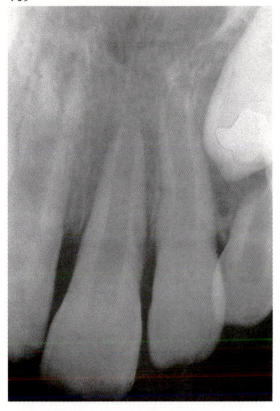

708 Shows the failure to erupt in conformity with neighbouring teeth as a result of ankylosis.

709 The patient was first seen two hours after the trauma and the tooth was replaced in the socket.

710 One week later the canal was prepared and filled with calcium hydroxide.

711 Seven months later formation of the apex is complete.

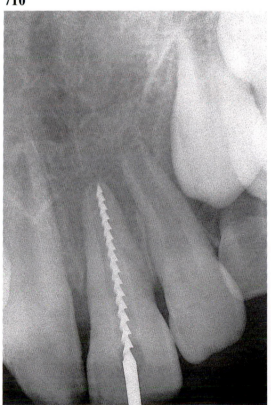

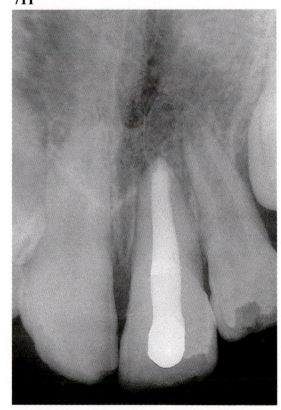

INDUCTION OF APICAL CLOSURE IN IMMATURE PULPLESS TEETH

Pulpotomy is indicated solely for teeth with vital pulps which are relatively uninflamed. However, where the root is incompletely formed and the pulp is partially or totally necrotic, dressings of calcium hydroxide can be used to provide the necessary environment for healing of periapical pathosis and induction of root-end formation. This technique has been referred to as 'Apexification' (**712**).

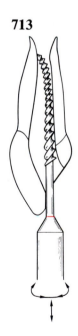

712

The steps in treatment of an immature root with necrotic pulp

FIRST VISIT
1. Apply rubber dam.
2. Gain access to the root canal.
3. Prepare coronal two thirds of canal with wide files, then irrigate and dry.
4. Place dressing of tricresol-formalin (a minute quantity on a cotton pellet) in the pulp chamber.
5. Seal access cavity with Cavit.
6. Make sure that the tooth is ground free from masticatory stress.

SECOND VISIT *2-4 days later.*
1. Remove dressing and irrigate canal.
2. Take diagnostic radiograph, using a large file and establish working length 1-2 mm short of the root end.
3. Bend tip of file to enable it to make contact with flared apex and file, wash and dress canal. Use a thick calcium hydroxide paste. Seal the access cavity with Cavit (**713**).

713

THIRD VISIT *7-14 days later.*
1. Remove dressing, irrigate canal and dry, using thick, inverted paper points, confining them within canal.
2. Fill canal with thick paste of calcium hydroxide and pack it home firmly with wide pluggers.
3. Seal the access cavity with silicophosphate cement.

FOURTH VISIT *Recall after six months.*
Repeat treatment of previous visit and recall at six-monthly intervals until the apical stop is palpable and there is radiographic evidence of healing. Duration of treatment usually varies from 12-18 months.

FINAL VISIT
The canal is filled with gutta percha, which is condensed, and coronal restoration is carried out.

NB. At the first recall visit, the canal is irrigated and the dressing is removed carefully with files. Inverted paper points, confined to the canal, are used to dry the walls prior to the insertion of a thick mix of calcium hydroxide.

If the preparation used does not contain a radiopacifier, approximately 5-10% w/w of barium sulphate or iodoform, well mixed into the paste, will render it visible on the radiograph. If voids are visible between the walls and the dressing, they can be corrected by the addition of further paste which is condensed firmly.

Calcium Hydroxide paste in the treatment of infected root canals

714 Patient aged 26 years. Maxillary left central incisor with necrotic pulp, periapical infection and apical resorption; ill-fitting gutta percha cone present in the root canal.

715 Gutta percha cone removed and canal re-prepared. Diagnostic radiograph prior to filling canal with calcium hydroxide paste.

716 Canal filled with gutta percha six months later and following three changes of dressing.

714

715

716

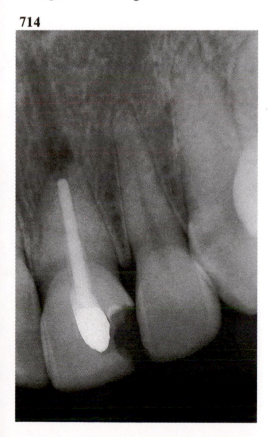
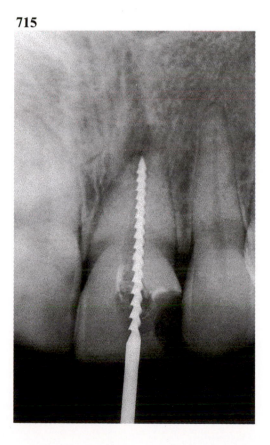
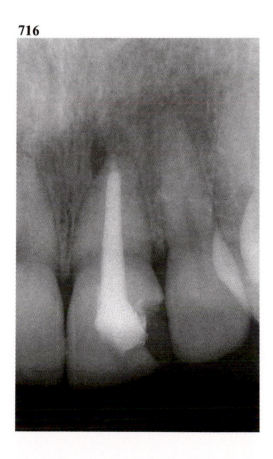

INTERNAL RESORPTION

Internal resorption is apt to occur following trauma, pulpotomy, pulp capping, deep caries and traumatogenic occlusal stress. Therefore it is essential to check the radiographic appearance of the pulp and its vital response at regular intervals, in such cases, in order to discover any sign of resorption before perforation can occur.

If internal resorption is found, the pulp must be removed and the canal prepared and irrigated, using a protein solvent, such as 5 per cent sodium hypochlorite. The cavity is dried and filled with a paste composed of calcium hydroxide, mixed to a thick consistency with either sterile water or anaesthetic solution (without vasoconstrictor). The paste is inserted into the canal with the aid of a pressure syringe or a 'Jiffy Tube' (717) and packed home firmly with a root canal plugger. The access cavity is sealed with a reinforced zinc eugenolate cement (with orthoethoxy benzoic acid and quartz) or silico-phosphate cement.

717

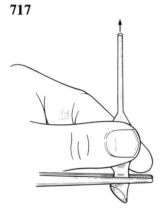

The patient is recalled after six weeks for the dressing to be changed. This is repeated subsequently at intervals of three months until the dressing is seen to be dry, at which time a gutta percha root canal filling is inserted and condensed simultaneously into the area of resorption. The McSpadden technique of thermatic compaction of GP is ideal for filling internal resorptive defects.

When the resorption has produced a perforation of the root, conservative treatment with calcium hydroxide has, in general, given better results than a surgical approach and repair with amalgam, provided the defect lies within the bone. However, should the defect lie coronal to the bony crest, a surgical repair offers a better prognosis. This is also the case when the cortical bone overlying the perforation has been destroyed.

At times there is intractable haemorrhage from a perforation, which interferes with placement of the calcium hydroxide dressing. This can be controlled by copious irrigation of the canal with isotonic saline, followed by careful drying, followed by the obliteration of the canal with a firmly condensed dressing of calcium hydroxide.

The dressing is changed after four weeks and thenceforward at intervals of six weeks, until an adequate calcific barrier has been laid down. At that time a gutta percha root filling can be inserted.

Apart from the treatment of resorptive perforations of internal or external origin, this technique can be used to treat iatrogenic perforations, however ideal results ensue solely when the perforated area of the root lies within the bone. Perforations located coronal to the bony crest are better repaired with amalgam or incorporated within a coronal restoration.

POST-ORTHODONTIC RESORPTION

Following orthodontic treatment, teeth which have been moved too rapidly can develop apical resorption, which produces a truncated effect, similar to an apicected tooth, initially without loss of vitality, although some pulps may die while others may undergo progressive dystrophic calcification. No treatment is indicated unless pulps become necrotic. Such resorptions can be caused by unduly rapid movement of teeth and certain individuals appear to be more prone to a resorptive response than others receiving similar treatment.

Such apical resorption removes the apical constriction, thus producing a wide apical foramen with the consequent problem of confining the root filling to the canal. Therefore, if a pulp should die, the canal can be prepared and filled to a point approximately 1.0 mm short of the apex. When the canal is wide, this may prove difficult, so it is preferable to use calcium hydroxide dressings to stimulate the formation of a calcific barrier in the manner described above.

BIOCALEX

A clinical variant on the use of calcium hydroxide, referred to as the 'Biocalex' or calcium oxide expansion technique, by Bernard[1], is a method devised for treating infected and purulent pulps.

Although the technique is supported by clinical and laboratory evidence, supplied largely by Bernard, the somewhat exaggerated claim of the expansive properties of Biocalex and the instruction that the preparation of canals to their apices is not only unnecessary but contra-indicated, has resulted in a general lack of interest by endodontic specialists throughout the world.

Notwithstanding, the author has experimented clinically with the material in otherwise unsavable teeth, obtaining a surprisingly high rate of success. This has led to the conclusion that there is scope for further independent clinical and laboratory investigation of the nature of the action of calcium oxide in infected root canals.

The basic concept, claimed by Bernard, is the chemical reaction between calcium oxide (in a chemically pure form) and water to produce calcium hydroxide and a release of chemical and physical energy. The reaction is slowed down by the admixture of four parts of ethylene glycol to one part of water, thus limiting the exotherm which accompanies the expansion of the mass and the chemical 'incineration' of necrotic tissue in the canal.

The original Biocalex 4 formulation, in which the powder consisted solely of calcium oxide, was reputed to expand 250-280 per cent, but it was replaced by Biocalex 6:9 which consisted of a heavy form of calcium oxide, to which was added zinc oxide. This combination, it was claimed, expands 600-900 per cent. Zinc oxide is incorporated with the calcium oxide in the ratio of 1:2, ostensibly to provide radiopacity so that the expanded mass can be left in situ as a radiographically visible root filling.

Bernard considers that the carbon dioxide given off as a result of the breakdown of complex protein molecules, reacts with calcium hydroxide to give calcium carbonate and water. The calcium carbonate aids in blocking the canal system while the water reacts with calcium oxide to provide further calcium hydroxide. Thus the expansive reaction, with dissemination of the hydroxide and carbonate throughout the canal system, is purported to sterilise and fill all the canals.

This dubious contention has not been proved by independent experimentation. The author, however, using the Biocalex as a canal medication and not as a filling, has achieved excellent results, especially in infected teeth which it was impossible to root treat by accepted methods, because the canals were not amenable to instrumentation to their apices.

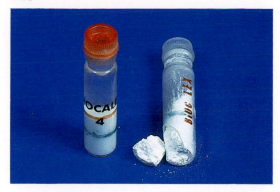

718 Experimental expansion of Biocalex in vitro, 24 hours. *left* Approximately 100 per cent expansion (Biocalex 4). *right* Approximately 150 per cent expansion, sufficient to fracture the fragile glass (Biocalex 6:9).

Biocalex—indications and contra-indications

1. When the whole pulp is necrotic, with or without a periapical lesion. However, Biocalex should never be used in canals in which there is vital pulp tissue, because there can be an acute inflammatory response. Furthermore, it should never be used during the acute phase of a periapical inflammation.
2. Because there is a risk of an acute reaction, the calcium oxide suspension should not be placed further apically than half way down the root canal. Thus, if the canal is wide initially and an instrument can be placed without hindrance to the apical foramen, Biocalex should not be used, unless a sinus is present.
3. Where a root canal appears to be blocked and the blockage is due to uncalcified organic tissue, Biocalex may facilitate subsequent instrumentation as a result of chemical breakdown of the necrotic debris.
4. Pronounced apical curvature of the roots can prevent adequate preparation and debridement of canals. Biocalex has proved to be invaluable for sterilising and rendering inert the apical necrotic pulp tissue. Clinical evidence to substantiate this statement is found in the early disappearance of a discharging sinus and rapid healing of a periapical area.

Although it has not proved possible to obtain the 600-900 per cent expansion, claimed by Bernard, there is a wealth of clinical evidence to substantiate his claims of success. In all probability, the most important factor in relation to healing is the high pH of calcium hydroxide which, following the expansive reaction, is deposited in the fine canals and secondary canaliculae. This exerts a bactericidal action and stimulates osteoblastic activity in areas of pathosis around the root. Thus it would appear to provide the conditions needed for the initiation and progress of healing.

A technique for the use of Biocalex

An acute apical periodontitis or periapical abscess must first be brought under control by means of drainage, antibiotic (oral or parenteral), and relief of masticatory stress. The canals are shaped and cleaned to a point approximately half way to the apices or to the point beyond which an instrument cannot be advanced, and it may be necessary, if symptoms are severe, to leave the canal open to the mouth for one or two days until the acute condition has been rendered chronic. At that stage, rubber dam is applied and all the canals are filed as far as the half way point, enlarging them to size 80, if possible. A wide canal will thus accommodate a large reservoir of Biocalex.

The canal is then irrigated with liberal quantities of a 2-5 per cent solution of sodium hypochlorite, and this is then washed away with distilled or boiled water. The canal is partly dried, leaving the walls moist so that the residual water can react with the calcium oxide. Water straight from the tap should not be used because it contains dissolved gas, which would come out of solution, thus reducing the volume of the expansion.

719

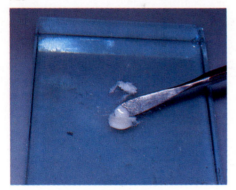

720

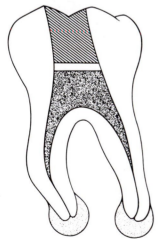

▨ Biocalex

▧ Cavit

Biocalex is prepared by incorporating sufficient powder into the liquid to produce a thick creamy paste (**719**), which is introduced into the canal on a spiral filler, operated at slow speed as it is withdrawn along one wall, and repeating the action until the prepared part of the canal and the pulp chamber are completely filled. The dressing is covered with a piece of pink denture wax and the access cavity is filled with polycarboxylate cement or Cavit (**720**). No cement which contains eugenol or oil of cloves should be used, because there would be a chelation with calcium oxide to produce calcium eugenolate, thus arresting the expansion on which the action of Biocalex depends.

It is important that the occlusal load on the cavity seal be checked before the patient is dismissed, because a severe apical periodontitis could result from a traumatogenic occlusion. Should there be an acute exacerbation between visits — a rare complication if this technique is followed carefully — the Biocalex should be replaced with a corticosteroid/antibiotic preparation.

The Biocalex is removed after 6-8 days and an attempt is made to prepare the remainder of each canal to the level of the apical constriction. If this can be done, the working lengths of the canals are calculated; they are then prepared and dressed with a calcium hydroxide suspension, and filled at the next visit if clean and free from symptoms. In the event that the canals are impassable, a second dressing of Biocalex should be inserted, and replaced finally by a well-condensed gutta percha and AH26 root filling, as far as the original limit of preparation. A radiographic check is made after six months and thenceforward annually.

Success, in the first instance, is demonstrated by the disappearance of a discharging sinus and the restoration of pain-free mastication, and ultimately by radiographic evidence of healing.

Although, in the event of failure, re-treatment with Biocalex is possible, there is no guarantee that the apical part of the canal has not been blocked by sealer, hence a surgical approach would be more appropriate.

Treatment with Biocalex offers no panacea, but it is worth reserving for those difficult teeth which defeat conventional, accepted procedures.

Treated Cases

721

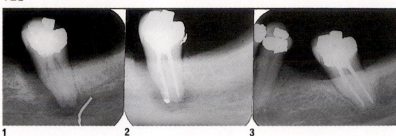

722

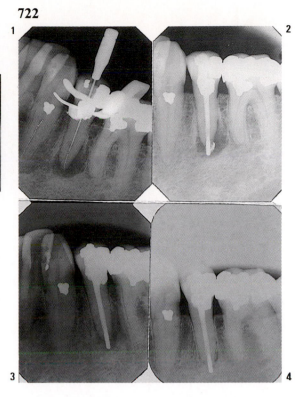

721
1. Periapical pathosis (treated with Biocalex 6:9).
2. Area diminishing 4 months later; some AH26 beyond the apex.
3. Final check two years later shows healing and resorption of excess sealer.

723

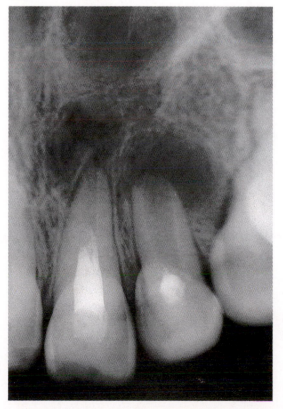

722 Treatment of open apex and acute periapical abscess, using Biocalex 6:9. Canal filled with AH26, silver apical tip and gutta percha.
1. Pre-treatment radiograph.
2. Post-treatment radiograph.
3. One year later.
4. Eleven years later . . . note the good toleration of a well-fitting silver cone by the periapical tissues.

The following cases, treated by W. L. Rumun of Hounslow, Middlesex, England, are typical examples of the use of Biocalex.

Case 1 An 11-year-old girl presented 18 months after trauma had resulted in fracture of her upper left incisor crowns with exposure of the pulps. Examination revealed the presence of a discharging sinus, labially, between the roots (**723**).

At the first visit, an access cavity to the canal of the central incisor was opened fully and a copious purulent discharge was noted. However, because a sinus was present, the canal was prepared to its full length and dressed with Biocalex.

Two days later, the adjacent lateral incisor was prepared similarly and dressed with Biocalex.

One week later, the sinus had disappeared, both canals were dry and the teeth were free from symptoms. Further filing was done and the canals were filled with a paste of monochlor-phenol-camphor/ calcium hydroxide. Temporary restorations were placed in the access cavities.

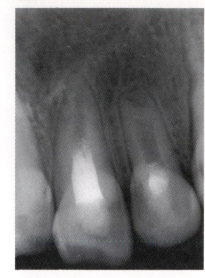

724 The patient was asked to return in three months, but did not do so for eighteen months. The canals were cleaned and the presence of positive apical stops was verified. Both canals were filled.

725 Four years later radiographic check shows healed periapical tissues.

726 Six years later, no adverse changes were observed.

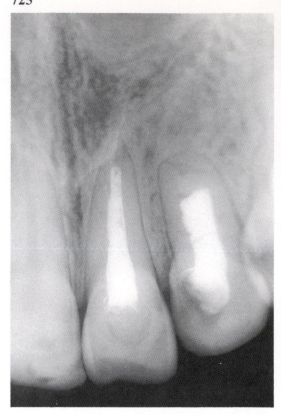

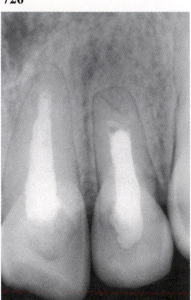

Case 2 **727** A 46-year-old lady complained of a constant vague ache in her upper right first premolar, which was tender to percussion. A radiograph showed the presence of a periapical area and two roots.

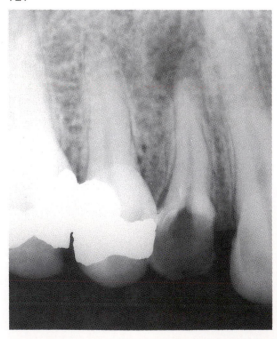

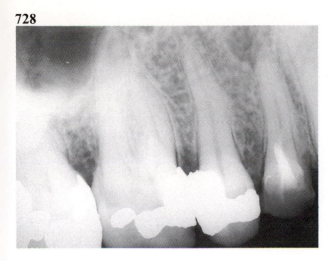

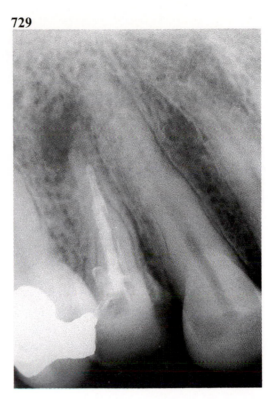

728 Despite a careful search, only one canal could be found. It was enlarged solely in its coronal half and filled with Biocalex.

729 Three weeks later the patient stated that all symptoms had disappeared. The canal was prepared to a point short of the apex, and root-filled with gutta percha and a sealer with a zinc eugenolate base.

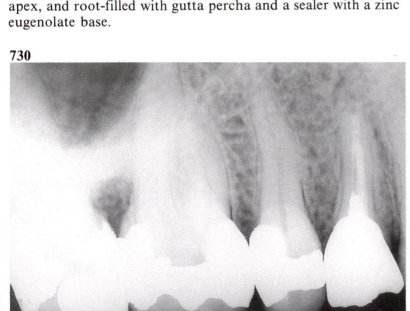

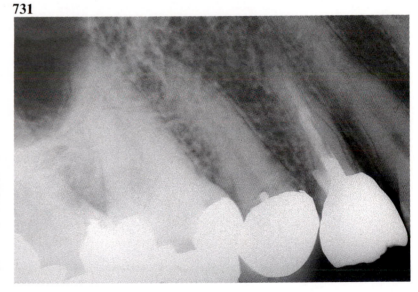

730 Six months later, the tooth was free from symptoms and the radiograph showed healing of the periapical tissues.

731 Nine years later, there were no changes, clinically or radiographically.

14　Primary Dentition　J R Goodman

Endodontics

Endodontic treatment of the primary dentition differs from that of the permanent teeth for two main reasons — pathology and morphology. Even the ultimate aim is different in that primary teeth need only be retained for limited periods until exfoliation occurs.

DIAGNOSIS OF PULP PATHOLOGY

It has been shown that inflammatory changes in the pulp occur more rapidly in the primary tooth in response to dentine caries than in the permanent tooth. Pathological changes within the pulp become irreversible early after the carious attack, and rapidly extend throughout the coronal pulp. It would be desirable to be able to diagnose the condition at this stage prior to the development of total pulpitis. However, an additional problem is that symptoms resulting from pulpal pathosis in primary teeth may not be severe, and often infection has spread to periradicular tissues before treatment is sought (**732**).

732

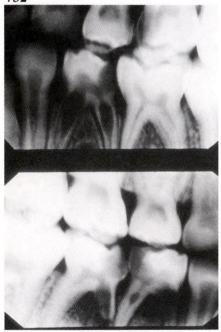

Diagnosis is also hampered because children are usually poor historians and respond unpredictably to subjective clinical tests. As a result, few useful conclusions concerning the condition of the pulp can be made from clinical findings.

Therefore, the diagnosis of early or partial pulpitis cannot be made on clinical grounds with any certainty, and the techniques chosen on those premises have no rational histological basis.

MORPHOLOGY OF THE PRIMARY TEETH

733 Buccal　　　　　Lingual

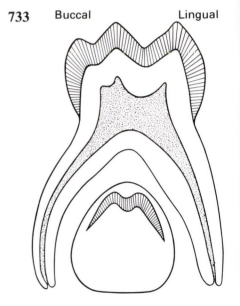

The morphology is such that the enamel and dentine are thinner and the pulp chamber, with its extended horns, larger in proportion, than in permanent teeth (**733**).

The molar teeth have irregularly shaped ribbon-like canals which become narrower with the deposition of secondary dentine, and there are numerous ramifications and lateral branches. In the inter-radicular area the floor of the pulp chamber is thin and there are numerous accessory canals. The resulting permeability of the dentine in this area often leads to inter-radicular rather than periapical bone loss around infected primary molars (**734**).

734

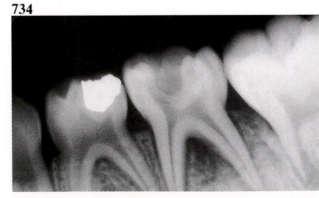

The roots of the primary teeth are in close relationship to the developing permanent successor and will, during exfoliation, undergo resorption. This therefore limits the materials which can be used in the canals, resorbable pastes being necessary.

In addition, trauma to or infection of primary teeth may lead to various types of damage to the successional teeth, including the arrested development of the permanent tooth germ. This consequence must be borne in mind.

735 The first premolar is seen sequestrating through the buccal alveolus and also has some enamel hypoplasia.

735

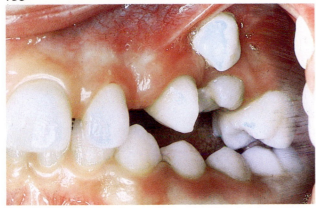

736 The radiograph indicates a lack of root development probably due to infection of the primary molar.

736

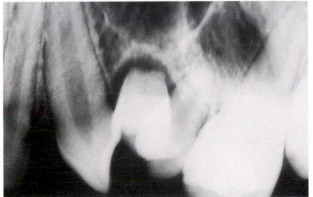

TECHNIQUES OF PULP THERAPY

(a) Indirect pulp capping

The deep carious lesion which is symptomless clinically and without radiographic change may be treated by intermittent excavation and indirect pulp capping. The treatment, which is carried out under local analgesia, involves the removal of all peripheral caries to provide sound cavity margins, and the careful excavation of deep soft caries overlying the pulp. A dressing of calcium hydroxide is applied to the remaining carious dentine and sealed effectively to prevent leakage of fluid or bacteria into the cavity. The treatment is considered to progress satisfactorily if, after a minimum period of 6 weeks, the tooth is symptomless, and on removal of the dressing there is evidence of arrest of the lesion and reparative dentine formation. The carious dentine will be darker in colour, less moist and harder. Any remaining soft dentine is removed with a large bur or excavator prior to a further dressing of calcium hydroxide, the insertion of a lining and a final restoration.

(b) Direct pulp capping

This has limited effectiveness in the primary dentition due to the rapid progress of pathological changes in the pulp, and its poor healing ability. The technique is only indicated in small traumatic exposures arising accidentally during cavity preparation in an area of otherwise sound dentine, in a symptomless tooth. The long term effectiveness of this treatment used in other circumstances, such as a carious exposure, compares poorly with pulpotomy procedures.

(c) One visit formol cresol pulpotomy

The rational basis for the use of this technique in the primary dentition is the existence of healthy pulp in the root canals, which is left following the removal of the inflamed coronal pulp tissue. The difficulties of diagnosing this situation from available clinical evidence have already been discussed, and have led some clinicians to favour a two visit devitalising technique, which makes no assumptions concerning the health of the radicular pulp tissue.

Those authorities who advocate a single visit method assume that after removal of the inflamed coronal tissue, healing may take place at the surface of the radicular pulp, which is essentially normal. However, previously, when calcium hydroxide was used widely in the vital pulpotomy technique in the primary dentition in the belief that healing would occur, internal resorption of the root canals was observed frequently. The use of the one visit formol cresol technique in carefully selected cases is considered by many clinicians as a useful treatment with a very good prognosis.

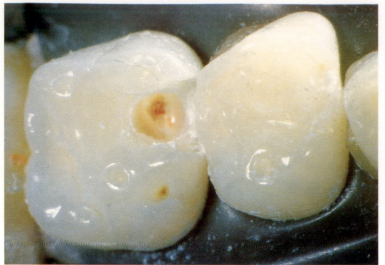

737

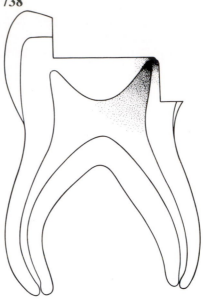

738

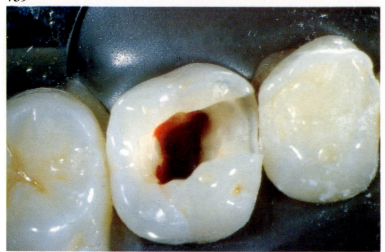

739

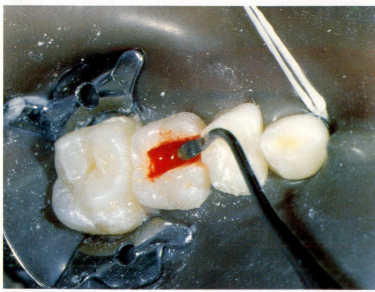

740

737, 738 The procedure is carried out using local analgesia and isolation is achieved preferably with rubber dam, or alternatively with the use of a saliva ejector and cotton wool rolls. Cavity preparation is completed with the removal of peripheral caries prior to the exposure of the pulp by removal of deep caries.

The entire roof of the pulp chamber is removed along with any overhanging dentine which may hinder the removal of fragments of coronal pulp (**739**).

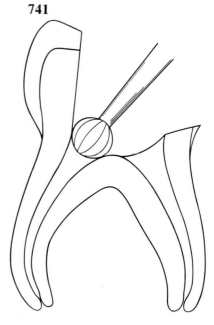

741

The coronal pulp tissue is then removed with either a sharp excavator (**740**) or a large round bur at slow speed (**741**) avoiding the weakening of the fragile walls of the tooth or perforation of the thin floor of the pulp chamber.

742 Irrigation of the pulp chamber with sterile water or normal saline dislodges the pulp and dentine debris. The cavity is dried with pledgets of cotton wool, to allow the haemorrhage to be controlled and the pulp stumps to be identified.

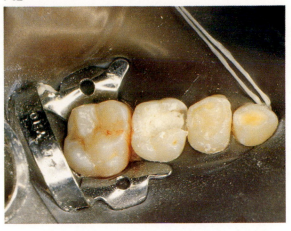

The natural cessation of bleeding of the radicular pulp is taken to indicate the presence of healthy tissue. The openings of the root canals are covered with a cotton wool pledget moistened in Buckley's formol cresol (35 per cent cresol, 19 per cent formalin in aqueous glycerine). After a five minute application the cotton wool is removed and the tissue at the entrance to the canals should have a dark brown appearance due to fixation (**743**).

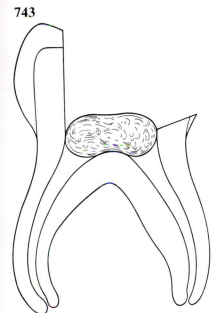

743

The Buckley's formol cresol is used in a 1:5 solution which has been shown to be as effective as the concentrated form. However, there is a risk of damage through spillage on the soft tissues; leakage into the interdental area, where it causes sloughing of the papilla; and diffusion into the periapical area. More recently a 2 per cent solution of glutaraldehyde has been investigated as an alternative medicament. The reactions following glutaraldehyde are irreversible, unlike those of formol cresol; it is less likely to penetrate the periapical foramen; and less solution is required to fix the tissues. It also appears that more vital tissue remains in the root canal following the use of glutaraldehyde.

In cases where the radicular pulp has undergone some inflammatory change, there will be an inability to control pulpal haemorrhage during this procedure, and a two visit technique may be required.

A thick cream of zinc oxide and eugenol in equal parts with formal cresol is placed in the floor of the chamber and over the radicular pulp, followed by a further layer of cement, placed without pressure. The tooth is finally restored, usually with a preformed nickel-chrome crown to prevent later cuspal fracture (**744**).

(d) Two visit formol cresol pulpotomy
Two visit paraformaldehyde pulpotomy

In both techniques the aim is to fix part of the remaining radicular pulp tissue by the application of either formol cresol or paraformaldehyde devitalising paste (Paraformaldehyde 1.00g, Lignocaine 0.06g, Propylene Glycol 0.5ml, Carbowax 1.3g and Carmine) for a period. The prognosis of these treatments is also favourable.

Following cavity preparation and removal of the coronal pulp, a dressing of either medicament is sealed into the pulp chamber for 7-10 days, after which the patient is questioned about any symptoms. The dressings are removed and the tooth is re-examined for signs of periradicular infection. If the radicular pulp appears fixed the tooth is restored as previously described. In addition, if complete anaesthesia cannot be obtained the devitalising paste may be applied to the exposure on a cotton wool pledget without amputation of the pulp. This seldom leads to complete pulpal devitalisation, but may reduce sensitivity to permit a pulpotomy and a further application of devitalising paste at the second visit.

744

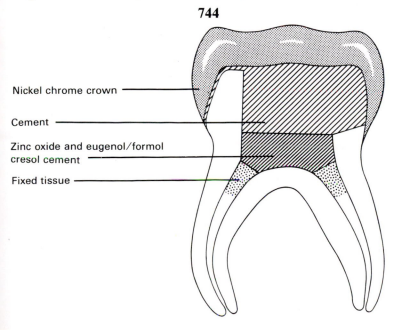

Nickel chrome crown

Cement

Zinc oxide and eugenol/formol cresol cement

Fixed tissue

However, when the pulp is infected, such that there is clinical or radiographic evidence of periradicular pathology, or the root canals contain necrotic tissue or pus, different techniques are required either to disinfect the pulp or to remove the radicular tissue.

(e) Beechwood creosote disinfection technique

The cavity preparation is carried out and the coronal pulp chamber is thoroughly cleaned to allow placement of a dressing of cotton wool moistened with Beechwood creosote. This is sealed in the cavity for 7-10 days, after which the tooth is re-examined for mobility, the presence of a sinus or any tenderness to pressure. If the tooth is satisfactory it is restored as for the previous pulpotomy procedure. If signs of infection persist a further period of disinfection is required.

The prognosis for this technique is much poorer than for the pulpotomy procedures, and recently a pulpectomy technique has been developed.

(f) Pulpectomy

In this method the infected tissue is removed from the canals mechanically in combination with pharmacological agents. Radicular pulp tissue and debris are removed with broaches and the canals prepared with files, using an estimated measurement of length from the diagnostic radiograph, and taking care not to instrument beyond the apex, or perforate the root, which may have a marked curvature. Access and the

morphology of the root limits the preparation and it may be necessary to use an antimicrobial dressing to aid disinfection. The roots are then filled with a resorbable paste, such as zinc oxide-eugenol, which is either syringed into the canal or condensed with amalgam pluggers (**745**).

745

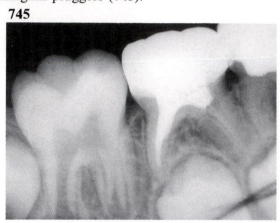

746

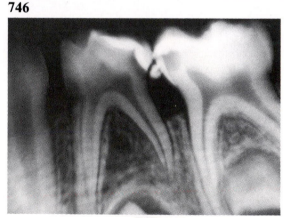

March 1979.

FOLLOW-UP. Any endodontically treated tooth requires regular clinical and radiographic assessment of the developing succeeding permanent tooth, or to observe any pathological sequelae which may occur.

This series shows the continued premolar development over a 4½ year period in the absence of pathology, associated with primary molars treated by the one visit formol cresol pulpotomy technique (**746-748**).

747

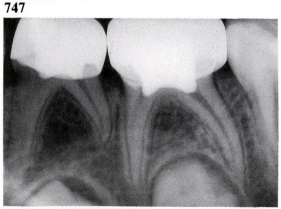

December 1979.

748

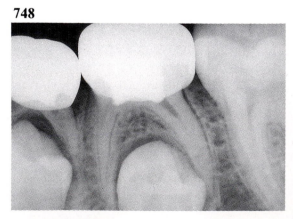

September 1983.

749

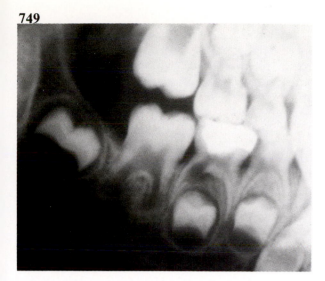

749 An inadequate two visit devitalising pulpotomy on a primary second molar shows internal resorption perforating the root, leading to an area of inter-radicular radiolucency.

750

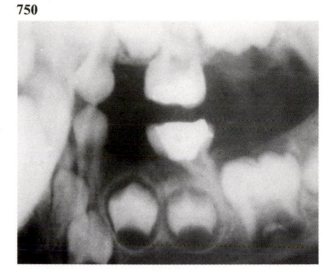

750 A Beechwood creosote disinfection technique on a primary second molar, which failed due to extensive external and internal resorption of the mesial root.

751

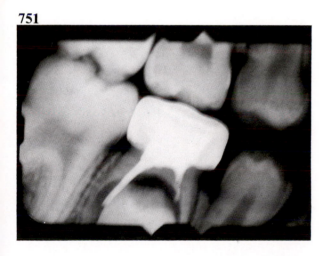

751 This primary molar was treated by the pulpectomy technique, but there is evidence of internal resorption around the filling material in the distal root.

752

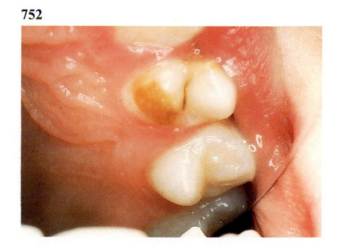

752 Infection of the primary molar may lead to disturbance of the enamel formation of the developing premolar, resulting in an hypoplastic defect.

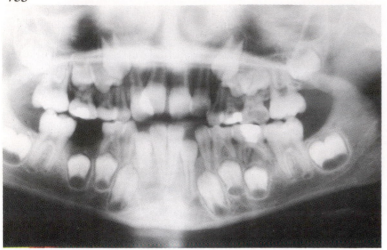

753 Chronically infected primary teeth, whether pulp treated or untreated, may occasionally be associated with the formation of infected follicular cysts around the successional teeth. A radiograph shortly after inadequate treatment has been carried out on a non-vital primary molar.

754

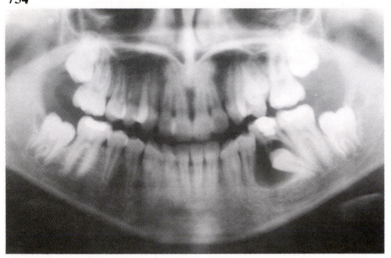

754 Four years later a cyst has developed and the premolar has been displaced.

755

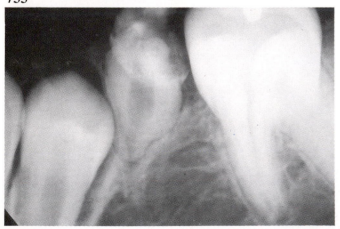

755 A long-standing untreated pulpal infection may lead to gross disturbance or cessation of the development of the underlying tooth germ. In this case when the patient was 5 years of age, a grossly carious primary molar was removed along with the associated granulation tissue. At 16 years of age the permanent tooth shows a stunted root and hypoplastic crown.

Trauma

In the primary dentition approximately 30 per cent of children sustain dentofacial injuries, with the maximum number occurring between 2 and 4 years of age. The most commonly affected area is the maxillary incisor region, and damage may involve the soft tissues, supporting bony structures and teeth.

756

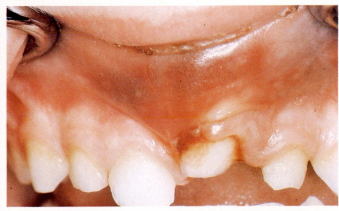

757

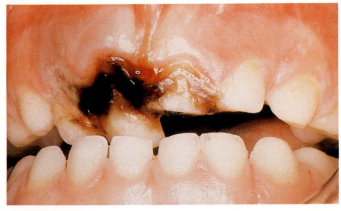

756 It is more usual for the supporting tissues to be injured, as in this 3½-year-old, with an intruded left central incisor, associated with a fracture of the alveolar bone. There is also extensive bruising of the lip.

757 Extrusive luxation may be severe and lead to problems of occlusal interference.

758

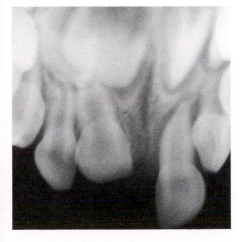

759

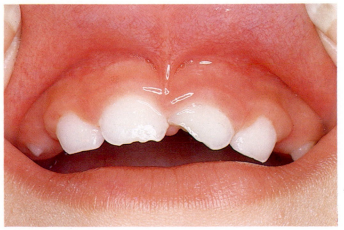

760

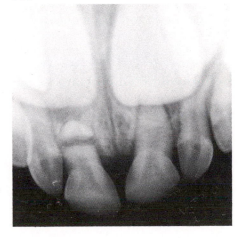

758 Alternatively, the force of the blow may drive the tooth into the alveolus, such that it is invisible on clinical examination, due to the displacement and associated swelling. The tooth may only be located following a radiograph of the area, which shows the intruded tooth in close relationship with the partly formed permanent incisor.

759 More unusually trauma may result in a fracture of the crown, which is, by contrast, a common finding in permanent incisors.

760 Root fracture may occur, often in the apical portion, as in this patient who fell against a concrete post.

SEQUELAE

(a) Primary dentition

Following trauma the primary tooth may change colour.

Calcification of the pulp chamber with retained vitality of the tooth leads to a yellowish discoloration of the crown.

Alternatively the tooth darkens to a grey colour due to necrosis of the pulp contents (**761**).

761

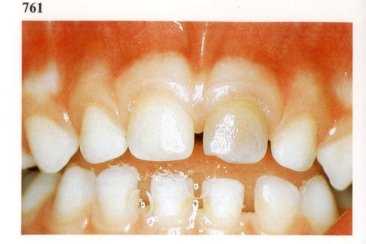

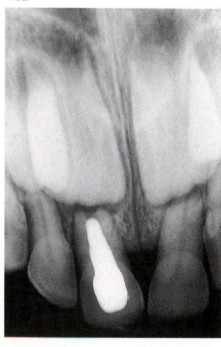

762

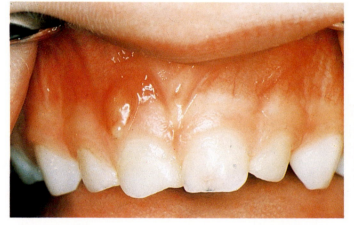

763

Inadequate treatment of non-vital pulp tissue may lead to periapical infection and sinus formation. In this case trauma has resulted in fracture of the crowns of the central incisors, with exposure of the pulp of the left tooth. A sinus is seen discharging through the labial plate above the right tooth (**763**).

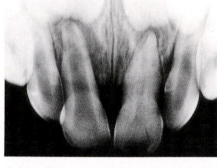

764 The radiograph shows evidence of bone loss in the periapical region of the right incisor with external resorption of the root. The left incisor has responded by partial obliteration of the pulp chamber and root canal.

762 The treatment of choice is endodontic therapy as demonstrated in this case, where the necrotic debris has been removed from the pulp chamber and root canal using a pulpectomy procedure.

765 Another reaction following loss of vitality of the pulp is shown, where the root of the tooth sequestrates through the labial alveolar plate.

765

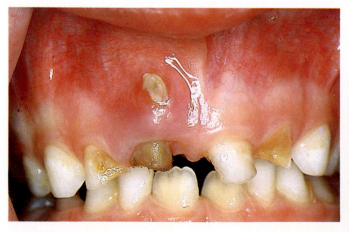

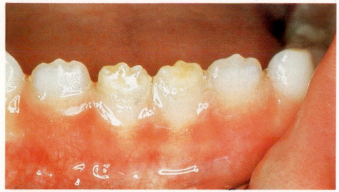

766

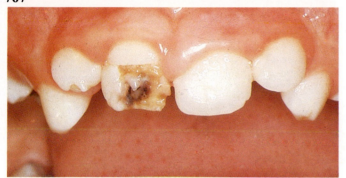

767

(b)   Permanent dentition

Because of the close developmental relationship between the primary teeth and their permanent successors, the latter are susceptible to damage. This may be due directly to the trauma to the primary tooth, or as a result of the subsequent infection which may develop on such a tooth. It is therefore important to review regularly traumatised primary teeth and intervene as soon as there is any clinical or radiographic evidence of infection developing, to prevent any disturbance in the odontogenic process, which may lead to a number of sequelae in permanent teeth. The patient's age at the time of injury is important in this respect.

766   The lower central primary incisors were dislocated at 7 months of age, but became firm again by 11 months. On eruption the permanent teeth showed a white/yellowish-brown discoloration of the incisal tips.

767   A more extensive disturbance in odontogenesis is demonstrated in the marked hypoplasia of this incisor, following trauma to the predecessor at a later stage of development.

769

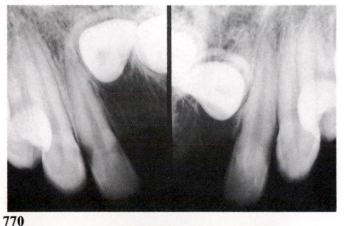

768

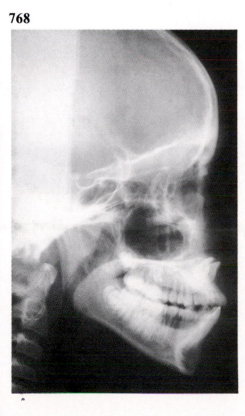

770

Dilaceration occurs as a result of a disturbance in the relationship between the uncalcified and already calcified portions of the developing tooth.

In this case the upper central incisors were traumatised at 4 years of age necessitating their removal. At 11 years of age the patient presented with unerupted permanent incisors, which were shown radiographically to be severely dilacerated. The teeth were removed surgically in multiple fragments which, when reassembled, show the extent of the distortion (**768, 769, 770**).

References

ANDREASEN, J.O. *Traumatic injuries of the teeth* (2nd edition) Munksgaard.
BROOK, A.H., WINTER, G.B. Developmental arrest of permanent tooth germs following pulpal infection of deciduous teeth. *Br. Dent.J.* 1975; 139: 9-11.
HILL, F.J. Cystic lesions associated with deciduous teeth. *Proc. Br. Paed. Soc.* 1978; 8: 9-12.
HOBSON, P. Pulp treatment of deciduous teeth. *Br. Dent. J.* 1970; 128: 275-282.
SHAW, W.C., SMITH, D.M.H., HILL, F.J. Inflammatory follicular cysts. *J. Dent. Child.* 1980; 47: 97-101.

15   Endodontic Surgery J. J. Messing

In recent years, recognition of the fact that dentists are exposed to the risk of contracting AIDS, herpes or hepatitis from contaminated blood or saliva has led to recommendations that protective gloves be worn. In this series, which was recorded over a period, gloves were not worn but the author recommends that they should be used routinely in the light of increased awareness of these conditions.

APICECTOMY

771

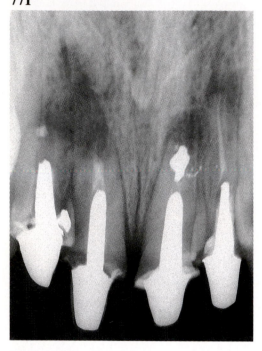

772

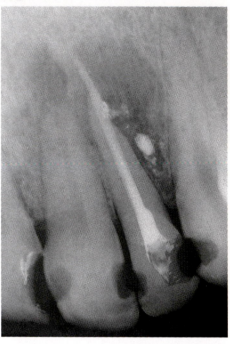

773

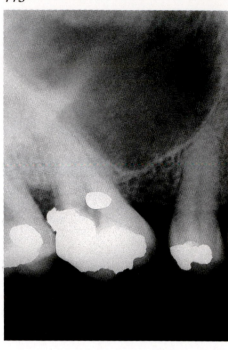

Indications

Apicectomy is indicated solely when a conservative approach is impossible or inadvisable eg:

(a)   Access to the root canal is prevented due to dystrophic calcification, an *irremovable post crown* (**771**) or severe curvature of the root.

(b)   The presence of a large periapical lesion, not responding to conservative treatment.

(c)   Chronic periapical infection associated with the introduction of a large quantity of root filling material into the periapical bone (**772**).

(d)   Fracture of the root with gross displacement of the apical portion. (It may be possible to treat such a condition with calcium hydroxide dressings, but surgery is often more predictable.)

(e)   Perforation of the root, resulting from injudicious instrumentation, internal or external resorption.

(f)   When time is limited, the endodontic and surgical treatments may be completed in one visit.

(g)   When conservative treatment has failed, eg when symptoms persist despite numerous dressings, or after a canal has been filled with an irremovable filling.

(h)   In order to confirm the presence of a suspected fracture of the root.

Contra-indications

(a)   Difficult access: eg palatal roots of some maxillary premolars and molars and lower molars, also individual anatomical problems, such as a small mouth, trismus, or severe facial scarring.

(b)   Proximity of inferior dental canal, mental nerve and maxillary antrum (**773**) when operating on the roots of premolars and molars. An experienced, confident oral surgeon would not necessarily consider such anatomical factors to be hazardous, although great care would be essential. Access to buccal roots of upper molars is not usually a problem (**774**).

(c)   Systemic factors: eg neurosis, history of rheumatic fever or chorea, pregnancy, haemorrhagic diatheses, cardiac disease, debilitating diseases.

(d)   Poor oral hygiene associated with periodontal disease or severe caries. If there is marginal bone loss associated with untreated marginal gingivitis, it should be treated prior to periapical surgery.

(e)   The strategic importance of the tooth and the subsequent possibility that it cannot be restored to full function.

Rationale

Treatment consists of gaining the best possible access to the bony lesion, with the aid of local or general anaesthesia; removing a small part of the apical portion of the root in order to obtain a clear view of the cut end of the root and locating all palpable orifices of the main canal and any accessible subsidiary canals.

It is then necessary to check for defects in an existing apical seal, or to place an amalgam seal in a root-end cavity, prepared so as to involve the apical 1-3 mm of the canal.

Granulation tissue should be eliminated whenever possible without damaging the neurovascular bundles of the adjacent teeth or involving the maxillary antrum or inferior dental canal. This is done so that the contents of the periapical lesion can be examined histologically, to establish the absence of cystic or malignant, neoplastic changes in the tissues. It is performed by gentle curettage and irrigation of the bone, the specimen for biopsy being dropped into a Bijou bottle of formol-saline before being sent to the laboratory.

Post-operative radiography, both immediate and at intervals over the subsequent 3-4 years, is necessary in order to check progress.

774

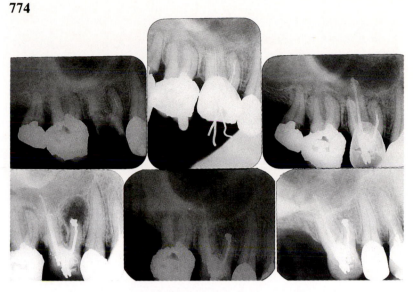

Review (6 months)   Review (12 months)

Armamentarium

The instruments required should be checked carefully against a list, and all cutting instruments sharpened before they are sterilised. When ready for use, they are laid out on a sterile towel and covered until required. It is helpful if the instruments are placed in order of use (**775**).

Top

Towel clips
Hunt's syringe
Syringe for L.A.
Aspirator tips
Mouse-tooth forceps
Fine forceps
College tweezer
Scissors
Suture needle holder
Curved needle holder
Handpiece (straight)
Burs
Angled flap retractor

Below

Galley pot
Cotton wool rolls
Cotton buds
Mirror
Briault probe
Straight probe
Scalpel handle & no. 15 blade
Periosteal elevator
2 Tungsten-carbide straight chisels
3 excavators & Mitchell trimmer
4 custom-made amalgam condensers
Baldwin amalgam burnisher
Double-ended flat plastic
K.G. retro-amalgam carrier
Messing amalgam gun

775

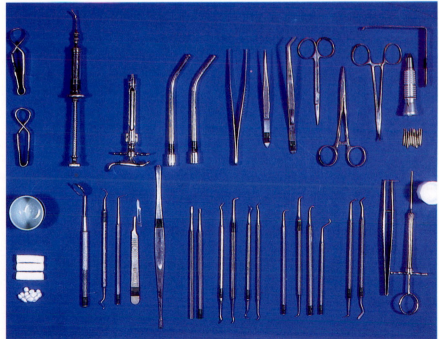

The apical seal

Amalgam is used most commonly as an apical seal, inserted by the retrograde approach and condensed into an apical cavity, prepared after resection of the apical tip.

If, following the failure of conservative treatment, surgical intervention is planned, some surgeons prefer to fill the canal by the orthograde route, using condensed gutta percha and a sealer, or alternatively to obliterate the apical 3-5 mm with silver amalgam, using an *endodontic amalgam carrier* (**776**), and condensing the amalgam either by hand or using a mechanical condenser via the coronal orifice (**777**).

The retrofilling technique is used primarily when direct access via the canal is impossible. Some operators prefer to fill the canal, if accessible, at the time of operation. After apicectomy the canal is coated with sealer and a gutta percha cone is forced through the end of the canal until it jams. The excess gutta percha projecting through the end of the root is excised with a sharp scalpel, thus minimising the lute of sealer at the root end. The remainder of the canal is then filled with gutta percha cones, using a lateral condensation technique. This technique is particularly useful when the apex is wide open.

When a canal is straight and the apical 3 mm can be reamed to a circular cross section, an apical titanium cone can be cemented. Provided a tight frictional fit is obtained, this method is eminently satisfactory.

This technique is of value when obliterating a lateral perforation with amalgam. The apex is sealed with the tip and the rest of the canal is filled with gutta percha, against which the amalgam can be condensed to fill the defect.

Of all these techniques, the retrofilling method is the most popular. Each technique has its advocates and, in the right hands, appears to achieve a good measure of success.

Design of the flap

So that the area to be anaesthetised can be visualised, the design of the flap should be planned prior to injecting the local anaesthetic.

In order to avoid 'keyhole' surgery with the attendant problems of inadequate access and trauma to the soft tissues, the design of flap must be planned with care. It has been found that a trapezoidal shape (**778a**) permits maximum access to the root. However, when there are porcelain crowns on the teeth the margins of which are well-fitting and aesthetically acceptable, it is better to avoid any cutting of the marginal gingivae, which would tend to recede while healing.

Alternative means of access may be obtained either with a semilunar incision (**778b**) or by producing an envelope-shaped (or modified semilunar) flap. In both techniques, the incision should not approach closer than 3.0 mm to the cervical margins of the teeth, otherwise serious impairment of the blood supply to the marginal gingiva could lead to its necrosis.

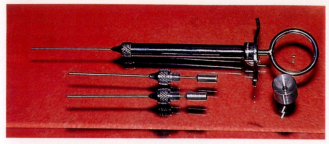

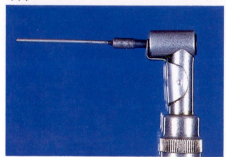

778

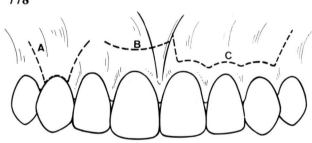

The horizontal component of the envelope (Ochsenbein-Luebke) flap (**778c**) may be a straight or scalloped incision. It is made at a right angle to the bone and, being in attached gingiva where there is an abundance of collagen, an increased rate of healing is promoted. The chief advantage of this flap is the lack of interference with the epithelial attachment. It should not be used, however, where the zone of epithelial attachment is small or where there is pocketing, because there is a risk that the blood supply to the marginal gingivae will be lost, with consequent dehiscence.

779

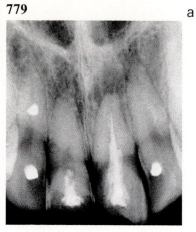
(a) before apicectomy

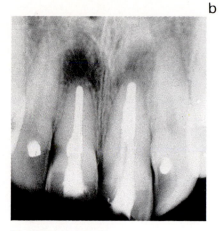
(b) after apicectomy

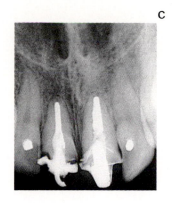
(c) 6 months postoperative

780

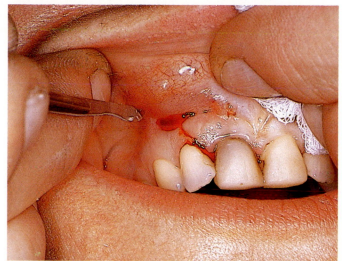

It is customary to extend the flap to one tooth on either side of the tooth involved. For the trapezoidal flap (**780, 781**), two vertical incisions are made through the interdental papillae, then along the gingival sulcus to produce a flap with a wide base. The height of the vertical incisions is dictated by the need for apical access.

A full thickness flap should be raised, incising down to the bone to facilitate a one-piece retraction of the mucoperiosteum. This is done with a periosteal elevator (**782**). In cases in which fibrous repair tissue has been laid down after previous surgery, the corner of a gauze square can be tucked under the flap. When pressed apically with the periosteal elevator, this materially facilitates the separation of periosteum from bone.

781

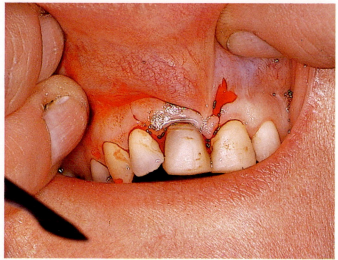

782

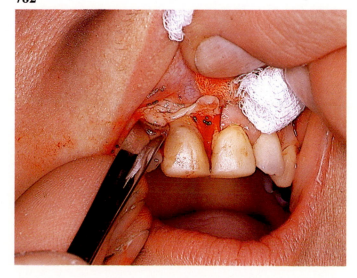

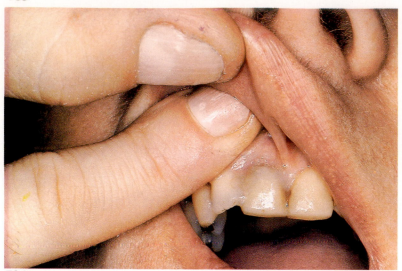

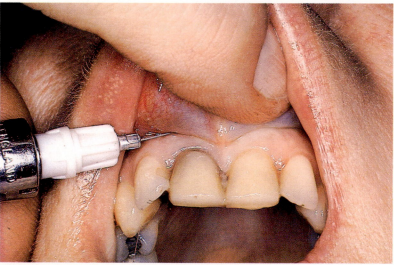

784

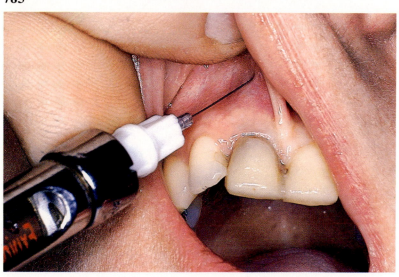

785

Anaesthesia

In the majority of cases, a local anaesthetic is used. However the administration of a general anaesthetic may be dictated by the patient's fear of surgery or by problems associated with difficulty of access. As a rule of thumb, it is advisable to administer a general anaesthetic when three or more apices are to be resected, because more time will be needed and local anaesthesia could wear off prematurely.

The ability to work on a conscious patient is enhanced by the complete absence of pain. Perfect anaesthesia cannot be assured in the presence of acute inflammation, apart from the risk of spreading infection by operating in an inflamed area. The condition must initially be rendered chronic through the use of drainage and antibiotics, if necessary, in order to contain the infection before embarking on surgery.

The psychological aspect of pain control should not be neglected. Surgery should be undertaken in a quiet, confident and unhurried manner with sufficient time allowed for the onset of anaesthesia. Nervous patients may need pre-operative medication, for which purpose Diazepam (2.0 mgm), or Meprobamate (400 mgm) have proved useful (taken the night before and 1 hour before the operation).

It is also essential to allay the patient's fears by explaining in lay terms what is to be done; how long it should take; what sensation will be felt — and that there should be no pain after the injection has become effective.

Before the hands are scrubbed, a topical anaesthetic (5% Lignocaine cream) should be smeared over the mucosa in those areas to be injected (**783**). While the surgeon is scrubbing up, the assistant should wipe the lips and circum-oral skin with a 2% solution of chlorhexidine on gauze in order to minimise contamination of the area.

The anaesthetic solution, warmed to body temperature is infiltrated slowly and massaged gently in advance of the needle as it is moved through the tissue (**784**). The solution should be deposited high above the apices of the roots (**785**). Then, after a suitable delay to allow the onset of superficial anaesthesia, the needle is advanced through the periosteum and deposited subperiosteally at a slow rate in the region of the apices.

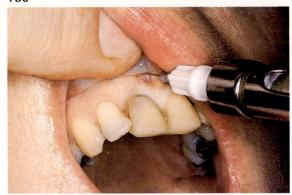

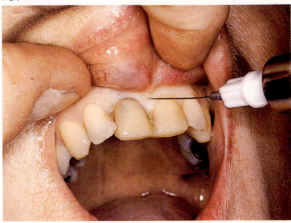

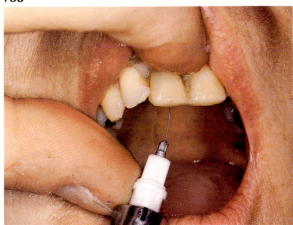

The anaesthetic solution is dispersed throughout the proposed area of the flap by gentle massage.

If the periapical bone destruction has involved the labial cortical plate, the needle may be advanced into the bone cavity and a small quantity of solution injected (786). This technique, taught by A. R. F. Thompson, has proved to be a valuable means of preventing pain when curetting an extensive granuloma or cyst close to the floor of the nose. If this is not done and curettage is found to cause pain, a strip of gauze soaked in a 10% solution of cocaine hydrochloride should be packed into the bone cavity for about 30 seconds in order to restore anaesthesia.

In the maxilla a palatal infiltration opposite the affected tooth is necessary. This tends to be somewhat painful, although it can be rendered more bearable if the patient is warned to expect a pressure sensation, and the solution is injected slowly. Movement of the plunger along the cartridge should be barely perceptible.

When anaesthetising the maxillary incisors, having given a submucous infiltration, an intra-papillary injection is made between the centrals; advancing the needle slowly while injecting, until the point enters the palatine papilla (787). When this is seen to blanch, the needle is re-inserted at the lateral margin of the papilla in a line parallel with the axes of the incisors (788) and carried up through the incisive foramen, depositing 0.5 ml in the canal (789). This injection is painless and anaesthetises the premaxillary area (2/2) of the palate.

Anaesthesia for apicectomy should never be inadequate because insufficient anaesthetic solution was injected. At least 3-4 ml is usually required and, when more than one tooth is treated, 6 ml may be needed.

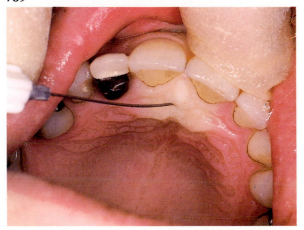

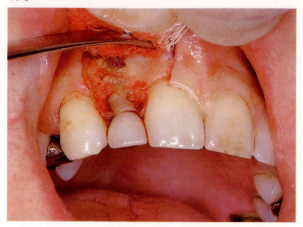

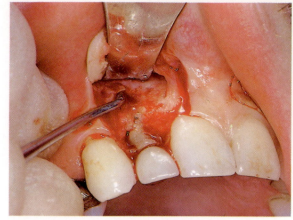

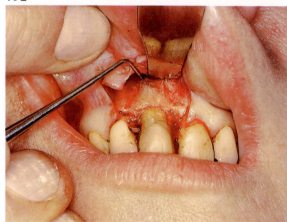

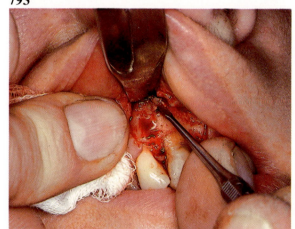

Location of the periapical lesion

After the muco-periosteal flap has been lifted from the bone, a retractor is positioned so that it rests on the bone and does not interfere with the operator's line of vision. The bone overlying the root is often destroyed and the inflammatory tissue is visible immediately when the flap is raised (790). A sinus, when present, is usually attached to the fenestration by fibrous tissue, enclosing the epithelium-line track. The sinus track may be excised as an aid to retraction of the flap. If it remains attached to the overlying mucosa, it does not delay healing; therefore, its removal is not essential.

In the absence of visible evidence of buccal bone loss (791), the area can be located with the aid of a sharp explorer (probe), used to find 'soft spots' where the cortical plate has been thinned by resorption related to the underlying periapical lesion (792).

Once it has been located, the bone cavity may be opened up with a pulling action around the perimeter with size 6-10 round steel bur, or by paring away the undermined cortical bone with a sharp, straight enamel chisel (793). The apex of the root is fully identified before any curettage of soft tissue is attempted.

With good access to the area established, soft tissue is curetted away from bone and root surfaces with a gentle teasing action (794, 795). Large and cystic lesions are best lifted away from the underlying bone by inserting a large spoon curette with the concavity facing the bone. This facilitates separation of the soft tissue. Where a large area of soft tissue appears to involve the apices of adjacent teeth, the vitality of which has been established, it is safer to avoid curettage in these areas so that the integrity of the apical vessels and nerves can be protected. The tissue is dropped into formol-saline solution in a specimen bottle and sent for histological examination (796).

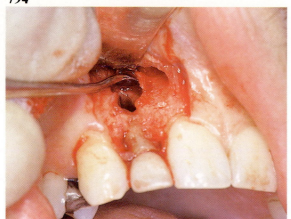

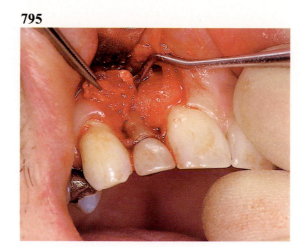

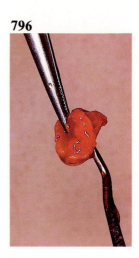

Resection of the apex

Previously, it was considered essential to remove the apical third of the root in order to eliminate the apical delta and the zone of 'infected' cementum. Contemporary attitudes favour minimum shortening of the root, consistent with the provision of access to the cut end, so that the apical seal can be verified or provided by cutting and filling an apical cavity. It should not be forgotten that, given a good apical seal, the majority of periapical lesions can be dealt with by the body's defences, thus obviating the need for a surgical approach.

There has been a tendency to remove an excessive length of root tip, thus leaving insufficient root support and, should a post-retained crown be needed subsequently, inadequate length of root canal.

In lieu of resecting a proportion of the root, with the attendant risk of displacing the apex and losing it in the tissues, the author prefers to place a small fissure bur on the apex at an angle of approximately 45° to the root axis and to drill away 1-2 mm from the apex until the canal can be located easily with a Briault probe (797). The end of the root can then be made smooth with a cylindrical diamond or carborundum bur (798).

Teeth with bifid roots, such as may be found in maxillary premolars and more rarely in mandibular canines and premolars present especial difficulty when attempting to gain access to the palatal or lingual apex. A larger amount of the buccal apex must be resected so that the lingual apex can be found and prepared for apical obturation.

The cut end of the root is inspected and probed in order to check for obvious defects in the existing seal, or large accessory or lateral canals, or for fractures of the root or perforations. Although the seal may appear to be satisfactory, it is good practice to prepare an apical cavity and seal the canal with amalgam as a routine procedure.

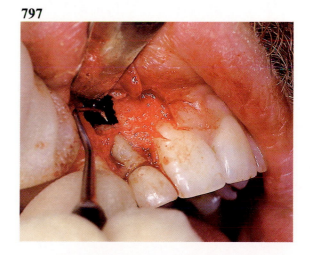

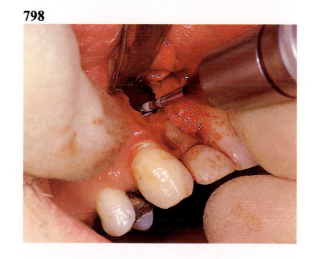

The apical cavity

The apical cavity usually can be prepared with a small round bur in a straight handpiece, provided the root face is adequately angulated and the root is not so long or the labial sulcus so shallow that access is thereby impeded. In such cases, a contra-angle handpiece should be used.

The bur is applied just labial to the canal orifice and, at slow speed, a cavity is prepared to involve the cross-sectional area of the canal and cut to a depth of 1.5-2.0 mm (**799**). This precaution is advised because roots tend to be narrow bucco-lingually at their apices which increases the risk of a lingual perforation if the cavity is started from the canal.

When the bur has reached the required depth, it is inclined a few degrees first mesially, then distally within the cavity in order to produce a retentive form (**800**). As an alternative, undercuts can be cut with a size 1 wheel bur.

When a combination of a shallow buccal sulcus, long roots and muscular lips is encountered, access to the apex can be gained with a (KaVo) microhandpiece (**801**). Alternatively a pedodontic handpiece may prove adequate.

When access to the apex is severely restricted, a cavity can be started at the labio-apical angle, in the form of a keyhole, and carried lingually to involve the canal (**802**).

799

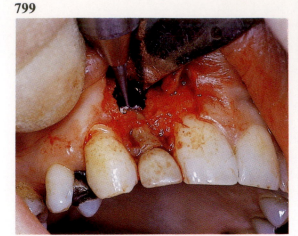

800

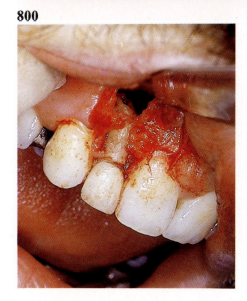

801

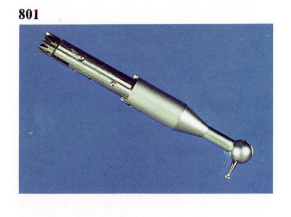

802

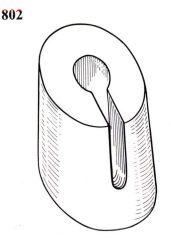

Filling the apical cavity

It is generally accepted that, as yet, the perfect filling material has not been found for retro-filling of apical cavities. Silver amalgam is the most commonly used material, but it may on occasion fail to produce satisfactory periapical healing. Whether this results from micro-leakage and bacterial contamination, or individual intolerance of the constituents or breakdown products of amalgam, has yet to be ascertained. Alternative materials, which have been used with varying degrees of success, are Cavit (a calcium sulphate cement), zinc eugenolate cement, polycarboxylate and glass-ionomer cements. Finne et al. (*Oral Surg.*, Apr. 1977) found that Cavit does not provide a perfect apical seal, especially when associated with a defective orthograde obturation. Despite varying reports of success, the most satisfactory results are obtained when silver amalgam is well condensed and finished in the apical cavity.

The greatest problem, when condensing the amalgam, is the exclusion of blood. It was taught, at one time, that the vasoconstrictor in the local anaesthetic, in conjunction with a strip of gauze soaked in 1/1000 adrenaline in the bone cavity, would produce a blood-free zone. Despite some degree of haemostasis, blood still tends to soak into the gauze strip used to line the periapical area, with the result that the contaminated amalgam, when hard, is porous and if it contains zinc, is expanded. Thus the seal is likely to be defective.

Seldin recommended the use of Horsley's bone wax, a combination of beeswax and phenol, as a temporary dam while inserting and condensing the amalgam. The author has used this technique, with gratitude to its inventor, for many years. The criticism that it is difficult to remove the wax *in toto* is invalid because there is no evidence that any residual film of wax interferes with healing.

A further advantage of using bone wax is the entrapment of particles of amalgam which become scattered during condensation and frequently prove impossible to locate during debridement of the wound. Although amalgam debris gives a 'snowstorm' pattern on the radiograph, there is no apparent interference with bony repair, because the particles become encapsulated in fibrous tissue and the wound will heal despite their presence (**803, 804**). Nevertheless, every attempt should be made to remove all debris from the operation area. As an alternative to bone wax, the cavity may be packed tightly with a strip of gauze.

803

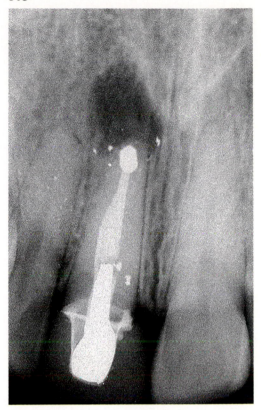

804

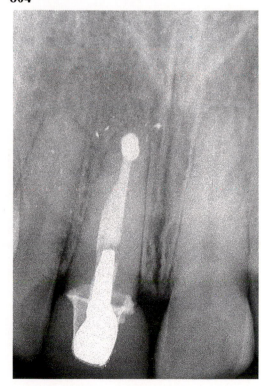

Use of Horsley's bone wax

The apical cavity is prepared, the bone cavity is irrigated with saline and aspirated and a tiny ball of cotton wool is packed into the apical cavity (**805, 806**). Then the bone cavity is filled with bone wax (**807**) and a small cave is excavated down to the apex of the root, using a large spoon excavator or Mitchell's trimmer (**808**). The assistant holds the aspirator tip at the perimeter of the wax, thus preventing contamination by blood from the incised mucoperiosteum. Care must be taken to avoid pressure on the wax by the retractor, which might force it back over the apex (**809**). The cotton is removed and the apical cavity is washed and dried, using inverted paper points.

805

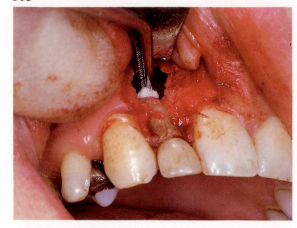

806

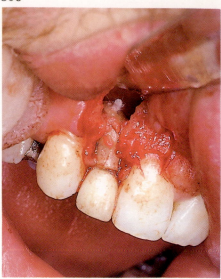

807

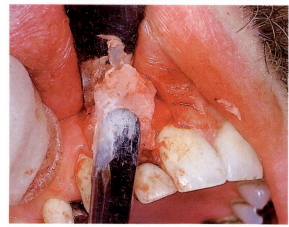

808

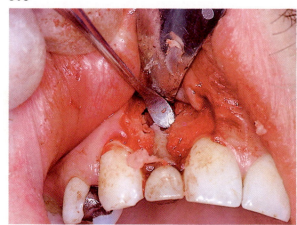

809

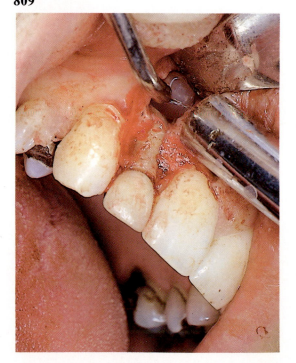

810

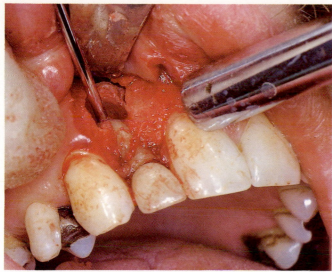

811

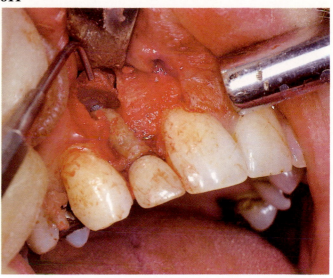

Small increments of amalgam are inserted (**810**) and condensed with small pluggers until slightly overbuilt (**811, 812, 813**). After 1-2 minutes, the amalgam is carved level with the root face, burnished (**814**) and wiped lightly with a cotton ball.

812

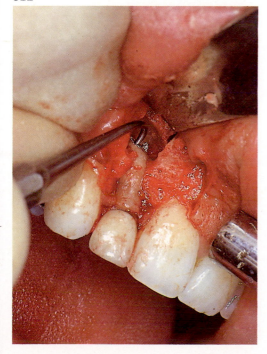

813

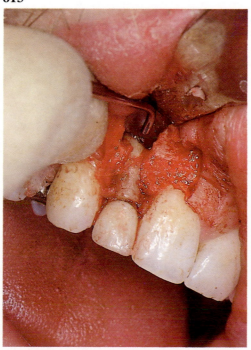

814

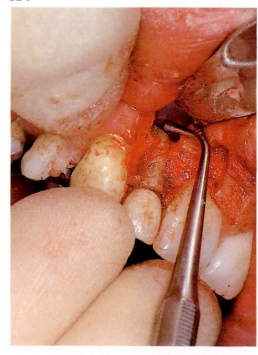

If there is doubt about the ability to eliminate moisture while condensing the amalgam, a zinc-free alloy should be used: however, the zinc-containing amalgams are cleaner to use and appear, in the author's experience, to produce a superior seal. Jorgensen (1972), found that zinc-free amalgam tends to corrode more than amalgam with zinc, hence the latter is preferable if isolated from moisture. Small increments of amalgam are inserted using an apical amalgam carrier (815) and considerable pressure is exerted, condensing the amalgam into the undercuts.

If a fast-setting amalgam is used, a good finish can be produced after a few minutes by means of several gentle strokes with a slightly blunt finishing bur (816, 817).

Instruments for condensation may be made from old probes and plastic instruments, the ends of which are ground to produce a flat surface. Various shapes can be fashioned to facilitate access in a variety of situations (818).

When access to the palatal apex of a maxillary premolar is so difficult that it proves to be impossible to manipulate amalgam without inordinate removal of bone, the author has achieved successful results using a polystyrene-bonded zinc eugenolate cement (Kalzinol) as an apical seal. The cavity is made retentive and the cement, mixed to a putty-like consistency, is packed into it with a flat plastic instrument. When hardened, which takes about 3 minutes, the surface of the seal is scraped smooth and all excess cement is washed out. Healing, which occurs in 6-12 months after operation, has been maintained for at least 7 years when followed up in the small number of cases thus treated by the author. Although hydrolysis of zinc eugenolate cement to zinc hydroxide and eugenol is found in cavities in contact with the saliva, it is probable that polystyrene hinders this reaction and the seal, soon covered with repair tissue, reaches equilibrium with its environment.

Nevertheless, because of its greater durability, silver amalgam is the material of choice, whereas zinc eugenolate cement can be reserved for those situations in which access is inadequate for proper manipulation of amalgam.

Ref. K. D. Jorgensen (1972). Amalgam in Dentistry no. 334 U.S. Department of Commerce D.M.R. National Bureau of Standards Special Publication, p.33.

815

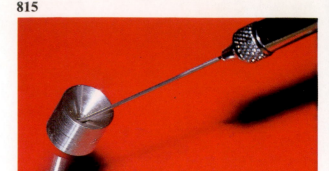

816

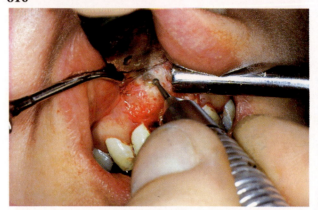

817

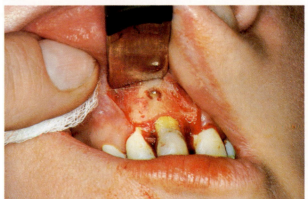

818

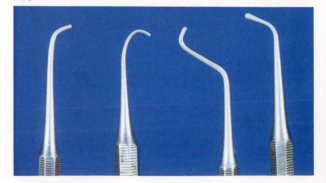

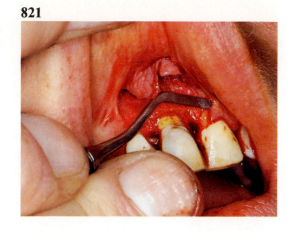
819

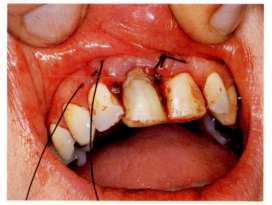
821

Apical curettage

The treatment of periapical lesions solely by curettage of the lesion, has been recommended by some authorities, and has found a place in numerous publications.

In this technique the fact is ignored that the lesion owes its origin to a defective seal, in the majority of cases, therefore curettage alone cannot be advocated.

Support for this view is evident when a lesion heals after satisfactory preparation and filling of the canal, without having recourse to surgical intervention.

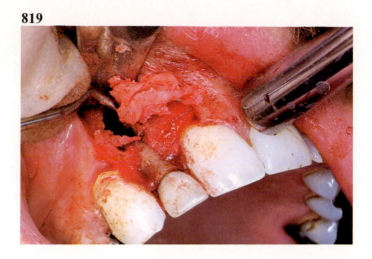
820

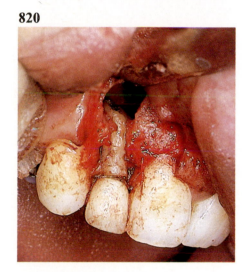
820

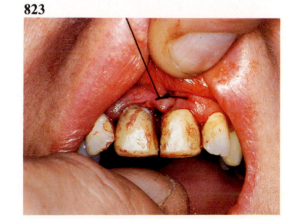
822

823

Debridement of the bone cavity

After the apical seal has been ensured, the gauze pack or bone wax is removed (819) and, using a liberal quantity of isotonic saline, the bony cavity is well irrigated. For this purpose, a Hunt's syringe or a Record Syringe with a wide bore needle can be used (820).

A careful check should be made with a back-action excavator, in order to eliminate residual debris which tends to be trapped in the bone, especially lingual to the end of the root.

Closure of the wound

Prior to suturing the flap back into position, a flat plastic instrument, should be insinuated beneath the mucoperiosteum at the fixed sides of the flap, in order to mobilise the tissues and thus facilitate the

insertion of the needle (821). A minimum number of nylon sutures is used, sufficient to hold the flap in position (822). Where a full flap has been reflected, it is essential that it be pulled well down to cover the surface of the root and not be allowed to ride up disclosing the enamel/cementum junction. To do this, a suture (823) is passed through the labial interdental papilla and then

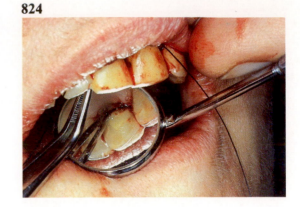
824

passed interproximally and carried below the cingulum bulge of the apicected tooth (**824**), through the other interproximal space and, piercing the interdental papilla from the lingual (**825, 826**), it is pulled through and tied off labially over the apicected tooth. This pulls the flap down coronally, maintaining it until it is stabilised by healing (**827**).

Laterally the flap is sutured and care is taken to ensure good adaptation of its margins.

Protection of the flap for the first day or so is obtained by placing a wafer of Stomahesive (Squibb) (**828**) 'Dental Bandage' over the suture lines. The mucosa is dried with gauze and the Stomahesive is pressed firmly into contact with the surface and brought over the cervical margins of the teeth, and held firmly for 30 seconds.

It tends to dissolve away slowly, being composed chiefly of Carboxymethyl cellulose and Pectin. The patient is warned that it will probably stay in place for 24-48 hours and, if swallowed while eating is harmless.

825

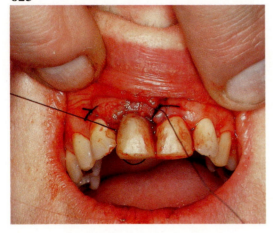

826

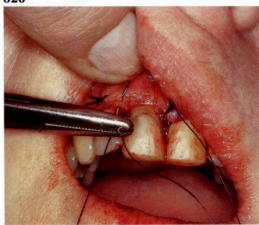

827

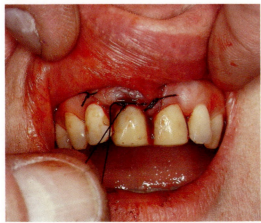

828

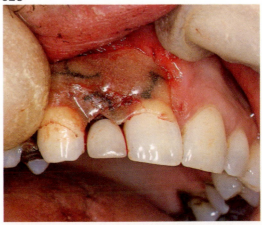

Radiological control

A periapical control radiograph is recorded before dismissing the patient. If there is any doubt about the seal, especially in multi-rooted teeth, a radiograph can be taken prior to suturing and developed in a rapid developer as an additional check.

Subsequent radiographs are recorded after six and twelve months and, thereafter, annually for at least four years.

Instructions to the patient

The patient is warned against disturbing the wound, eg by lifting the lip to view the incisions in a mirror, especially while the tissues are anaesthetised, and also to avoid hot food and liquids during the same period. He should expect tenderness and swelling for a few days and, rarely, some patients exhibit varying degrees of bruising of the skin in the region (**829**).

If these signs should increase in intensity or be accompanied by a foul discharge and a rise in temperature or a sudden onset of haemorrhage, the patient should return immediately for treatment with antibiotics. In the author's experience such sequelae are extremely rare.

Supportive measures should be recommended. Hot, hypertonic saline (a teaspoonful of salt in a glass of hot water) makes an ideal mouthwash and should be used hourly for the first two days and, subsequently after meals until the sutures have been removed. It should be stressed that hot mouthwashes must not be used while the tissues are anaesthetised.

Swelling may be diminished by hourly application of crushed ice in a polythene bag on to the skin overlying the wound. Used for about two minutes at a time, it is only of value for the first three hours after operation. The tooth should be relieved from occlusal contact so that physiological rest will aid healing (**830**).

Removal of sutures

After a minimum of four days, the sutures can be removed. At the same time, the continued vitality of teeth adjacent to the periapical lesion should be checked, if their apices were in close proximity to the bony lesion.

Failure to observe this precaution and subsequent contamination of the wound by toxins and bacteria from a neighbouring tooth can lead to breakdown of healing.

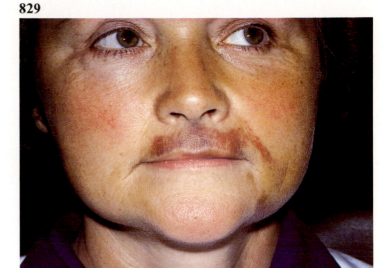

829

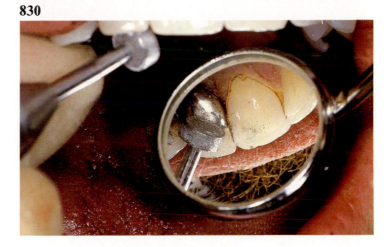

830

The radiographic check-up

After an interval of six months, the patient is recalled. Clinical evidence of failure to heal will be apparent if a discharging sinus is visible or if the patient complains of any tenderness or swelling. The radiograph should show evidence of bony repair, although complete restoration of bone and establishment of lamina dura may take up to two years. Palatal defects found at the time of apicectomy are repaired by fibrous tissue and a sharply defined radiolucency remains on the radiograph — it is of no consequence (**831, 832, 833**).

Such defects are found most commonly in areas associated with lateral incisors. This is due to the proximity of the apex to the palatal cortical plate which may be resorbed or perforated at the time of operation.

Otherwise, some large areas shrink down to a small size and remain constant for many years. In the absence of symptoms, such a situation is acceptable.

831

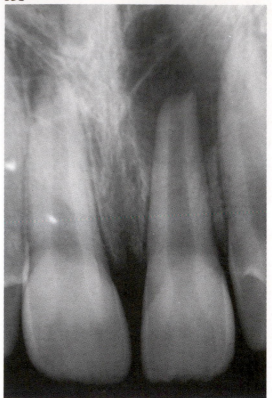

832

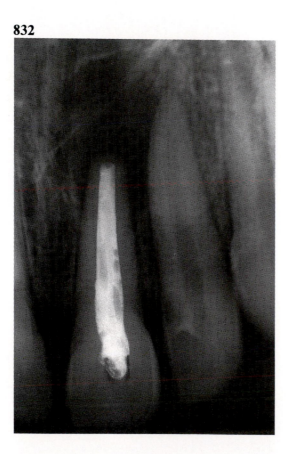

833

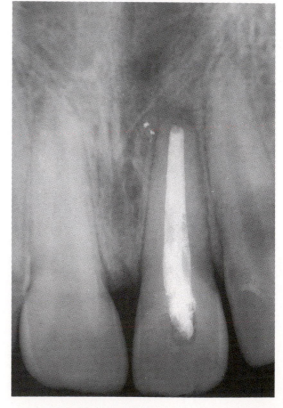

Replantation

Endodontic treatment on posterior teeth may not be feasible for a variety of reasons and, whereas apicectomy can be performed on the majority of anterior teeth, anatomical considerations limit its use on many posterior teeth. Should there be an unmanageable perforation of a root, canals blocked by dystrophic calcification, or any gross anatomical variations of canal morphology, endodontic preparation may prove to be impossible. A conservative approach is similarly negated if the mouth is too small or the tooth grossly malaligned.

When the sole treatment is extraction, replantation may offer a valid alternative as a last resort.

In order that a tooth be replanted, the following criteria must be fulfilled:

(a) The tooth should be firm without gingival or infra-bony pocketing.
(b) The patient should not be suffering from any systemic condition which might interfere with healing or place him at risk.
(c) Extraction of the tooth in one piece should be feasible.
(d) The operation must be completed at high speed and with minimum trauma.
(e) The surface of the root and attached periodontal fibres must not be unduly traumatised by the extraction and no caustic drugs should be applied to it.
(f) After replantation, the tooth should be relieved from occlusal stress, function being restored when the tooth becomes firm in its socket.
(g) Some form of splinting will be indicated if, after replantation, the tooth is loose in its socket.
(h) The root canals should be prepared as far as possible and, if feasible, filled before extraction or dressed with calcium hydroxide and filled after replantation.

Because there is a risk that the tooth could fracture when extracted (**834, 835, 836**), no promise of success should be made to the patient. It should be pointed out that, due to circumstances, the tooth is unsavable and should be extracted. Then, provided the patient accepts the proposed treatment plan and its implications, a replantation can be undertaken.

834

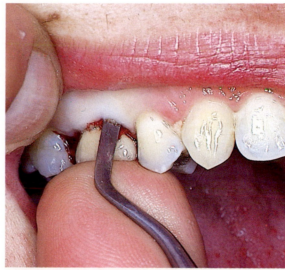

835

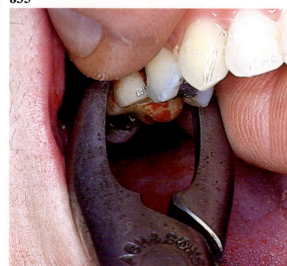

836

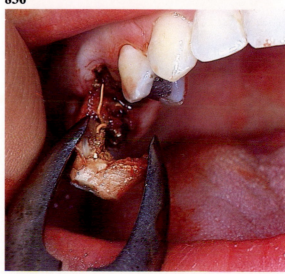

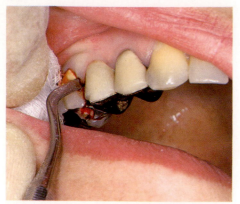

837

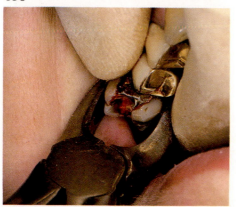

838

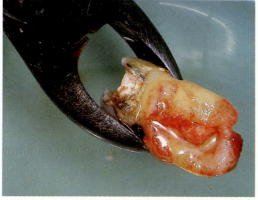

839

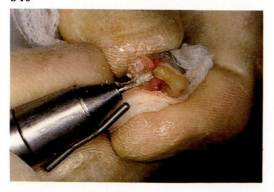

840

TECHNIQUE FOR REPLANTATION

In order that the roots may be prepared and sealed with minimum delay, it is essential that all the instruments which could be needed are sterilised and set out in the proposed order of use.

After the area has been anaesthetised, the gingival crevice is painted with a solution of Povidone-Iodine. The gingival attachment is severed from the crown, using either a number 12 Bard-Parker scalpel or a sharp Hollenback carver (**837**), thus minimising the risk of gingival laceration during extraction.

Root forceps are used. They are applied to the tooth with a slow, deliberate pressure, directed apically, alternating the pressure from buccal to lingual until a firm grasp can be obtained on the roots (**838**). Any premature attempt to exert pressure on the crown or coronal aspect of the roots will tend to cause the tooth to fracture through the already weakened furcation area. If the tooth were to fracture at this stage, surgical removal of the roots would be necessary. However, if an apex is fractured and can be removed from its socket without undue loss of bone, replantation can still be carried out. If the apex is loose, a root canal file can be engaged in the canal and used to pull it out.

839   After extraction, the tooth is inspected and any attached gingiva is removed gently. The tooth is placed in isotonic saline and the socket is packed with a strip of ribbon gauze, soaked with saline.

All contact with the periodontal remnants on the root surface should be kept to a minimum. The crown is held in a gauze swab, impregnated with isotonic saline. The apical 1-2 mm of each root is resected using either rongeur forceps or a fissure bur or diamond drill to pare down the apex (**840**). The tooth is held in the path of a powerful beam of light which creates a pinpoint shadow, denoting the position of the orifice of the root canal. Small cavities are prepared, using a size 2 round bur to drill to a depth of about 2 mm along each canal, and angulating the bur to undercut the cavities (**841**). The periodontal ligament which remains attached to the root should not be allowed to dehydrate, nor should it be traumatised if re-attachment, rather than ankylosis, is to occur.

841

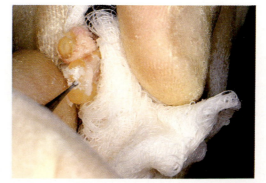

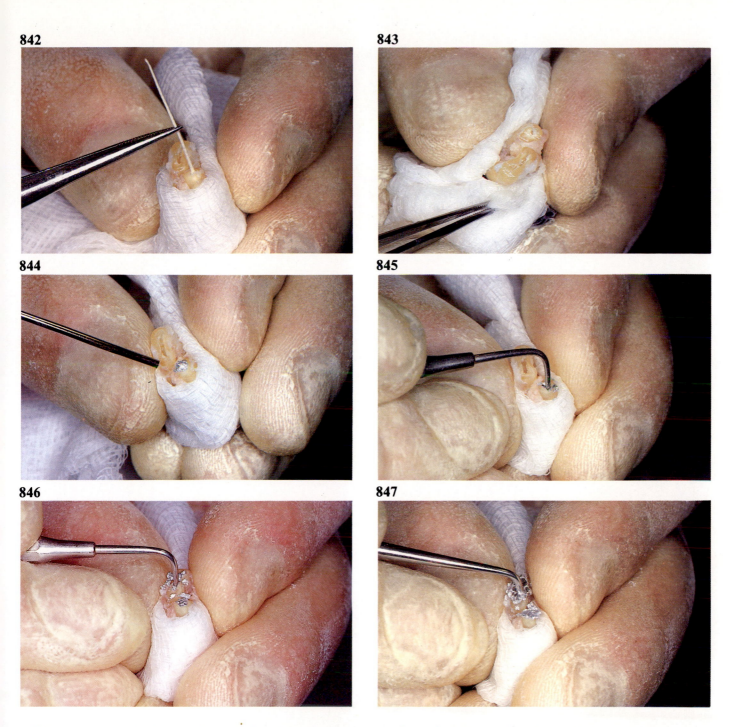

842

843

844

845

846

847

When completed, the cavities are dried out, using inverted, absorbent paper points (**842**), then painted with copal-ether varnish, in order to ensure a good seal against micro-leakage (**843**). Amalgam, with a high alloy:mercury ratio, is triturated by the assistant, and dropped into a sterilised amalgam well. Such a well is supplied with the Produits Dentaires Apical

Amalgam Carrier which can be used to deposit small increments of amalgam in the apical cavities (**844**). The same pluggers which are used to condense retrograde amalgam can be used to condense solid, over-built apical plugs of amalgam (**845, 846, 847**).

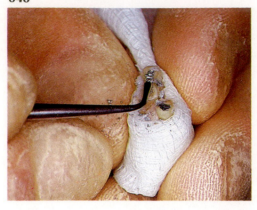

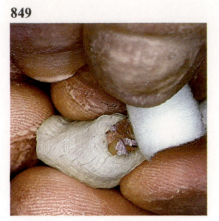

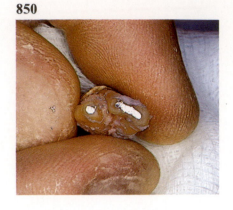

As they start to harden, the amalgam plugs can be carved flush with the root end, burnished and wiped with a cotton roll (**848, 849, 850**) to remove vestiges of mercury-rich, excess amalgam. While this is being done, the end of the root must be kept dry, whereas the surface of the root must be kept moistened with saline. Finally, prior to replanting the tooth, any particles of amalgam, adherent to the roots, should be washed off by agitating the tooth in a bowl of saline maintained at body temperature.

851

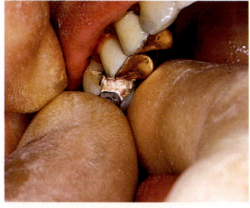

The gauze is now removed from the socket, which is also irrigated with warm saline, and the tooth is replaced in the socket, taking care to avoid entrapment of the gingivae, and employing a side to side rotatory movement, it is pressed firmly home (**851**). This can be aided by having the patient bite hard on the tooth. The expansion of the walls of the socket, resulting from the extraction, is reduced by the exertion of digital pressure on the buccal and lingual walls (**852**).

853 Using articulating paper or ribbon, the occlusion is checked and the tooth is ground out of occlusion.

852

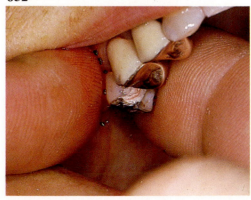

853

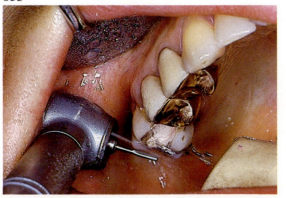

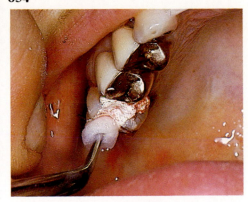

854

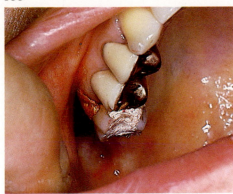

855

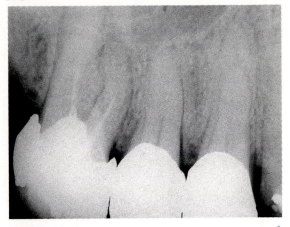

856

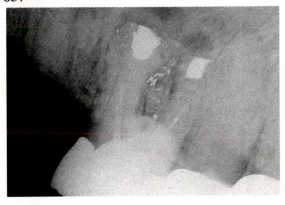

857

In a small number of cases, especially teeth with divergent roots, splinting is unnecessary. However, when the tooth is seen to be loose after replantation, it should be splinted. This may be effected most easily, when there are contiguous enamel surfaces, by etching the enamel and joining the teeth with a 'posterior' composite resin. Where the replanted tooth and adjacent surfaces have existing restorations, they can be replaced by composite resin, used to join the teeth together as a means of temporary splinting. A dressing of polystyrene-bonded, zinc eugenolate cement, made into a pack with a few fibres of cotton wool, and placed in a mesio-occluso-distal cavity in the replanted tooth and extended into the neighbouring cervical areas, also affords excellent immobilisation when hard (**854**). Protection for the detached gingival cuff is provided by the extension of the pack or placement of a periodontal pack (eg Coepak), around the circumference of the tooth (**855**). Whatever form of splinting is used, a final check must be made to ensure the elimination of any occlusal prematurities, which if missed could lead to severe pain.

Instructions are given to avoid chewing on the tooth for a few days and to keep the toothbrush away from it until the pack has been removed, but cleaning the other teeth as usual. Cleansing of the mouth can be aided by the control of plaque with a chlorhexidine mouthwash (Corsodyl—ICI), used once or twice daily for 7-10 days after replantation.

A mild analgesic, such as aspirin or paracetamol, should be prescribed, to combat minor discomfort, and the patient is asked to report any severe pain, swelling or discharge without delay. Thus, premature signs of sepsis and rejection can be dealt with by giving a suitable antibiotic or by extracting the tooth.

Usually, after 10-14 days, the tooth becomes firm and, within 21 days, the splint can be removed and a restoration placed in the cavity (**856**, before replantation; **857**, three weeks after replantation).

When it can be seen, radiographically, that there is re-attachment, whether it be ankylosis (absence of periodontal ligament space), or reconstitution of the suspensory ligament, and if the tooth is comfortable and firm, without pocketing, a full or partial veneer crown should be constructed. A radiograph should be taken each year to check for evidence of resorption of the root.

Such replacement resorption tends to progress at a slow rate, usually without signs or symptoms, and the tooth remains firm until the roots have undergone considerable resorption. Several teeth treated by the author, have remained firm and comfortable for up to 17 years, although those which gave trouble during the early stages were more likely to fail within the first year.

858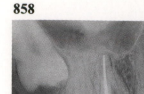

859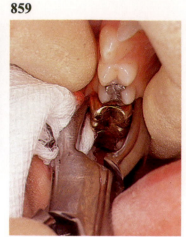

860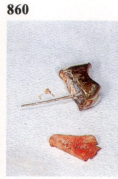

858 The patient was complaining of pain in her upper right molar. An attempt to gain access to the buccal canals was frustrated by total blockage of their orifices, therefore extraction was felt to be the only alternative.

While removing the tooth, the fragile mesio-buccal root fractured but was removed without difficulty. A decision was made to replant the remainder of the tooth (**859**).

Preparation and apical obturation were carried out as described above, despite the absence of the crown, which had broken off, and the root which had fractured during extraction.

The roots were then replanted and covered with Coepak and zinc oxide (**860-869**).

861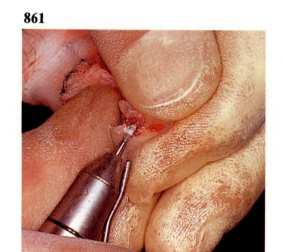

862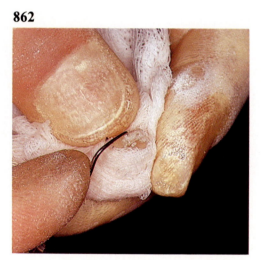

863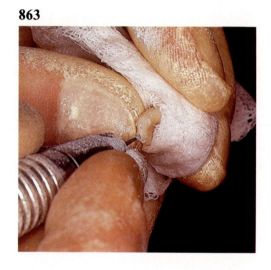

864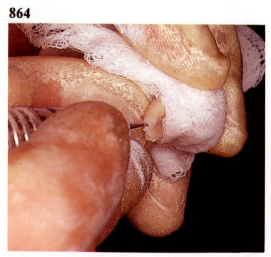

865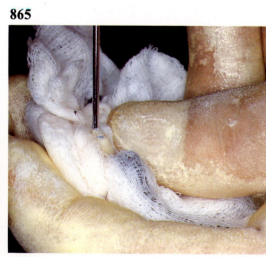

866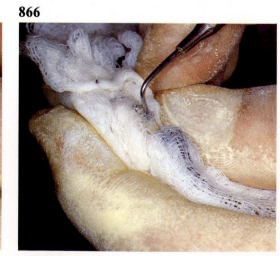

867

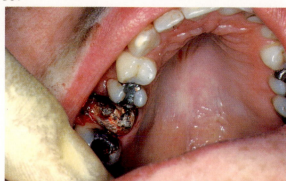

868

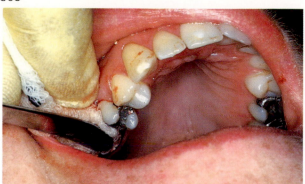

869

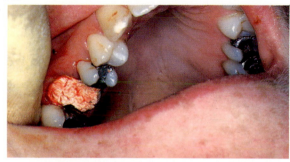

After four months, the tooth having remained symptomless, a composite core was constructed on cemented pins in the dentine and a retention screw, cemented into the palatal canal. Figure **870** shows a radiograph illustrating the use of a periodontal pack to afford protection to the socket.

In **871**, three months later, a composite resin core was constructed, and **872** shows the modified gold crown, immediately after cementation.

Subsequent use of toothbrush and floss brought about a speedy return of healthy marginal gingivae around the tooth.

870

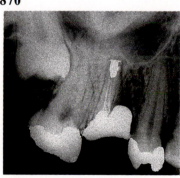

871

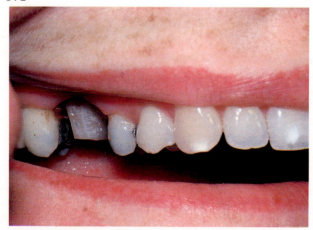

872

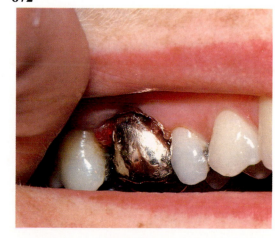

Root resection

When a multi-rooted tooth is not amenable to either conservative or surgical endodontic treatment, one line of treatment which is often successful is the resection of one root, while the other root (or roots) is filled. This technique is most commonly used for the elimination of furcation involvements, primarily of periodontal origin, but also those which stem from endodontic infections and do not respond to conservative treatment. Root resection is more applicable to maxillary molars, whereas hemisection, either accompanied by removal of one half of the tooth, or conversion to two premolars ('bicuspidisation'), tends to be the method of choice for mandibular molars. In view of the periodontal relationship of root resection, the technique has been covered in Chapter 16 on 'Endo Perio Lesion'.

HEMISECTION

Lower molars, the majority of which have two separate roots, can be treated as two teeth from an endodontic viewpoint when the need arises. The commonest reason for this eventuality is an infra-bony pocket involving the bifurcation which is not amenable to plaque control. This is often associated with pulp pathosis due to bacterial contamination of the pulp via lateral canals which communicate with the pocket. Provided sufficient bone remains around the roots, it is possible to hemisect the crown through the bifurcation and extract one root, having filled the canal system in the other. As an alternative, provided it is possible to treat the canals in both roots and that there is sufficient space between the roots, the tooth can be divided bucco-lingually, eliminating the furcation, and subsequently constructing two premolars. This technique of bicuspidisation is more likely to succeed when one or both neighbouring teeth are missing because, the roots, following hemisection, lose their transeptal fibres and tend to drift apart. If there is no room for this drift to occur, the proximity of the resected roots, one to the other, allows insufficient space for satisfactory contour of the interdental papilla, and predisposes to a chronic gingivitis.

Hemisection followed by removal of one root is indicated for the following conditions:
(a) Perforation of a root, or bifurcation, by a drill or endodontic instrument.
(b) Internal or external resorption of one root (when conservative treatment fails).
(c) An irremovable fractured instrument in a canal, associated with a periapical area and giving rise to symptoms (873).
(d) Inability to locate or negotiate canals in a root with a periapical lesion.
(e) A deep infra-bony pocket around one root or in the furcation.
(f) Deep caries or a fracture extending sub-gingivally, in relation to one root only.
(g) A vertical fracture through the crown, involving the furcation (874).
(h) A radiolucent area around one root, which is increasing in size despite root canal therapy, and where it is impossible to remove the root filling.

Roots which are to be retained should possess sufficient length of canal to allow preparation for a post-retained crown.

873

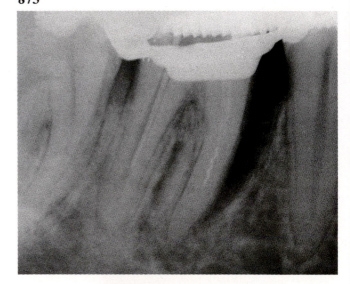

874

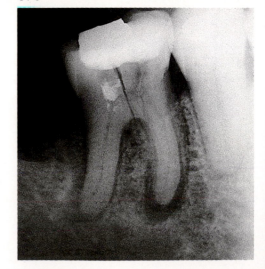

When it has become obvious that one root of a lower molar cannot be treated, attention should be diverted to the other root, making certain that its periodontium is sound or can be made healthy and that the canal system in that root is treatable. There must also be sufficient tooth, at the end of treatment to permit the making of a satisfactory restoration.

Some surgeons favour resection of one root of a molar, but leave the crown in its entirety. If the crown can be locked firmly to an adjacent tooth, so that the latter acts as a splint, and the undersurface of the crown is rendered easily cleansible, the technique is acceptable. However, a crown carried on a single root would transmit excessive stresses to the alveolar bone and periodontal ligament, leading to resorption of bone and loosening of the tooth. Therefore, a pontic may be slung between two retainers, either fixed at both ends or stress-broken at one end, or cantilevered from two or more soldered retainers (875).

Technique for hemisection

Rubber dam is applied and the root canal system of the savable root is prepared and filled. The orifices of any canals in the other root are restored temporarily. A pre-operative radiograph is taken.

875

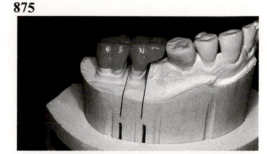

876

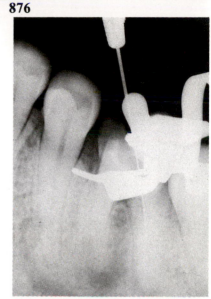

876-882 Preparation and filling of savable distal root of mandibular molar using AH26 sealer and lateral condensation of gutta percha cones.

877

878

879

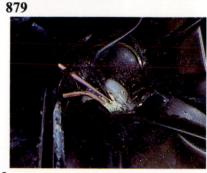

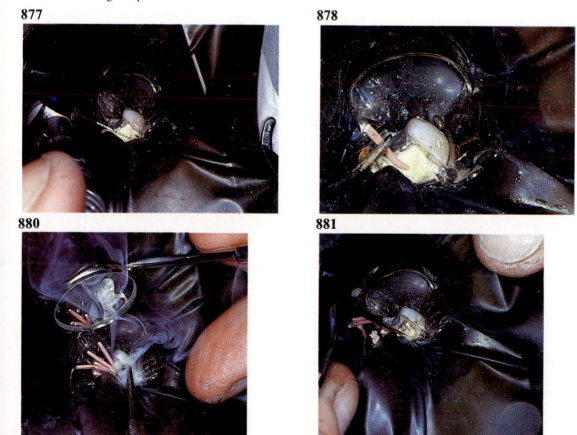

880

881

882

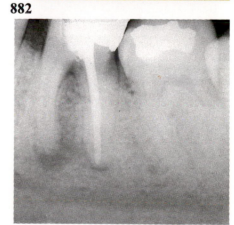

883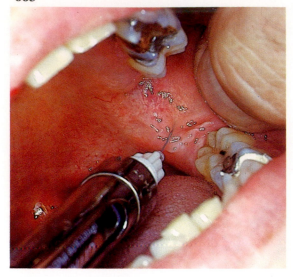

884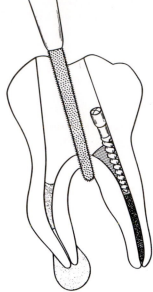

885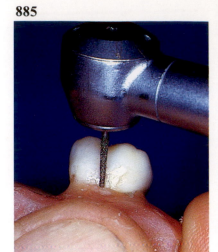

▨ temporary filling

▨ phosphate cement

▨ root filling

886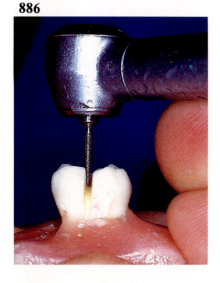

Surgical technique

Hemisection can be carried out either under local or general anaesthesia. Local anaesthesia is best achieved by means of an inferior dental nerve block plus a buccal infiltration (ie long buccal) of 2% lignocaine HCl (**883**).

Unless there is sufficient gingival recession to expose the bifurcation, it is advisable to reflect a flap, buccally. The cut should be made at the expense of that part of the crown which is to be removed, and it is made with a long tapered diamond bur, with a copious spray of coolant in the turbine handpiece.

Starting at the bifurcation, a vertical groove is cut in the buccal enamel and then, checking constantly the horizontal and vertical alignment, the cut is continued across the crown by means of a gentle sawing action (**884-889**).

887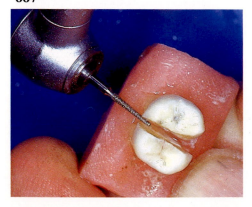

888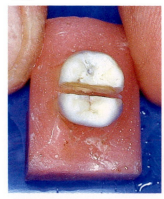

889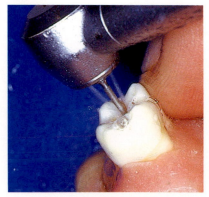

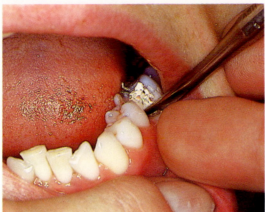

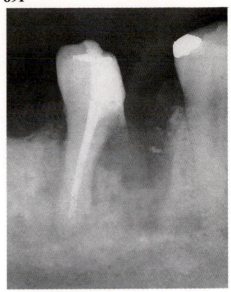

When it is possible to pass a probe between the halves of the tooth, and they can be seen to move slightly when an instrument is interposed and twisted gently (**890**), a check is made with a probe to ensure the elimination of the furcal arch from the filled root. This, if left, would serve as a plaque trap and be impossible to keep clean (**891**). It can be removed by further grinding with the diamond bur, which is used also to round off any sharp margins thus preventing trauma to the soft tissues.

Defects in the crown are filled with cement or a fast hardening amalgam. The other root is now extracted, using either forceps or elevators, and exercising great care to avoid trauma to the remaining root (**892**).

The socket is inspected and any loose fragments of bone are removed and rough alveolar margins smoothed. If a flap has been reflected, it is now replaced and sutured, and a protective wafer of Stomahesive Intra-oral Bandage (Squibb) can be pressed over the socket and sutures. Alternatively, the socket can be insufflated with iodoform powder, having previously ruled out any history of an idiosyncrasy to iodine. Iodoform provides excellent protection against alveolar osteitis or dry socket (**893**). A control radiograph is taken (**894**).

When the socket has healed superficially, the crown is restored, gaining retention from a cemented canal post or cemented dentine pins, and building a premolariform contour in amalgam or composite resin. After a further 8-12 weeks, and in the absence of clinical or radiological signs of pathosis, a crown or onlay can be made.

892

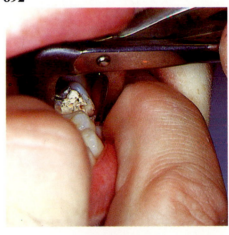

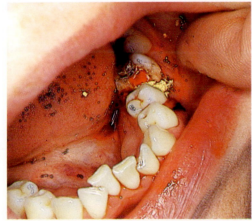

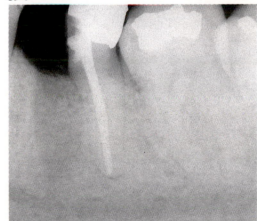

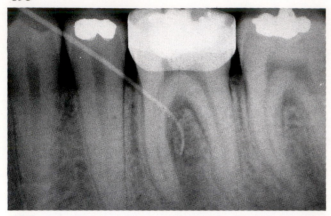

895 Lower molar fractured vertically through the crown. Gutta percha cone placed in the sinus track and copper band cemented as a splint.

896

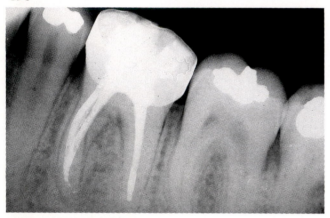

896 Canals root filled.

BICUSPIDISATION

Elimination of the furcation and conversion of a lower molar to two premolars is a sound technique for dealing with the problem of plaque control in furcal, periodontal, infra-bony pockets. It is axiomatic that both roots should have canals which are suitable for root treatment. Therefore, after definitive periodontal treatment, the canals are prepared and filled. Ultimate success of this technique depends also on the mesio-distal width of the furcation, ie the degree of separation of the roots.

Where indicated, a flap is reflected as for hemisection and the crown is divided through the bifurcation, but in this case any residual flare of the furcal area of the roots is ground away. Sharp margins are rounded and a periodontal pack, such as Coepak, is placed between the roots for 6-8 days. The patient is asked to be extra careful about oral hygiene, so that the tissues can heal as rapidly as possible with the formation of a gingival col between the roots.

At this stage, if the furcal arch is narrow, an orthodontic appliance can be used to increase the separation of the roots, provided there is sufficient room in the arch. Finally, if there is adequate bulk of coronal dentine, the roots are built up with amalgam, otherwise cast cores with post retention are cemented. Gold or bonded porcelain crowns are made in the form of premolars with good clearance gingivally to aid marginal cleansing. It is also possible to restore the tooth as a molar with a high furcation to permit easy insertion of a floss threader.

Case presentation (895-907)

897

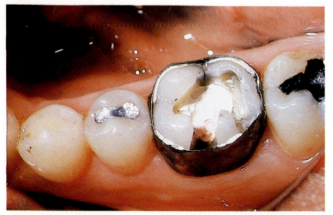

897 Root treatment completed. The fracture line is visible.

898

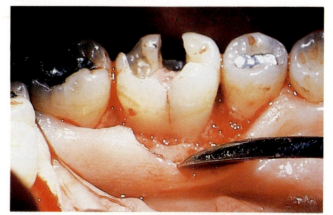

898 Reflection of a buccal flap.

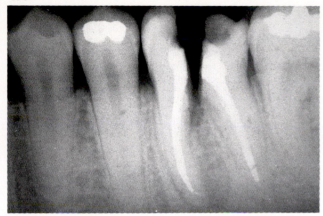

899 Crown hemisected.

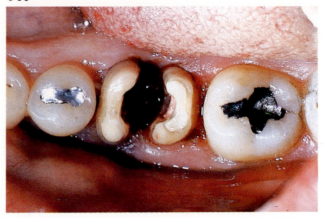

900 Separation of the roots.

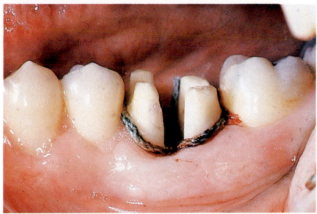

901 Retraction of the gingivae with cord and an astringent solution.

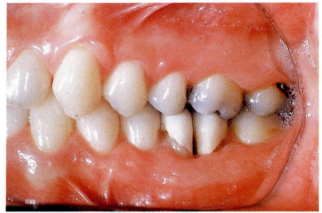

902 Temporary acrylic crowns cemented (buccal aspect).

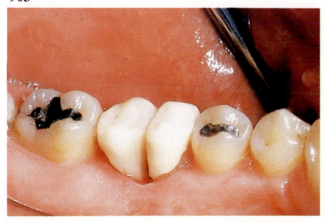

903 Temporary acrylic crowns cemented (lingual aspect).

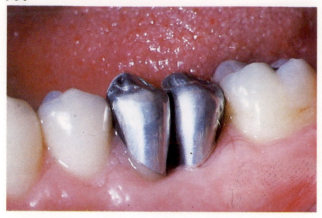

904

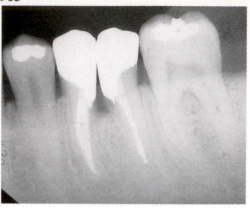

905

904, 905 Amalgam cores constructed when the soft tissues have healed.

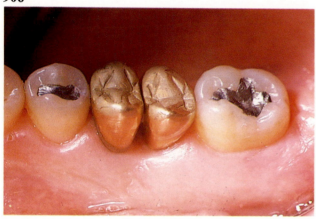

906

906, 907 Gold crowns cemented (Note wide proximal embrasure).

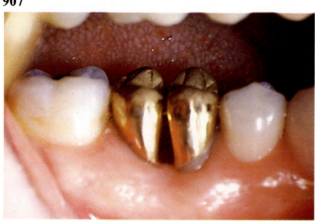

907

INSTRUMENTS FOR PLANNED REPLANTATION OR HEMISECTION

Local anaesthetic, syringe and needle
Sterile towels (disposable)
Absorbent gauze swabs
Paper points
Straight handpiece and cover for flexible drive
Bowl of isotonic saline and irrigation syringe
Scalpel with no 15 blade (Bard-Parker)
A selection of excavators (caries) for curettage
Curved mosquito forceps
Needle and suture
Fine straight scissors
Straight probe no 6
Briault probe
Flat plastic instrument (Ash no 56)
Burnisher (Baldwin) and an assortment of amalgam condensers
Mouth mirror
Dressing forceps
Steel burs   round I, 3
             fissure 2
             1.5 mm cylindrical diamond or carborundum stone
Apical amalgam carrier — Produits Dentaires
Amalgam well; alloy and mercury
Extraction forceps
Root elevators
Copal-ether varnish
Insufflator with iodoform powder or Stomahesive

16　The Endo Perio Lesion C J Stock

Classification

Periodontology and endodontology are often considered as two separate entities yet clinically they are closely related and this must influence our diagnosis and treatment. There is no doubt that either inflammation or necrosis of the pulp will affect the periodontal tissues, but there is some dispute concerning the degree of influence that periodontal disease may have on a vital pulp. Communication between the periodontal and pulpal tissues may be via the apical foramina, lateral canals, root fractures or perforations. The incidence of lateral canals is shown in the table below. Lateral canals should be considered channels of communication which are capable of allowing noxious material or micro-organisms to pass in either direction.

There are several ways of classifying endo perio lesions so that the primary aetiological factors can be identified. The classification given below is a modification of Simon, Glick and Franks classification (1972).

INCIDENCE OF LATERAL CANALS

		Teeth	Number of Teeth	% Lateral Canals
Rubach and Mitchell	(1965)	All teeth	74	45
Lowman et al	(1973)	Maxillary and mandibular molars	46	59
Vertucci and Williams	(1985)	Mandibular 1st Molars	100	46
Burch and Hulen	(1974)	Furcation of Maxillary and mandibular molars	195	76
Kirkham	(1975)	Teeth with Accessory Canals in perio pockets	100	23
De Deus	(1975)	All teeth	1140	27.4
Guttman	(1978)	Furcation of Molars	102	28.4
Vertucci and Gegauff	(1979)	Maxillary 1st Molars	400	49

CLASS 1 — PRIMARY ENDODONTIC LESION DRAINING THROUGH THE PERIODONTAL LIGAMENT

908

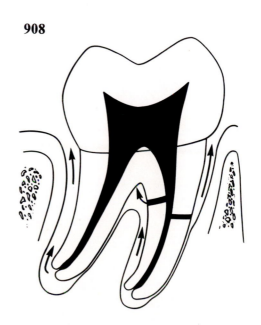

These lesions present as an isolated periodontal pocket or swelling on the side of the tooth (**908**). The patient rarely complains of pain although there will usually be a history of an acute episode. The tooth concerned will not respond to vitality tests. The lesions are caused by a necrotic pulp draining through the periodontal ligament. A sinus tract may occur from an apical foramen and/or a lateral canal. The furcation area of both premolar and molar teeth may be involved, diagnostically one should suspect a pulpally induced lesion when the crestal bone levels on the mesial and distal aspects of the tooth appear normal and only the furcation area is radiolucent. The prognosis following root treatment is good.

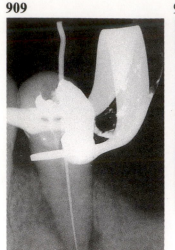

909

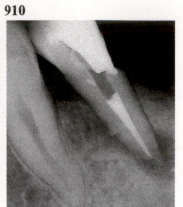

910

Three cases are shown to illustrate the Class 1 lesion.

Case 1 (**909, 910**). Notice the periapical radiolucent area and the area associated with the mesial aspect of the root. There is good crestal bone level on both the mesial and distal aspects of the tooth. The patient had an acute episode of pain and swelling but had taken antibiotics. On examination there was a discharge from the gingival crevice buccally. The second radiograph of the completed root treatment shows a lateral canal which has been filled with sealer.

912

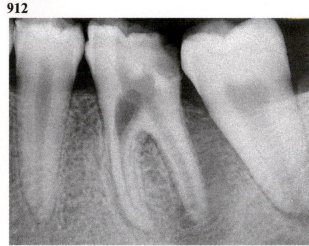

911

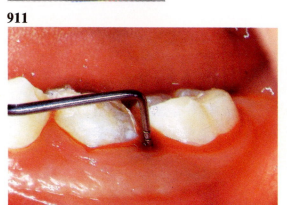

Case 2 (**911, 912**). A grossly broken down pulpless lower left first molar with internal resorption and a pocket to the apex on the distal aspect of the distal root. The radiograph shows considerable bone loss associated with the distal root. The canals were cleaned, prepared and filled with calcium hydroxide. The patient returned in six weeks (**913, 914**) and the tooth was root filled. The gingival condition was healthy with no pocketing and the post-operative radiograph shows evidence of bony healing.

914

913

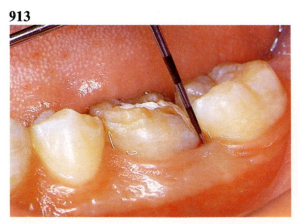

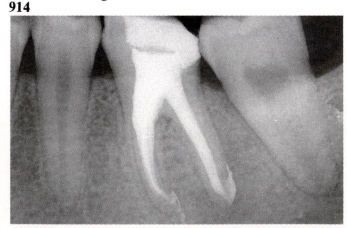

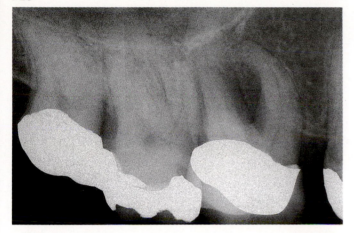

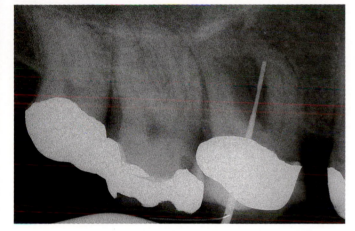

Case 3 (**915, 916**). The maxillary molar has a full crown which makes testing the vitality of the pulp difficult. There is a trifurcation involvement which can be probed from the buccal aspect. Palpating the buccal gingivae and the buccal roots produced a discharge of pus. Careful examination of the first and second radiographs show a widened periodontal ligament space around the apical portion of the mesio-buccal root. Bone levels mesially and distally were normal and the lesion was isolated. A test cavity revealed that the tooth was pulpless. The postoperative radiograph (**917**) shows a lateral canal on the mesial aspect of the disto-buccal root (arrow). A follow-up 5 months later (**918**) shows bony healing in the furcation.

CLASS 1: PRIMARY ENDODONTIC LESION DRAINING THROUGH THE PERIODONTAL LIGAMENT

Diagnosis	*Treatment*
1 Necrotic pulp with discharge via pdl space.	1 Root canal treatment.
2 Isolated lesion.	2 Review 4-6/12 for healing of periodontal pocketing and bone repair.
3 Good crestal bone levels on both the mesial and distal aspects of tooth.	3 Prognosis good.
4 Root surface in pocket contains minimal plaque or calculus.	

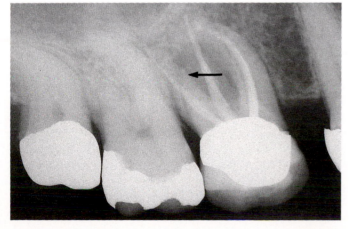

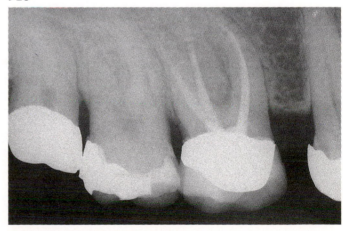

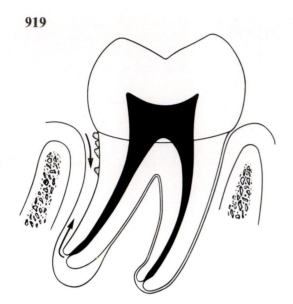

CLASS 2 — PRIMARY ENDODONTIC LESION WITH SECONDARY PERIODONTAL INVOLVEMENT

If left untreated the primary endodontic lesion may become secondarily involved with periodontal breakdown (919). Endodontic treatment will heal part of the lesion but complete repair will involve periodontal therapy. The prognosis is generally good.

920

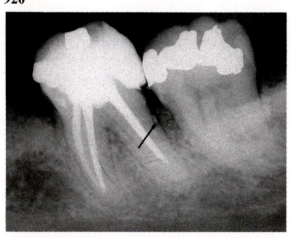

Case 1 (920). 5.00 mm pocketing found between molar teeth. The mesial molar had been inadequately root treated. There was inter-proximal gingival inflammation which was isolated to the area between the molars. Re-root treatment of the molar demonstrated the lateral canal (arrow) in the distal root opening near the base of the pocket on the distal root surface. Periodontal treatment in the form of a deep scale and oral hygiene instruction was carried out.

921

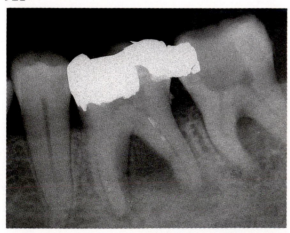

Case 2 (921). Both molar teeth had been left open to drain due to periapical abscesses. There was generalised periodontal involvement. Note calculus on the distal root surface of the first molar. Molar root treatment demonstrated the primary cause of the furcation area was probably of endodontic origin (922). The final radiograph taken one year later showed healing had taken place (923). The patient had improved her oral hygiene but had not returned as advised to her dentist for permanent restoration of the molar teeth. Note that calculus still remains on the distal aspect of the first molar and must be removed before complete healing of the periodontal tissues can occur.

922

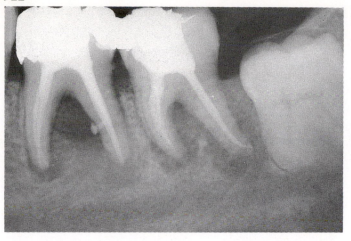

923

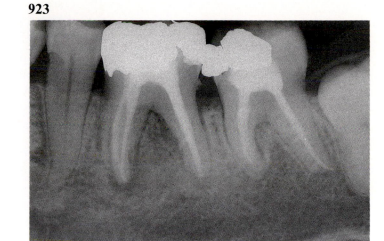

924

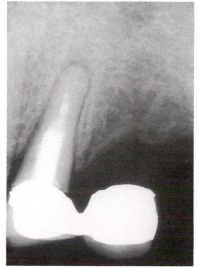

925

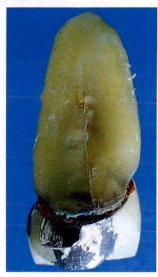

Case 3 (924). The tooth had been tender to touch since the post crown was fitted 8 months previously. The generalised widened periodontal ligament space and large post suggested a possible vertical fracture in the root. The fracture is visible in the distal aspect of the extracted root (925).

CLASS 2: PRIMARY ENDODONTIC LESION WITH SECONDARY PERIODONTAL INVOLVEMENT

Diagnosis	*Treatment*
1 Necrotic pulp or other source of irritation to the periodontium from the root such as a poorly obturated root filling or root fracture.	1 Root treatment or re-root treatment.
2 Isolated deep pocket although there may be generalised periodontal disease.	2 Periodontal treatment will be required.
3 Periodontal breakdown with calculus or plaque present in the pocket.	3 Vertical fractures are invariably untreatable and the tooth is extracted.
	4 Prognosis generally good.

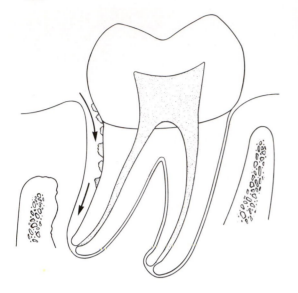

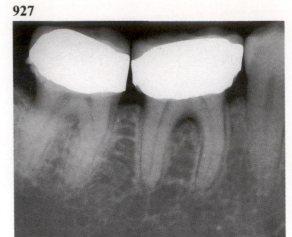

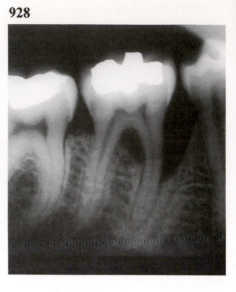

CLASS 3 — PRIMARY PERIODONTAL LESIONS

These lesions are caused by periodontal disease (926). Periodontitis slowly advances down the root surface until the apex is reached. The pulp will be vital in the early stages but may become affected as the disease progresses (see Class 4 below). The tooth will become mobile as the attachment apparatus and surrounding bone are destroyed leaving deep periodontal pocketing. Probing may detect calculus and plaque within the periodontal pocket. The periodontal involvement will not be confined in general to one tooth, except in the case of a palatal developmental groove. The prognosis for primary periodontal lesions becomes worse as the disease advances.

Case 1 (927). The patient complained of discomfort in the first molar area. A radiograph shows a furcation radiolucency. Oral hygiene was poor and the crowns were bulbous and contained ledges. A test cavity cut through the crown into dentine produced a vital pulp response. The furcation area could be probed. The treatment consisted of oral hygiene instruction and replacement of both the crowns.

Case 2 (928). The periodontal lesion involving the mesial root of a vital lower right first molar (928). The pulp was removed and the distal root canal prepared and filled (929). Amalgam was placed in the pulp chamber and the entrance to the mesial root canals. The mesial root was then resected leaving a smooth surface easily cleaned by the patient (930). The final radiograph taken three months later shows some healing of the bone (931).

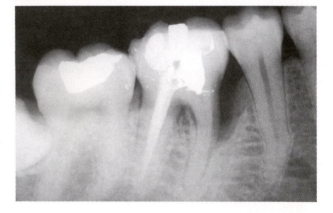

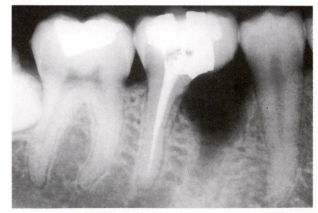

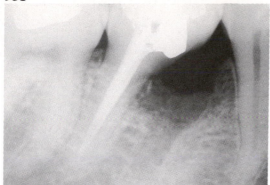

931

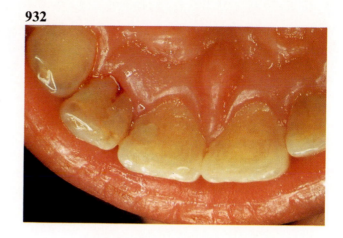

932

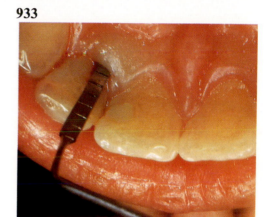

933

Case 3 (**932**).   The lateral incisor was painful to touch. Oral hygiene was barely adequate. The palatal gingivae around the lateral incisor were inflamed (**932, 933**). A 6.0 mm pocket was evident and a cingulum groove noted. The tooth was vital to the pulp test. The radiograph showed a deep groove with an apparent vestigial root mesial to the main root (**934**). These cases present considerable problems in treatment. A palatal flap was reflected and the groove cleaned thoroughly. The prognosis is poor if the groove travels the full length of the root. Sometimes the groove disappears well short of the apex and in these cases it may be possible to reposition the gingival tissues so that the entire groove is exposed.

CLASS 3: PRIMARY PERIODONTAL LESIONS

Diagnosis	*Treatment*
1 Pulp is vital.	1 Oral hygiene advice, scaling and root planing.
2 Description of the pain is periodontal rather than pulpal. It is a chronic localised discomfort sometimes relieved by biting on the tooth.	2 Removal of cause such as a poor restoration. Developmental grooves once they are periodontally involved are difficult to treat successfully.
3 Periodontal breakdown with calculus or plaque present within the pocket.	3 Periodontal surgery may be indicated.
	4 Prognosis becomes worse as the disease advances.

934

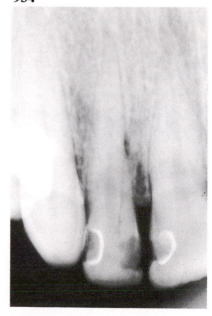

CLASS 4: PRIMARY PERIODONTAL LESIONS WITH SECONDARY ENDODONTIC INVOLVEMENT (935)

There is considerable controversy concerning the extent of pulpal involvement. Langeland's view (1974) is that the tooth will remain vital until all the main foramina are involved with dental plaque. Despite this view there is evidence (Rubach and Mitchell 1964) that the pulps of periodontally involved teeth may become inflamed. The periodontal procedure of root planing may interfere with the blood supply to part of the pulp through lateral canals or may remove cementum from previously sealed lateral canals. There is also evidence to suggest that root treatment of terminal cases of periodontal disease which have not responded to periodontal therapy is recommended. The prognosis for these lesions is poor.

935

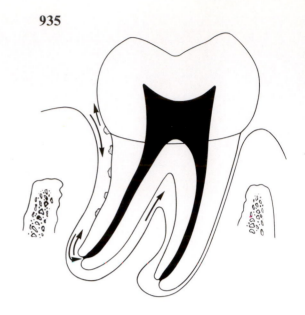

Case 1 (**936**). The patient complained of discomfort from distal abutment of bridge. Finger pressure on the gingival tissue around the tooth produced a frank discharge of pus. Deep pocketing to the apex, demonstrated by the insertion of a gutta percha point (**937**) was present both buccally and mesially. The electric pulp tester indicated a necrotic pulp. On removal of the bridge the tooth was very loose (mobility 3). The tooth was extracted.

936

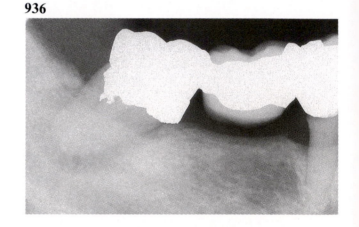

937

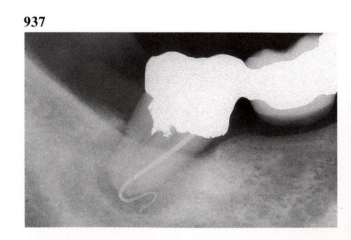

Case 2 (**938**). Long history of mild discomfort with upper left first molar. On examination there was a palatal discharge of pus. The tooth gave an indeterminate response to vitality and the radiograph shows a gutta percha point in a periodontal pocket to the apex of the palatal root. The tooth was root treated; the pulp in the buccal canals was found to be vital and that in the palatal canal was necrotic. The palatal root was amputated (**939**). A follow-up radiograph three months later showed good healing of both bone and periodontal tissues (**940**). The clinical appearance (**941**) was satisfactory. The depth of sulcus on the palatal aspect was normal.

938

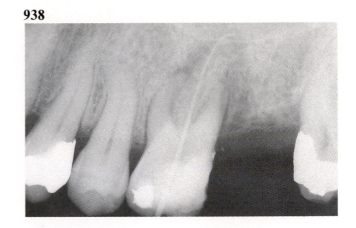

939

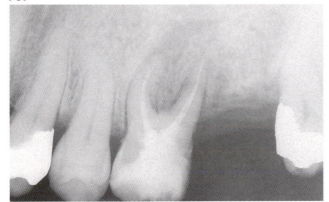

940

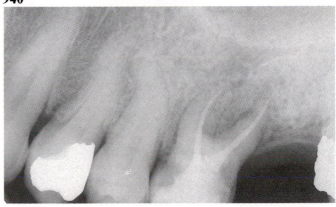

941

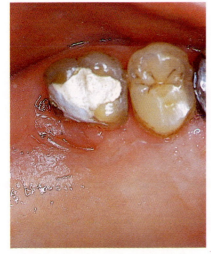

CLASS 4: PRIMARY PERIODONTAL LESIONS WITH SECONDARY ENDODONTIC INVOLVEMENT

Diagnosis

1 Non-vital pulp.

2 Long standing periodontal involvement with deep pocketing to the root apex. Plaque and calculus present in the pocket.

3 Discharge usually present from the pocket on palpation.

4 Tooth mobile in the majority of cases.

5 Generalised periodontal disease will often be present except in the case of a palatal groove or root fracture.

Treatment

1 Root treatment or re-root treatment.

2 Periodontal treatment will be required in some cases with surgery.

3 Prognosis poor.

233

942

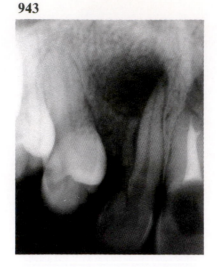

943

Case 3 (**942, 943**). The patient had a history of recurrent pain and swelling associated with upper right lateral incisor. The tooth had a developmental groove and the pulp was non-vital. Root canal therapy was carried out to no avail (**944**) and the tooth was extracted (**945**).

944

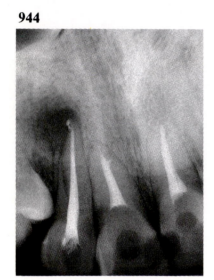

945

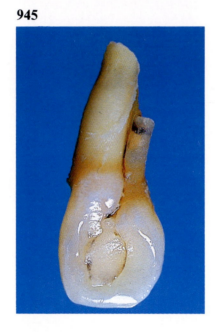

Simon's classification describes a Class 5 termed the true combined lesion. In the author's opinion it is difficult to distinguish between a lesion of periodontal origin with endodontic involvement and a true combined lesion. In addition clinically it is not necessary to distinguish between the two classes as the treatment is the same. It is for these reasons that the Class 5 has been omitted. Despite this there are many cases when it is difficult to determine whether the primary aetiology was periodontal or endodontic in origin, that is Class 2 or Class 4.

946

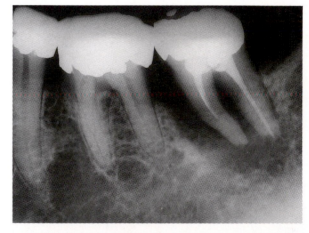

946 illustrates the difficulty in diagnosing the primary aetiology. In this case the patient, aged 48, had poor oral hygiene with several areas of alveolar bone loss. The lower left second molar had been poorly root treated four years ago.

Root Canal Treatment and Root Removal

In cases where there is advanced periodontal disease associated with multi-rooted teeth, treatment may involve the removal of one or occasionally two roots. Root canal treatment will be required in all cases of root removal. Before embarking on this form of treatment the operator should consider carefully the obvious alternative which is to extract the tooth and provide some form of fixed or removable prosthesis. Teeth with resected roots are difficult to maintain by the patient and require considerable skill by the operator to restore. As a guide the following factors should be considered before root resection.

(1) Functional tooth. The tooth should be a functional member of the dentition.

(2) Root filling. It should be possible to provide root canal treatment which has a good prognosis. In other words the root canals must be fully negotiable.

(3) Anatomy. The roots should be separate with some inter-radicular bone so that the removal of one root will not damage the remaining root(s). Access to the tooth must be sufficient to allow the correct angulation of the handpiece to remove the root. A small mouth may contra-indicate the procedure.

(4) Restorable. Sufficient tooth structure must remain to allow the tooth to be restored. The finishing line of the restoration must be envisaged to ensure that it can be cleaned by the patient.

(5) Patient suitability. The patient must be a suitable candidate for the lengthy operative procedures and be able to maintain a high standard of oral cleanliness around the sectioned tooth. The surgical removal of a root must be planned with care, particularly the timing of the root treatment. The problem arises when it is not always possible to decide which root should be removed until a flap has been reflected and a clinical assessment made of the extent of the bone loss around each root.

TIMING OF ROOT CANAL TREATMENT

1 When it is decided prior to surgery which root is to be removed.

Root canal treatment is carried out on the root or roots which are to be retained. The canal in the root(s) which is to be removed is briefly instrumented and then the coronal 2-3 mm are widened with a round bur or large Gates Glidden bur. The coronal portion of the canal is filled with amalgam as shown (**947**).

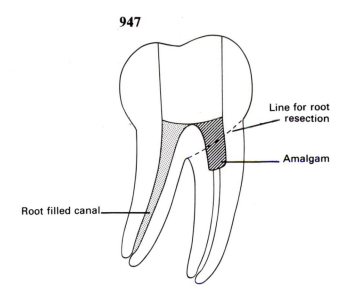

947

Line for root resection

Amalgam

Root filled canal

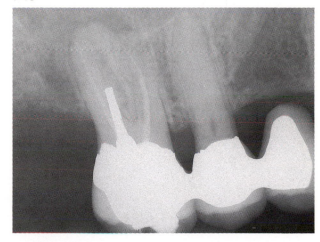

948 Root canal therapy of the first molar has been completed in the buccal canals. Amalgam has been packed several millimetres into the palatal canal ready for its resection.

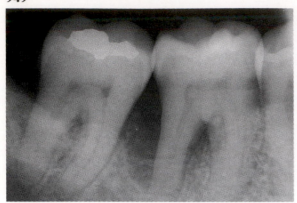

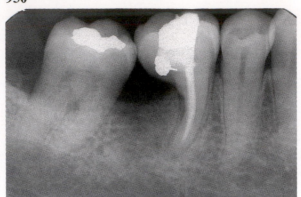

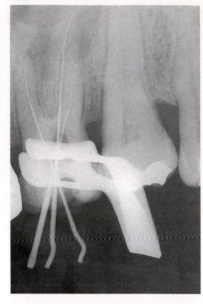

2   When it is decided during surgery which root is to be removed.

949, 950   The distal root is periodontally involved and the tooth is vital (Class 3). The mesial canals have been filled and amalgam placed in the entrance to the distal canal. The root was then resected.

Vital pulp   When the pulp is vital (Class 3) the root is removed leaving the pulp exposed (Tagger and Smukler 1977). The root canal treatment should be started in 10-14 days. An alternative is to extirpate the pulp prior to surgery and place a retrograde temporary dressing of zinc oxide at the time of operation.

Necrotic pulp   Prior to surgery all the canals are cleaned and prepared and a coronal seal inserted. A temporary retrograde seal is placed during surgery and the root treatment completed after periodontal healing in 2-3 months. A permanent seal with amalgam is placed by cutting a cavity within the canal orifice as described in 1 (page 235).

3   When the removal of the root is delayed.

In some cases the root canal treatment is carried out and the endodontic surgery delayed for 4-6 months so that the degree of healing may be assessed. This is the treatment of choice when it is not clear how much bone regeneration will occur after root canal treatment. This is often the case in Class 4 cases. On occasion healing progresses to such an extent that root removal is no longer necessary. All the root canals are prepared and filled and then part of the root filling is removed from the coronal portion of the canal in the suspect root and replaced with amalgam (**951, 952**).

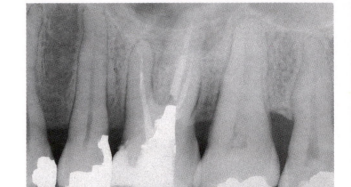

17   Root Resorption C J Stock

DEFINITION

Root resorption is either a physiologic or pathologic process which results in the loss of cementum or dentine. The process is initiated either outside the tooth giving rise to external resorption or from within the pulp where it is termed internal resorption.

TYPES OF RESORPTION

There are several different types of both internal and external resorption recognised clinically but no classification has been recognised universally. At a histological level there is little difference between the various types.

EXTERNAL RESORPTION

There are many factors both general and local which cause external resorption (Pindborg 1970). In the area of the periodontal ligament any alteration of the delicate balance between osteoblastic and osteoclastic action will initiate a build-up of cementum on the root surface (hypercementosis) or its removal together with dentine. Osteoclastic activity will predominate in an acid environment and this will occur in the presence of trauma or infection. External resorption may be found in the following conditions:

Periodontal disease	Calcinosis
Luxation injuries	Gauchers disease
Radiation therapy	Turner's syndrome
Hypoparathyroidism	Paget's disease
Hyperparathyroidism	

953

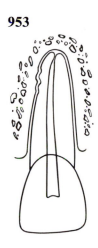

Surface resorption is a common pathological occurrence (Massler and Malone 1972) (**953**). The root surface shows superficial resorption lacunae repaired with new cementum. These lacunae have been termed surface resorption and presumably occur as a response to localised injury to the periodontal ligament or cementum. The condition is self limiting and shows spontaneous repair. It is not usually visible on a radiograph.

954

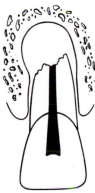

Inflammatory resorption is thought to be caused by the presence of infected or necrotic pulp tissue in the root canal (**954**). The cementum, dentine and adjacent periodontal tissue are affected and appear radiographically as a radiolucent area. The main sites affected will be around the apical foramina and lateral canal openings. It may occur in any tooth with a necrotic pulp (**955**).

955

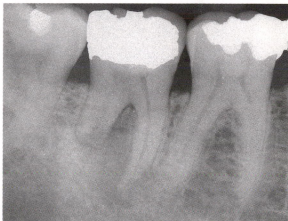

955 History of discomfort after the crown was fitted 4 years previously. Tooth now symptomless. The pulp was necrotic and both the mesial and distal roots show resorption.

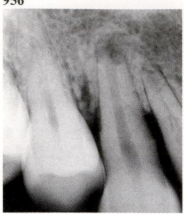

956 The canine had been auto transplanted 18 months previously but no root treatment had been carried out. The canal is wider than normal and does not narrow near the root apex. There is obvious apical resorption with a radiolucent area.

957 In some cases, particularly maxillary posteriors, resorption may be difficult to detect on the radiograph. The first molar had a history of pain on hot and cold and an intermittent dull ache. The tooth was root filled but the dull ache continued (**958**). An area of radiolucency is discernable on the palatal root and this was resected. The external resorptive area is evident on the buccal aspect of the palatal root (**959**).

959

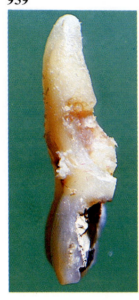

957

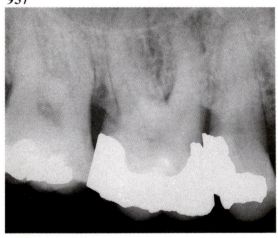

958

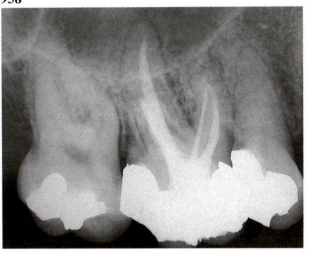

960

Replacement is also referred to as ankylosis. There is a direct union between bone and root substance. The bone gradually replaces the tooth substance (**960**). The condition occurs as a response to trauma and is diagnosed radiographically by a progressive disappearance of the periodontal ligament space and the root substance. This type of resorption has been well described by Andreasen (1981).

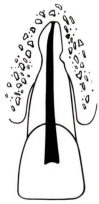

961 This case shows the result of two separate incidents of trauma. At the age of 7 years the upper left central crown was fractured in a fall, the tooth subsequently became abscessed and was root treated. Follow-up radiographs over 3 years show no evidence of breakdown (**962, 963**).

The upper right central was avulsed at age 8 years and replanted 2 hours later. The tooth was then root filled and a postoperative radiograph taken (**961**). A check radiograph (**962**) taken 2½ years later. Note the onset of replacement resorption in upper right central shows an almost complete loss of the middle portion of the root. The tooth was infra occluded by 2 mm.

The final radiograph (**963**) was taken 3 years after replantation. The tooth was extracted and is seen with almost no root substance remaining (**964**).

961

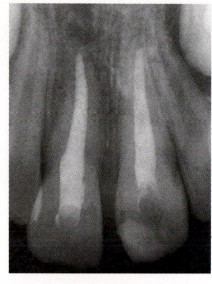

962

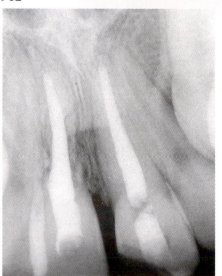

963

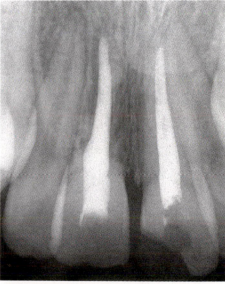

964

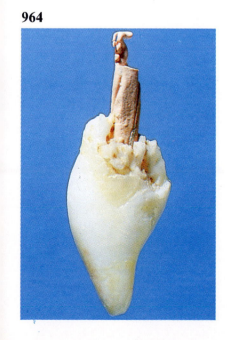

965

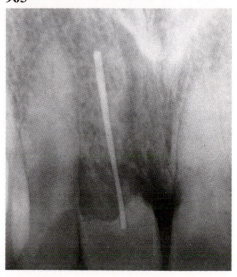

965 Patient aged 22 years had a history of avulsion of upper right central some 10 years previously. The tooth had been root filled probably before replanting as there is no access cavity and the shape of the cone is broader at the apex. Almost total replacement resorption has occurred.

Pressure Resorption due to pressure (966) may be caused by:

Erupting or impacted teeth
Orthodontic movement
Trauma from occlusion
Pathologic tissue eg slow growing cysts or neoplasms.

966

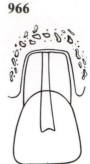

967

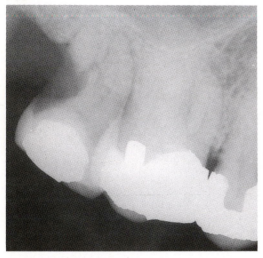

968

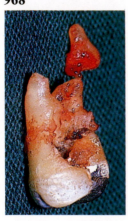

967, 968 The distal aspect of the maxillary second molar has been resorbed by the impacted third molar, and was extracted. The resorption extended into the pulp chamber as may be seen in the photograph of the extracted tooth.

969 Pressure resorption which is due to orthodontic movement, is a relatively rare occurrence. The root tends to have a cut off appearance at the apex.

970 Orthodontic treatment to retrocline the four incisor teeth had recently been completed. All the apices show typical blunting seen in resorption due to pressure.

969

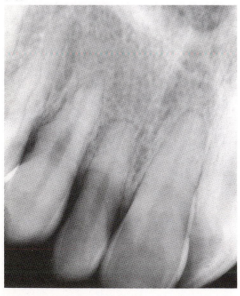

970

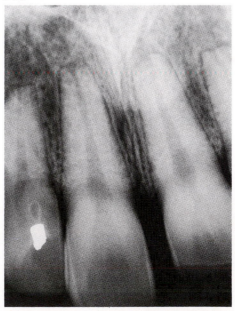

Idiopathic In some cases of external resorption neither a local nor systemic cause can be found. The root apices may be rounded and the teeth shorter than normal with several teeth affected. Another variety occurs which is more aggressive and affects the cervical aspect of the root. Two different types of idiopathic resorption have been described. Apical resorption is usually slow and may arrest spontaneously. One or several teeth may be affected with a gradual shortening of the root. The apices remain rounded and the periodontal ligament space is normal in width.

971, 972, 973 Female aged 34 years with no symptoms. Radiographs show a generalised shortening of the roots. The patient was healthy with no systemic disease. The only possible cause was that the patient was a bruxist. An occlusal splint was constructed.

971

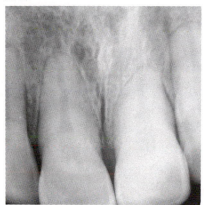

972

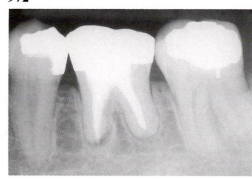

973

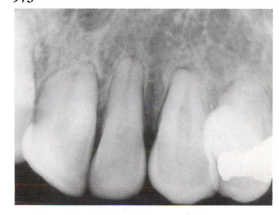

Cervical resorption is initiated in the cervical area of the tooth and may present clinically in two different forms. The defect occurs as either a wide shallow crater or conversely a burrowing type of resorption. In the crater form the resorption may be aggressive involving several teeth with the destruction of large amounts of dentine, or slow with only one tooth being involved.

974, 975, 976 Female aged 18 years with aggressive widespread external idiopathic cervical resorption. The premolars on the left side show resorption in both arches but the right side is unaffected. Some attempt at repair has been made. The mandibular incisors are the worst and the right side of the mouth the least affected.

974

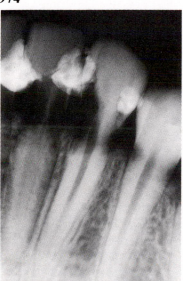

975

976

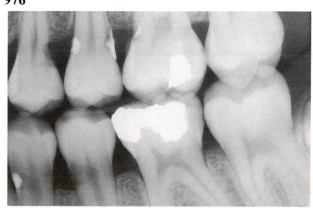

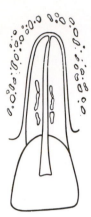

977

The burrowing type of cervical resorption has been described variously as peripheral cervical resorption, burrowing resorption, pseudo pink spot, resorption extra camerale and, more recently extra canal invasive (**977**). The resorption is characterised by a small defect on the surface of the root in the cervical area which then burrows deep into the dentine causing extensive tunnel-shaped ramifications. It does not as a rule affect the dentine and predentine surrounding the pulp which is left intact. The lesion is easily mistaken radiographically for internal resorption. The cause of cervical resorption is unknown but may be due to either chronic inflammation of the periodontal ligament or trauma.

978 The lower right second premolar shows an area of radiolucency overlying the root canal. No external root resorption could be detected and pocketing was minimal. Burrowing cervical resorption was diagnosed.

978

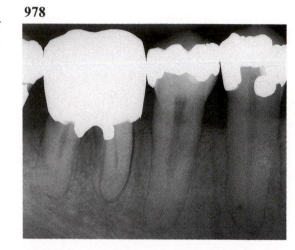

979

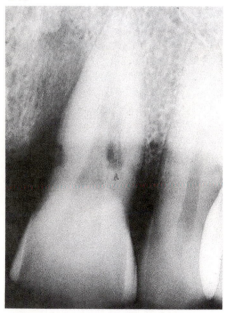

980

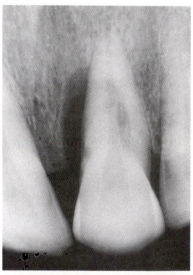

981

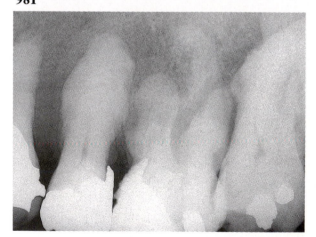

979, 980 Male aged 44 years complained of occasional episodes of pain and swelling associated with the palatal gingivae overlying the upper left central. There was an isolated 8.0 mm pocket. The radiograph shows the typical appearance of burrowing resorption.

Systemic Some systemic conditions are listed at the beginning of this chapter. The resorption will usually occur at the apices of several teeth and its appearance will vary according to the condition.

981 The radiograph shows a typical 'cotton wool' appearance of the bone and hypercementosis in Paget's disease. In addition there is resorption of the mesio-buccal and palatal roots of the first molar.

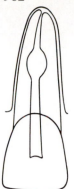

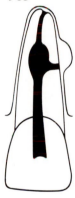

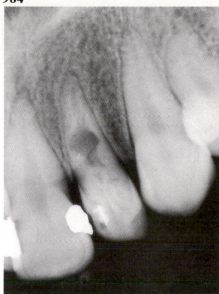

984

985

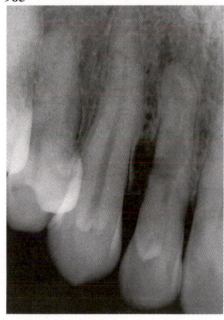

INTERNAL RESORPTION

The aetiology of internal resorption is not known but is the result of a chronic pulpitis. The resorption may be idiopathic or follow trauma, caries or iatrogenic procedures such as tooth preparation.

The typical radiographic appearance is a smooth widening of the root canal walls (**982**). When the pulp chamber is affected it may appear as 'pink spot' as the enlarged pulp is visible through the thin wall of the crown. Any tooth may be affected. The pulp usually remains vital and symptomless until the root has been perforated when it will rapidly become necrotic (**983**).

984 Upper left lateral showing internal resorption in the middle third of the root. The tooth gave a vital response to pulp tests.

985 Upper right lateral incisor with extensive internal resorption in the apical and middle thirds of the canal. The radiolucent area in the distal aspect of the root suggests that the resorption has perforated. There was no response to pulp testing.

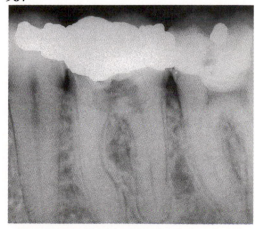

987

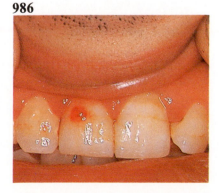

986

986 Clinical appearance of pink spot.

987 The pulp chamber in the lower left first molar is abnormally enlarged due to internal resorption. The tooth gave a vital response to the electric pulp tester and there were no symptoms. Note the irregular star shaped appearance of the resorption in contrast to **984** where it is smooth.

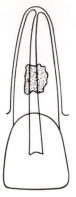

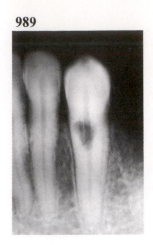

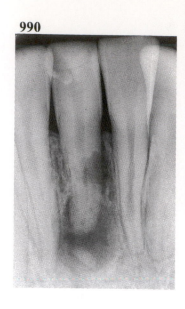

DIFFERENTIAL DIAGNOSIS

It is usually simple to differentiate between external and internal resorption. The diagram and radiograph (988, 989) show external resorption as an irregular radiolucent area overlying the root canal. The canal outline remains visible and intact. In internal resorption the outline of the canal is interrupted.

The radiograph (990) shows both internal and external resorption in adjacent teeth. The lower right central shows external resorption in the mesial aspect of the apical third of the root and some apical resorption. A history of trauma to these teeth suggests the cause, the apex of the lower right central appears to have been fractured. The lower right central is non-vital to the pulp tester and the lower left central is vital. There are two distinct areas of canal widening in the root suggesting internal resorption.

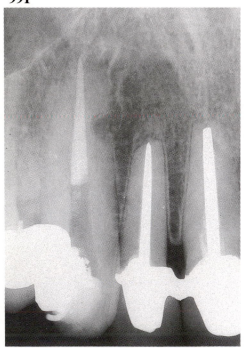

Differential diagnosis between external resorption and damage due to a bur may be more difficult. The case shown in 991 is easier because on close examination of the radiograph the periodontal ligament space is intact around the defect in the mesial aspect of the canine. The damage was inflicted when the upper left lateral was apicected some years previously.

992 The damage inflicted by a bur on both these central incisors is more difficult to differentiate from resorption. A careful case history left no doubt about the cause of the damage.

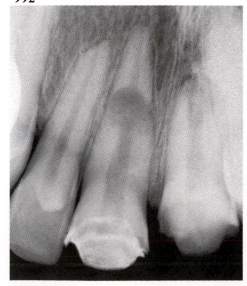

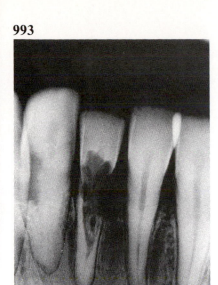

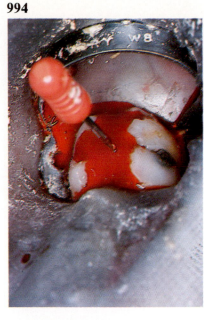

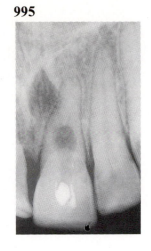

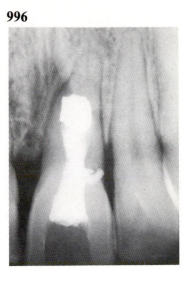

TREATMENT OF INTERNAL RESORPTION

When a chronically inflamed pulp is removed the internal resorption stops. If left untreated internal resorption will progress slowly or rapidly until the root is perforated. As soon as internal resorption has been diagnosed the pulp must be removed and the tooth root filled.

993 shows the amount of tooth destruction that can occur with internal resorption. As the condition is usually symptomless the patient does not attend seeking treatment.

The treatment of internal resorption follows the established aims of clean shape and fill. In cases where the resorption has perforated it is necessary to seal the defect. If the perforation is large and accessible to a surgical approach this will be the best form of treatment in addition to root filling.

Treatment Suggestions for Internal Resorption

(1) *Access.* It may be necessary to use burs or Gates Glidden drills to widen the access into the canal to reach as much of the canal walls as possible. A compromise must be made between weakening the tooth and providing access to a resorptive space.

(2) *Debridement.* Pulp tissue is removed both mechanically and by the use of copious amounts of Sodium hypochlorite. A 5 per cent solution of Sodium hypochlorite may be used so that organic material inaccessible to instrumentation may be dissolved. Endosonic agitation of the solution would be useful. Haemorrhage is a feature of internal resorptive tissue and can be difficult to control (**994**). Ledermix is a useful haemostat but complete cessation will be achieved only when all the pulp tissue has been removed.

(3) *Perforation.* The canal should be checked to see if there is a perforation. An electronic measuring device is helpful to explore the walls of the canal using an apically curved small file. Any perforation may be detected and its position and size noted. This is important in deciding if surgery is possible.

(4) *Canal Medication.* An inter appointment root canal dressing of calcium hydroxide should be used. If there is no perforation or only a small one the root may be filled at the second visit after the canal has been fully prepared.

When a large perforation is present and is inaccessible to surgical repair long term $Ca(OH)_2$ therapy is instituted. The regime for $Ca(OH)_2$ therapy is given in Chapter 13. The repair of the perforation will not be complete but the area of bone loss adjacent to it should have healed so that there will be minimum extrusion of filling material.

(5) *Root Filling.* There are several techniques for root filling the irregular root canal spaces. Compaction of warm gutta percha using a thermo-mechanical condensation technique has been employed by the author with success. The technique is described in Chapter 12.

(6) *Surgery.* A surgical approach is used when it is not possible to control the haemorrhage or the perforation is large and inaccessible to surgery. In **995, 996** the defect was situated buccally providing easy access for surgery.

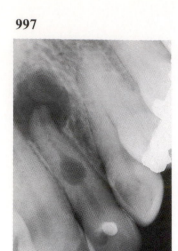

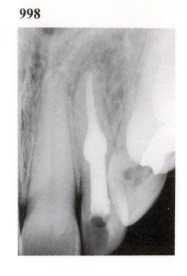

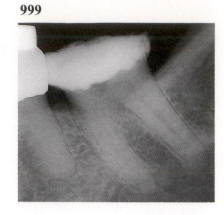

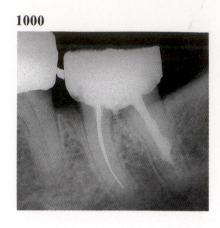

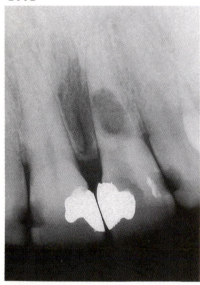

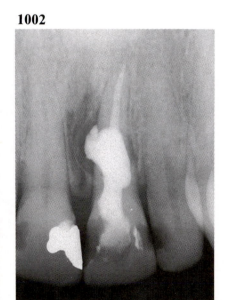

Five cases are shown of root canal treatment used to fill internal resorptive defects. **997/998** and **999/1000** were not perforated and were relatively simple to fill. **1001/1002** and **1003/1004** presented problems of initially arresting the haemorrhage and then achieving a dry canal.

The defects were sited on the lateral surface of the roots making it difficult to achieve a seal using the surgical approach. Ca(OH)$_2$ was used in both cases for 6-8 months prior to filling. The technique used was thermo-mechanical condensation. The final radiograph (**1004**) was taken 1 year later.

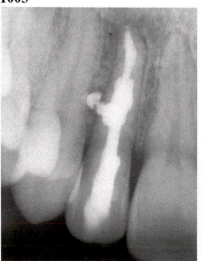

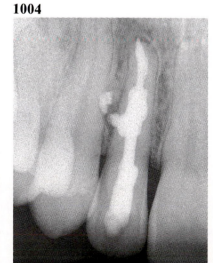

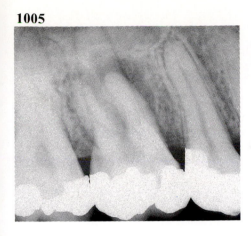

1005

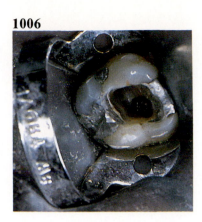

1006

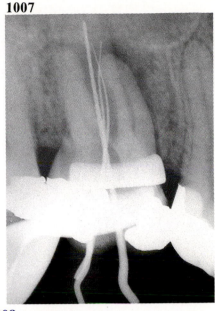

1007

1005, 1006 The upper right first molar had a large resorptive defect perforating the floor of the pulp chamber. The initial diagnostic instruments are through the perforation (**1007**). The pulp was extirpated and Ca(OH)$_2$ used for 3 weeks to dry the pulp chamber. A glass ionomer cement was used to repair the defect and the final radiograph (**1008**) was taken 3 months later. There were no symptoms or sinus and bony healing is evident.

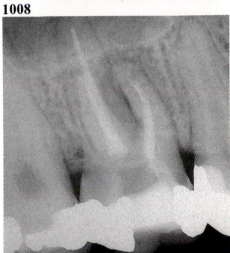

1008

TREATMENT OF EXTERNAL RESORPTION

The type of treatment will depend upon the cause of the resorption. If several teeth are affected a systemic or general cause is suspected. A history and clinical examination may reveal the systemic cause in which case local treatment may not be indicated unless the patient has symptoms. An obvious general cause should be treated, for example periodontal disease.

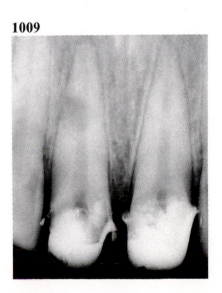

1009

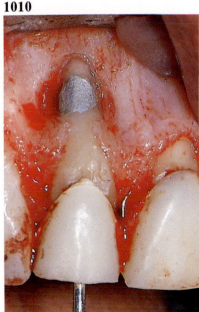

1010

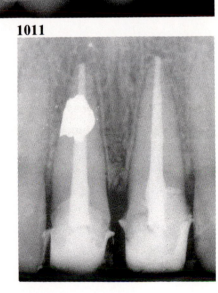

1011

247

When the resorption is restricted to one or two teeth then possible local causes are investigated. If there is any doubt about the vitality of the pulp in the affected tooth it should be extirpated and Ca(OH)$_2$ placed. This treatment will apply to all cases of inflammatory and replacement resorption and in many cases caused by pressure. Idiopathic cases may also benefit by placing Ca(OH)$_2$ in the root canal. The best treatment for external resorption in most cases is by prevention. Calcium hydroxide should be used in all cases of trauma such as avulsion, subluxation, intrusion and transplantation where root canal treatment is indicated.

Calcium hydroxide renders the pH more alkaline, favouring deposition rather than removal of hard tissue.

A surgical approach to external resorption is not usually indicated unless there is a communication with the oral cavity. The case shown (**1009, 1010, 1011**) may have been caused by a bur used by the operator in an attempt to relieve pain from an abscess in the upper right central, iatrogenic external resorption. In this case an external surgical repair in addition to root canal treatment was required.

1012

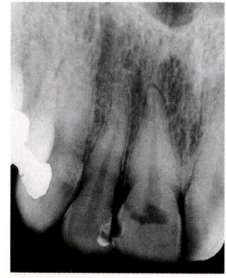

1013

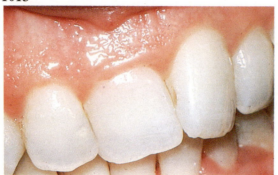

1014

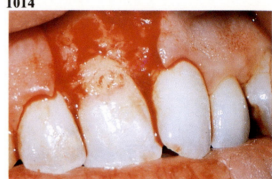

Cervical resorption may communicate with the oral cavity (**1012, 1013**). In these cases a surgical approach will be necessary to reflect a flap, clean the resorptive crater on the root surface, and repair with a restorative material (**1014**). The material used in the case shown was a glass ionomer cement (**1015, 1016**). The pulp reacted normally to pulp testing and so was retained. A calcium hydroxide liner was used to protect the pulp at the base of the defect.

1015

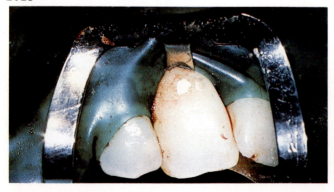

1016

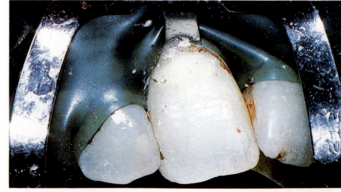

18 Removal of Root Canal Obstructions J. J. Messing

FRACTURED INSTRUMENTS — PREVENTION AND RETRIEVAL

One of the most time-consuming and frustrating side effects of endodontic treatment is the fracture of an endodontic instrument within a root canal. Prevention of such an accident is preferable to the effort, frequently abortive, expended in the retrieval of fractured portions.

1017

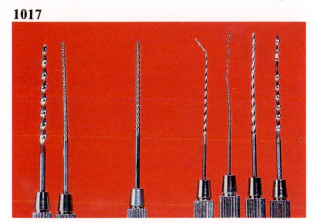

(a) unused instruments (b) blunt file... note shiny blades (c) distorted reamers and files — DISCARD.

Causes of Fracture
1. Over-use of the instrument.
2. Sterilisation at temperatures above 170°C (excepting the use of a glass bead steriliser, in which immersion of the instrument is solely for a period of 10-15 seconds).
3. Mishandling the instrument in the canal.
4. Faulty access cavity.
5. Faults in manufacture.

1 Over-use. The small diameter instruments are most at risk and should be used *once or twice* only and then discarded. As a rough guide, sizes 8-25 should be used once or twice, sizes 30-50 may be used twice and the larger sizes should be inspected after use for signs of bluntness or distortion, and rejected if either factor is apparent. Flaming of endodontic instruments is to be condemned out of hand, because it leaves them brittle and apt to fracture.

2 Sterilisation. When instruments are sterilised by dry heat, a temperature of 160°C for one hour is acceptable from a metallurgical viewpoint. After numerous repeated sterilisations, there is a tendency for the metal of some makes of instrument to become slightly brown in colour. This does not materially affect the properties of the large sizes, but an increased brittleness in the fine diameter reamers and files negates their further usefulness. Ideally, instruments should be stored sterile in glass phials, so that those not used will not suffer repeated thermal cycling. (See Chapter 5).

3 Mishandling. This constitutes the major cause of fracture. No endodontic instrument should be forced into a narrow canal. Barbed broaches and spiral fillers are especially prone to fracture and engine driven reamers invariably fracture, if they jam in a fine canal. No barbed broach or spiral filler should be used unless it can be inserted freely to the end of the canal.

Reamers and files, especially the finest sizes, should never be rotated more than one quarter turn in the first application, before being withdrawn, cleaned and reinserted. When the apical constriction has been reached, and it becomes possible to rotate the instrument without binding, the canal is irrigated and the next size of instrument is inserted. Filing is continued using a pulling action, whereas reamers operate only when rotated in a clockwise direction.
N.B. *Never miss out the next larger size.* Any attempt to rotate a reamer in a curved canal can lead to fracture of the reamer or perforation of the root.

If an instrument is jammed, great care must be taken to avoid reverse rotation because the distortion of the flutes leads quickly to fracture (**1017c**). The canal should be irrigated and then, using a pulling action coupled with a gentle, quarter turn, reciprocatory movement, disengagement can usually be achieved. Clockwise rotation of a jammed reamer or K type file tends to unwind the flutes (**1017c**), resulting ultimately in fracture. Such stresses are set up also in Hedstroem and similar files.

1018

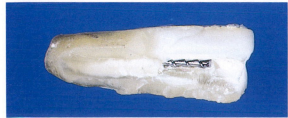

1018 Hedstroem file fractured in a root canal.

After each application of an endodontic instrument, it is mandatory that the flutes or blades of the instrument be checked for signs of damage. If any damage is found, immediate rejection is necessary.

Exerting excessive force when using fine instruments may lead to bending or kinking (**1017c**). Unless this is minimal, they should not be straightened, but replaced. Blunt endodontic instruments (**1017b**) are useless. Their continued use is false economy and the tendency to make them work by the application of greater force may lead to fracture (**1018**).

For endodontic preparation, a reciprocating handpiece has become increasingly popular. However, it should be used at speeds in the region of 1-2,000 rpm and with minimum force, otherwise fracture of instruments can occur. Peeso reamers and Gates Glidden drills similarly require a gentle touch. Their use for the total preparation of canals is to be condemned. They must fit the canal loosely before the engine is operated and be used for flaring the canals with a gentle circumferential pulling movement. They can also be used for removing gutta percha root fillings.

4 *Faulty access cavity.* It is a *sine qua non* that the access cavity must be prepared in a direct line with the root canal. In a multi-rooted tooth, extension of the cavity for each canal alignment is mandatory. In lower incisors, this will often result in involvement of part of the incisal margin lingually or even labially (**1019b, c**). Failure to observe this rule may lead to bending of the instrument with consequent risk of perforation of the root or fracture of an instrument, the flutes of which have undergone deformation due to jamming (**1019a**).

5 *Faults in manufacture.* Although rare, it is possible to have a flaw in a file or reamer which can lead to its fracture. It is difficult to assess whether such is the case when an instrument fractures in use. However, misuse is more likely to stress the defect, resulting in fracture.

It is salutary to note that the more experienced the operator, the lower the incidence of fractured files and reamers. Some endodontic instruments may vary in length by ∓ 1.0mm: this should be checked before root canal stops are adjusted.

1019

a   b   c

Retrieval of fractured instruments. When an instrument has been fractured near to the apex of the root, the ability to remove it is related to how closely it fits the canal and how tightly it has been forced against the walls, especially when the canal is curved. Grossman (1968) and Crump and Natkin (1970) have shown that, provided there is no rarefaction periapically, filling the canal as far as the obstruction will lead to a successful result in the majority of cases.

The old technique of dressing the canal with a strong solution of iodine, to corrode the steel, works only when the instrument is made of carbon steel. It is not effective with the vast majority of contemporary instruments which are manufactured in stainless steel. Consequently, the technique is out-dated.

1020

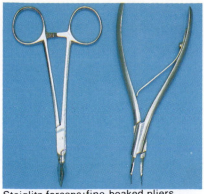

Steiglitz forceps: fine-beaked pliers

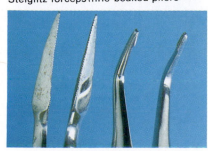

When the fractured part extends coronally into a flared portion of the canal, its removal is made easier. If it reaches the pulp chamber it may be possible to grasp it with Steiglitz forceps (**1020**) or tease it out with a fine sharp excavator or by wedging a Hedstroem file against it and pulling. If this is ineffective, a sharp tap on the beaks of pliers grasping the handle of the file, may dislodge the fragment (**1021**).

Frequently it is possible to insinuate a fine file past the fragment and reach the apical constriction. Then, by enlarging the space with ascending sizes of file, the canal may be prepared and filled, incorporating the fragment into the root filling (**1022**).

When such measures fail in known cases of periapical infection, the canal should be enlarged as wide as feasible up to the obstruction and filled with gutta percha and a sealer. Should symptoms persist or develop subsequently, surgical treatment will be indicated. As an alternative, the enlarged canal can be dressed with Biocalex.

The expansive effect of the reaction when the oxide is slaked — ($CaO + H_2O \rightarrow Ca(OH)_2$) may carry the calcium hydroxide beyond the obstruction and overcome the infection. After one or two dressings, the disappearance of symptoms and any existing sinus will indicate success, and the remainder of the canal can be filled forthwith.

The fracture of barbed broaches. The barbed broach was devised for extirpation of a vital pulp and its sole alternative function is the removal of entrapped fragments of cotton wool or paper points from a root canal. The most likely reason for fracture of a barbed broach is attempting to remove it from the canal when it has become lodged, and this occurs because it has been used in a canal which is the same size or smaller than the broach.

As a precautionary measure, barbed broaches should be used only in canals in which they do not bind against the walls. Otherwise, it is safer to eliminate pulpal tissue with files.

Removal of a fragment of a fractured barbed broach may be extremely difficult but it is best accomplished by attempting to bypass the fragment with fine files.

Alternatively, by widening the canal as far as the obstruction, so that a trephine can be inserted, it may be possible to cut away the dentine surrounding the fragment and thus release it.

1021

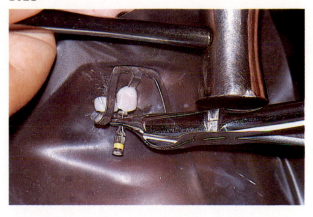

1022

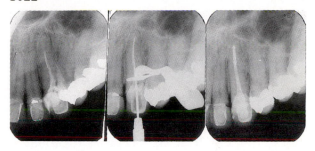

The Masseran technique. The mechanical removal of a fragment can be accomplished with the aid of a Masseran kit. A channel is cut around the fragment, extending approximately half its length, so that it may be grasped and removed. A fair amount of dentine is lost in the process and the instruments must be confined to the straight part of the canal. The Masseran kit is especially useful for the removal of fractured posts, instruments and metal points which are lodged within the coronal part of the canal.

1023

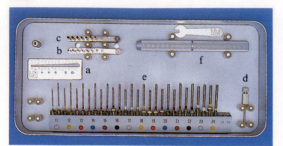

a flat gauge
b gauge 11-17
c gauge 18-24

d extractor
e trepan (long and short) 11-24
f handle

1024

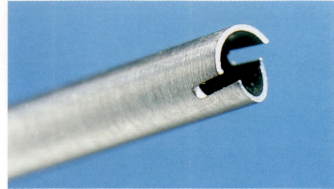

1025

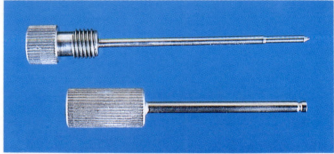

1026

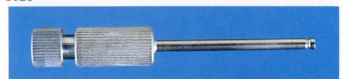

There are 14 different diameters of trepan (**1023**), varying from 1.1mm to 2.4mm, colour-coded for easy identification. There are two trepans of each diameter, one short and one long. The wall of the trepan is less than 0.25mm thick. Either the trepans may be screwed into the milled handle or mounted in a speed-reducing handpiece. The author recommends the use of the handle because greater control can be exercised than with a handpiece.

The smallest trepan that will fit around the fragment is selected by using one of the gauges provided. The trepan is pressed over the end of the fragment and turned in an anti-clockwise direction. Irrigation fluid or some other lubricant will facilitate this procedure. The trepan should be withdrawn from the canal after a few turns and the accumulated debris removed. Trepan burs (**1024**) are thin and easily damaged. However, they can be sharpened by the operator, following the instructions provided.

Removal of the fragment. The method of removal depends upon the site of the fragment. In the case of larger instruments, points and posts, a trepan one size smaller than that used to cut the channel is selected. The end of the trepan has to grip on to the metal until it is sufficiently secured to allow its removal by means of a twisting action combined with apically directed pressure.

If the fragment is sufficiently small an extractor may be used (**1025, 1026**). This consists of a rod which is screwed into a tube. Close to the end of the tube, internally, is a ridge against which the rod engages. The extractor is pushed over the partially freed fragment and the rod is screwed home, thus gripping the end of the fragment against the ridge and permitting its removal.

1027

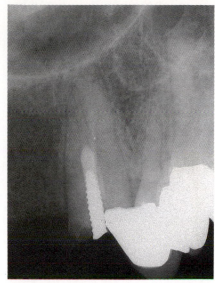

The series of illustrations (**1027-1034**) shows the removal of a fractured post.

1027 A fractured post in an upper left canine with an inadequate root filling.

1028 Clinical view of the post which has fractured at the level of the root face.

1029 A gauge is used to assess the size of trepan bur required.

1030 The trepan is fitted into the handle and a channel is cut by rotating it anti-clockwise.

1031 A narrow channel has been cut along half the length of the post.

1032, 1033 Fine beaked pliers were used to grip the end of the post which was then removed.

1034 Final radiograph showing the root treatment completed.

1028

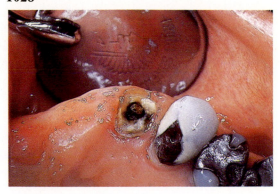

1029

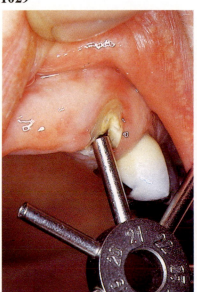

1030

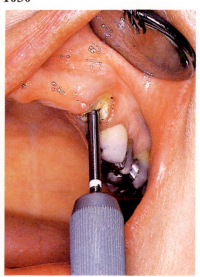

1031

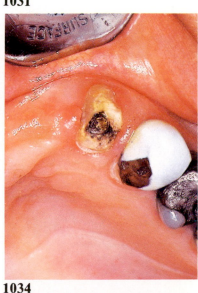

1032

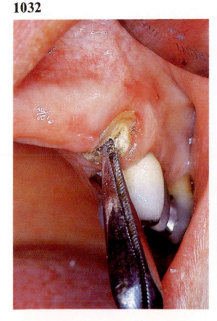

1033

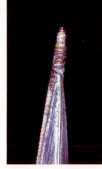

Note. Failure to remove or bypass the fragment, coupled with subsequent evidence of periapical pathosis will indicate the adoption of a surgical approach. Either extraction of the tooth, apicectomy or root resection (in a multi-rooted tooth) is indicated.

1034

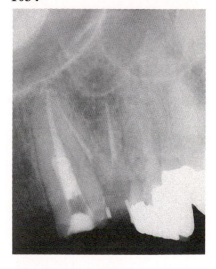

Apicectomy. After resection of the apex and disclosure of the fragment, it may be possible to remove it apically or push it coronally. If the latter approach is used, it may be removed from the tooth or, if this is impossible because a crown or bridge impedes access to the pulp chamber, it can be isolated by apical obturation with amalgam.

It cannot be over-emphasised that the patient must be informed immediately if an instrument is separated within the canal, and details should be recorded in his notes of the exact nature, position and length of the retained fragment. Thus, if litigation ensues, the facts are available.

REMOVAL OF POSTS

Situations occur in which posts and cores have to be removed. There are many reasons why this may be necessary but most frequently it is because the root canals have been inadequately filled. There are four ways in which a firmly cemented post can be removed.

(a) A post remover, such as the Eggler, may be used, provided there is a sufficient length of post or core protruding from the root. The Eggler consists of a knurled wheel which, when turned, tightens the jaws on to the coronal extension of the post or core. The flattened knob at the end of the instrument controls two feet which are lowered on to the shoulders of the root face on either side of the post. Because of the length of the instrument it is only suitable for use in the anterior part of the mouth.

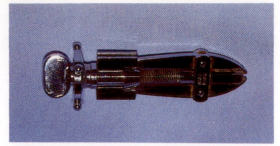

1035 The Eggler post remover.

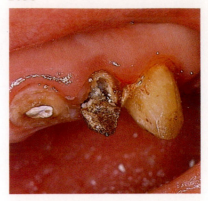

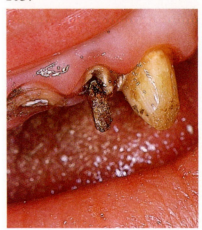

1036, 1037 The core must be reduced so that the mesial and distal aspects are parallel and do not overhang the shoulders of the preparation. Moreover, the buccal and lingual surfaces of the core must be adjusted so that the jaws can be aligned over them.

1038, 1039 The flattened knob is turned so that the two feet are lowered on to the shoulders of the preparation. It may be necessary to adjust the height of the shoulders to allow both feet to make simultaneous contact with the root face on either side of the post. Otherwise a non-axial force would be exerted, which could result in fracture of the root.

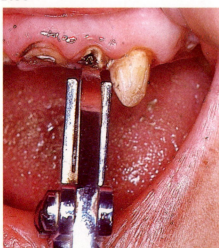

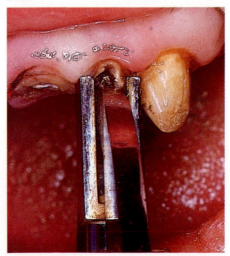

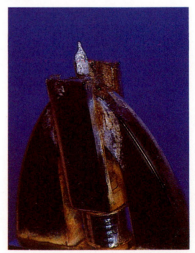

1040 The post is removed.

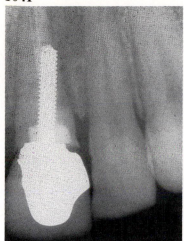

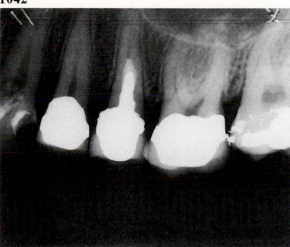

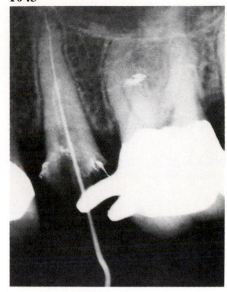

It is important to note that a post remover must never be used on a threaded post.

(b) A threaded post (**1041**) is usually simple to remove by gripping the coronal end with pliers and rotating it in an anti-clockwise direction. Occasionally, it may be necessary to cut a groove in the end of the post, thus converting it into a screw head so that it can be removed with a screwdriver.

(c) When it is not possible to use methods (a) or (b), the Masseran kit may be employed (see page 251).

(d) When access is poor or other methods ineffectual, it is necessary to drill out the post, using a tungsten carbide bur.

1042 A one-piece casting of nickel-chrome alloy. Great care must be exercised not to touch the dentine, but to keep the turbine-driven bur in contact with the post alone.

1043 The canal ready for preparation following removal of the post.

As an aid to visibility, the canal should be transilluminated using a fibre optic light in contact with the labial gingivae.

ROOT CANAL FILLING MATERIALS

The most important aspect, when considering the removal of a root filling material, is to decide which type of material has been used. It is essential, therefore, to recognise the radiographic appearance of those in common use.

1044 Three different types of root filling material.

The apex of the palatal canal has been filled with amalgam, the rest of the canal with gutta percha. The buccal canals contain silver points.

1044

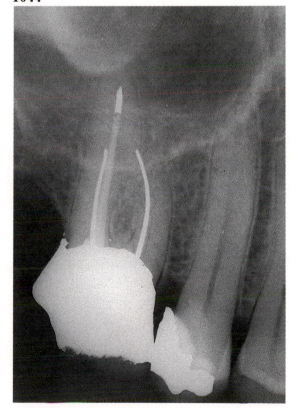

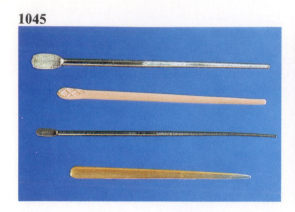

1045

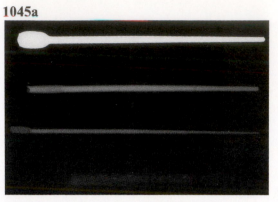

1045a

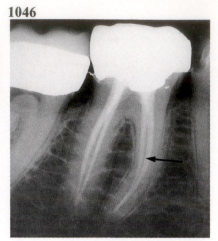

1046

1045a Radiograph of the four cones shown in **1045**.

It is important to note that there is no discernible radiographic difference between titanium and gutta percha.

1046 The mesio-buccal canal (*arrowed*) has been filled with a titanium point; the other three canals have been filled with gutta percha.

After a careful examination of the pre-operative radiograph, removal of the filling material is planned accordingly.

Metal cones. When re-opening an access cavity, caution must be exercised to avoid the accidental disturbance or removal of any metal cone left protruding into the pulp chamber. This can be difficult if the cones have been embedded in an amalgam core. Provided a sufficient length of a cone which is to be removed can be seen projecting from the orifice of the canal, it can be gripped with Steiglitz forceps, fine beaked pliers or artery forceps.

A straight, slow pulling action is aided by tapping the handle of the gripping instrument. When the cone lies within the canal without protruding into the chamber, files are used with solvents to edge down gradually alongside the cone. Occasionally a cone can be bypassed and incorporated into the new filling.

From the top:
Silver
Gutta percha
Titanium
Plastic

Gutta percha. This is simple to remove and many techniques are available. Chloroform or xylol will soften gutta percha rapidly. Gates Glidden burs, which should be slightly narrower than the canals in which they are to be used, will remove gutta percha from the coronal two-thirds of the canal.

Hedstroem files may be screwed into the body of the gutta percha. **1047** Three Hedstroem files have been embedded within the gutta percha and then the root filling has been removed by pulling on all three handles together (**1048**).

It is possible to retrieve a gutta percha cone that has been extruded beyond the apex. Ascending sizes of Hedstroem files are used to make a gap between the root canal wall and the gutta percha. At least two files are then 'screwed' along the gutta percha, almost to the length of the canal, before the handles are pulled together.

Pastes. A wide variety of pastes are used, and some of them are soluble in chloroform or xylol.

The pulp chamber is flooded with solvent and Hedstroem files are used to penetrate and remove the filling material. Care should be taken to prevent solvent penetrating the periapical tissues. The apical few millimetres of paste are removed using copious irrigation but without solvent.

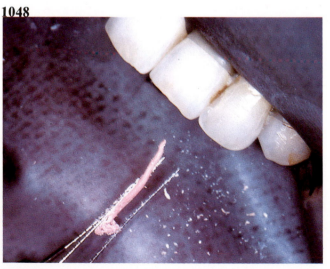

1047

1048

19 Bleaching J. J. Messing

CRITERIA FOR BLEACHING

Bleaching of discoloured teeth is best reserved for those which have darkened after death of the pulp has allowed the release of red blood corpuscles and their breakdown products (haemoglobin$\longrightarrow$iron sulphide) into the dentinal tubules (**1049**). Under the influence of the bleaching agent, the ferric sulphide, which is black and insoluble, is converted into white, soluble ferrous oxide.

Following trauma to a tooth and to the apical blood vessels, the crown may turn crimson, slowly changing colour to purple, bluish-black, brown or grey. Failure to remove all pulp remnants, eg in the pulp cornua, may produce varying degrees of discoloration of the crown. The greater the degree of discoloration, the greater the likelihood that some subsequent darkening will occur after bleaching. However, a considerable improvement can be obtained.

Colour changes resulting from chemicals used in endodontic treatments, such as iodine and silver salts, are resistant to attempts at bleaching and only minor improvements may be obtained.

Tetracycline-stained teeth have been treated with acidic peroxide solutions superficially but results are variable and usually temporary. To obtain satisfactory elimination of stain, it is necessary first to remove the pulp and fill the canal prior to bleaching the dentine from within the crown.

TECHNIQUE FOR BLEACHING

(a) Ensure the presence of a sound root filling without signs or symptoms of periapical pathosis.
(b) Remove all vestiges of restorative materials from the crown and eliminate root filling from the pulp chamber and canal(s) to a line 1-2mm apical to the gingival margin. (Similarly, any residue of cornual pulp tissue must be eradicated). There must be a good seal at that level, in order to prevent leakage of the bleaching agents alongside the root filling and thence, possibly, into the periapical region. As a precaution, a small plug of phosphate or polycarboxylate cement may be applied, keeping it away from the labial dentine of the crown.

The rubber dam is applied (preferably, to the affected tooth only) inverting the margins around the cervix to ensure a snug, water-tight fit. This will protect the gingivae from leakage of bleaching agent, which can cause a chemical burn (**1050**). Gingival tissue around the crown is given further protection with a coating of petroleum jelly.

ARMAMENTARIUM

(a) **A bleaching lamp.** For this purpose, to provide a source of uv. light, a no. 2 photoflood lamp may be used in a photographic reflector, in front of which a metal protective disc is mounted (**1051**). This is needed to protect the patient from heat and the risk, albeit uncommon, that the lamp may shatter. A short metal tube (measuring 6in. in length and 2in. diameter) is soldered to a hole in the centre of the disc. The tube transmits the beam of light to the tooth.

1049

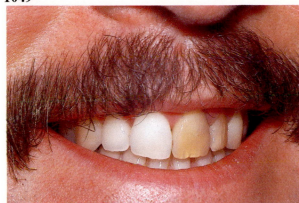

1050

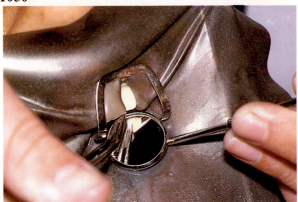

1051

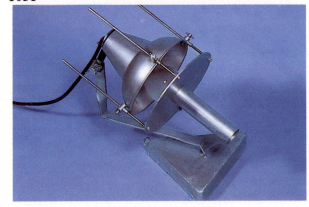

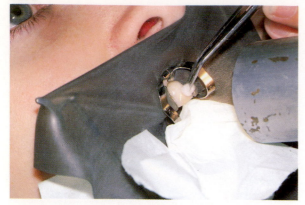

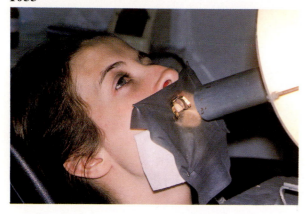

(b) **The bleaching agent.** For this purpose, a 30 per cent (100 vols.) solution of hydrogen peroxide (Superoxol) may be used. This should be stored in a cool place (preferably refrigerated), because a high ambient temperature can cause evolution of oxygen in a well-stoppered container and cause an explosion. Approximately 28-56ml should be stored.

(c) As an alternative to the use of uv. light, a 2-4 per cent solution of sodium hypochlorite may be used.

(d) Sodium perborate powder.

(e) An 80 per cent solution of chloral hydrate.

(f) Clear acrylic dissolved in chloroform.

(g) A surfactant liquid.

The crown and pulp chamber are washed and dried respectively with water spray and air jet. Dehydration of the dentine and removal of any fatty substances can be achieved by swabbing the dentine with a pledget of cotton soaked with ether. Increased potency of the dentinal tubules may be obtained by application of a solution or gel of 37-50% phosphoric acid, followed by thorough irrigation with water. One drop of surfactant is added to 1.0ml of Superoxol in a Dappens glass and a cotton pledget, soaked in the solution, is applied to wet the labial surface and then inserted in the pulp chamber (**1052**). The surfactant, by reducing the surface energy, allows the Superoxol to spread evenly over the enamel and dentine, thus facilitating the bleaching process. The lamp is adjusted to bring the beam of light on to the tooth, the tube being placed a few centimetres from the tooth (**1053**).

When the bleaching lamp is used, frequent augmentation of the peroxide in the pulp chamber and on the surface of the enamel is carried out. Bubbles of oxygen can be seen being evolved as the peroxide is broken down by the uv. light.

ALTERNATIVE TECHNIQUES

(a) When a bleaching lamp is not available, a similar result may be obtained by using a heated Baldwin burnisher to dissociate the Superoxol held in suspension in a pledget of cotton in the pulp chamber. ($2H_2O_2 \xrightarrow{heat} 2H_2O + O_2$) The process is repeated with a layer of cotton, similarly soaked in Superoxol, on the labial surface. This process is facilitated if a commercially available, electrically activated heat source is used (**1054**).

(b) Alternating applications of Superoxol and a 2-4 per cent solution of sodium hypochlorite ($H_2O_2 + NaOCl \longrightarrow NaCl + H_2O + O_2$).

(c) Inter-visit bleaching. This is effected by placing a slurry of sodium perborate in Superoxol into the pulp chamber, packing it in with a cotton pledget, and sealing it with polycarboxylate cement or 'Cavit'. Two or three dressings may be needed to produce the desired improvement.

Whichever technique is carried out in the surgery, the average duration of the bleaching should be about 20 minutes, and the inter-visit use of perborate slurry, often called 'the walking bleach', is recommended. The number of sessions will depend primarily upon the severity of the initial discoloration.

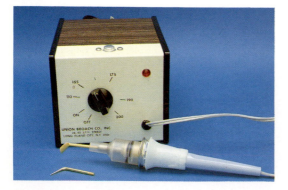

1055

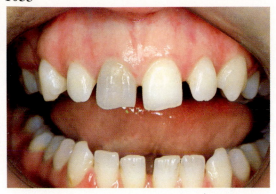

1056

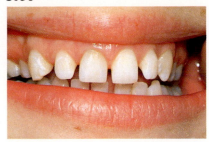

1057

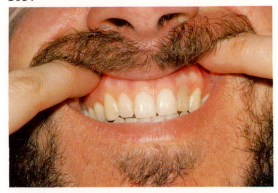

1058

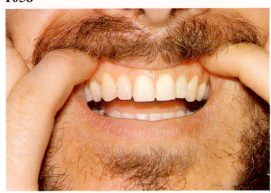

1059

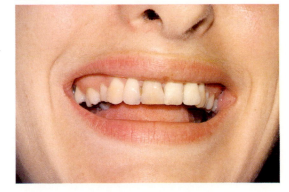

1060

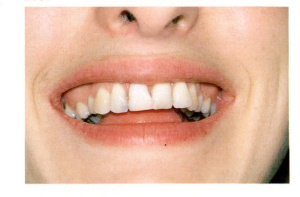

RESTORATION AFTER BLEACHING

At a subsequent visit, when the tooth has lightened enough to match the neighbouring teeth, or has become even lighter in colour, a final restoration can be inserted. The illustrations (**1055-1060**) show 3 cases of bleaching.

The pulpal cavity is washed thoroughly and dried with warm air. A partial restoration of the original translucency of the dentine can be achieved by wetting the dentine with an 80 per cent solution of chloral hydrate. It is left *in situ* for about 5 minutes.

After drying the tooth, the lingual cavity is painted with a protective varnish to help in the prevention of contamination and consequent discoloration as a result of microleakage. For this purpose, a solution of clear methyl methacrylate in chloroform is ideal. When the varnish has dried, bevel and etch the margins of the access cavity, and restore the surface contour with a composite resin.

It is important that the patient be informed that, in a percentage of treatments, the teeth may discolour slightly but further bleaching can then be carried out. If the result of bleaching proves to be unsatisfactory, cosmetic success may be achieved by facing the enamel with a composite resin, or a crown may be constructed.

PREVENTION OF DISCOLORATION

It is essential to emphasize the application of preventive measures to avoid discoloration. After endodontic treatment, in which every effort has been made to avoid contamination of coronal dentine by blood and the products of pulpal breakdown, it is unusual to have more than minor changes in the colour of the tooth.

When such changes are minimal, bleaching may consist solely of the application of a peroxide/perborate slurry, changed at weekly intervals until a satisfactory shade has been obtained.

20 Restoration of the treated tooth J. J. Messing

There is greater deformation of a pulpless tooth with an extensive cavity than in a sound tooth under a similar load, because a dead tooth contains about 9 per cent less water, which diminishes the elastic recoil of the dentine. Therefore, there is a potential risk that a tooth which has undergone root treatment can fracture under stress (**1061**). This is, in general, more apt to occur in posterior teeth. Incisors and canines are less likely to fracture, unless there has been extensive loss of tooth substance due to caries, erosion, abrasion or over-preparation. This is because the loss of tooth tissue from a correctly prepared access cavity need not weaken the tooth appreciably. Discoloration in anterior teeth, however, may indicate a need for bleaching or crowning.

A posterior tooth, in which there exists already a mesio-occluso-distal restoration, is rendered extremely friable following removal of the roof of the pulp chamber, because the buccal and lingual coronal remnants are united by a thin dentine arch at the furcation. Thus, bucco-lingual stresses on the cusps lead frequently to a total vertical fracture, and the patient becomes aware of severe tenderness when chewing, while mobility of the fragments becomes apparent with worsening of the symptoms. Unless endodontic treatment has been carried out in an otherwise unrestored posterior tooth, subsequent restoration should be done with an onlay or crown so that the whole biting surface is replaced (**1062, 1063**).

It is imperative that the risk of fracture be foreseen and prevented, both during endodontic treatment and subsequently.

ANTERIOR TEETH

If a tooth has lost a considerable amount of dentine, it will be advisable to make a crown as soon as there is clinical and radiographic evidence that any periapical lesion is healing.

Provided the cervical dentine is reasonably sound, the tooth is cut down to a conventional jacket crown preparation, which is then reduced in length by 1-2mm. The canal is then prepared and a wrought-gold or chrome/cobalt alloy post is fitted to a point 3-5mm from the apex, finishing about 1.0mm short of the proposed tip of the core and aligned within its labio-lingual contour, the coronal extension being angled, if required, by bending (**1064**). This post is then built up with inlay wax or acrylic resin (see Wiptam technique), to produce an incisal tip which is then cast in yellow or white gold.

If there is severe loss of tooth structure cervically or the access cavity is unduly wide, it will be necessary to reduce the dentine core to the gingival margin (**1065**). As much crown should be kept as is feasible, because thereby the crown to post-ratio is more favourable for retention.

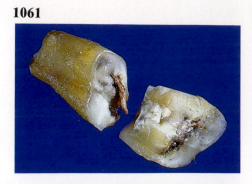

1061

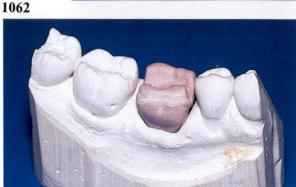

1062

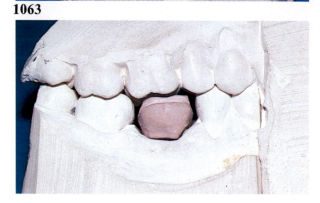

1063

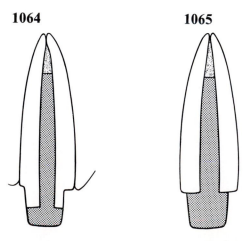

1064   1065

PREPARATION OF A ROOT CANAL FOR A POST

In order to use a root canal for the retention of a post crown, there must be a sound apical seal and the filling in the coronal two-thirds of the root must be removed, without damaging the walls or disturbing the apical seal.

As a rough guide, the length of the post should be at least that of the crown, and preferably longer. The post should have a good frictional fit with the greater part of the canal. This can be obtained by the use of matching drills and wrought wire posts, or by casting metal on to a length of post wire, so that the casting, produced from a wax matrix removed from the canal, is an exact replica of the space.

Gutta percha can be removed from a root canal in three ways:
(a) by inserting a heated spreader to soften the filling, which is then removed by reaming and filing.
(b) by flooding the canal with chloroform or acetone to soften the filling, prior to filing it out of the canal.
(c) by using Gates Glidden drills (**1066**). When rotating in contact with the gutta percha, they generate heat which softens it, facilitating its removal. The drills should be operated at about 8,000 rpm, with very light pressure, ensuring that the size of drill is less than the diameter of the canal. Gates Glidden drills are supplied in six sizes and should be used in sequence, starting with the smallest. They have cutting blades only on their sides, thus minimising the risk of lateral perforation.

If helical drills are used, such as 'Beutelrock' or engine reamers, there is a high risk, when the gutta percha is hard or the angle of preparation is wrong, that a false passage or perforation can be made (**1067, 1068**).

When a patient requests a post crown for a tooth with a poor root filling it is safer, despite the absence of signs or symptoms of pathology, to remove the filling, replacing it with a silver or titanium tip (**1069**). When the sealer has hardened, the risk of disturbing the apical seal is avoided, thus eliminating the attendant hazard of an acute apical periodontitis.

POST/CORE SYSTEMS

It is widely accepted that a gold core, either cast in one piece with the post, or cast on to a well-fitting wrought post, is ideal for single rooted teeth. Many variations of technique and types of post have been recommended, three of which will be described.

1066

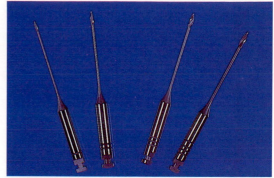

1067

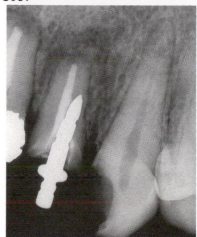

1068

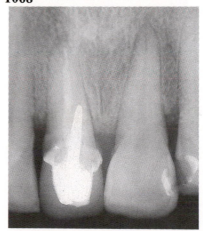

1069

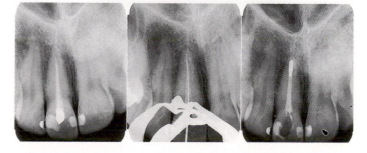

THE APICAL SEAL FOR POST CROWNS

A tooth which has an apparently satisfactory gutta percha root filling, may develop acute apical symptoms following the removal of a part of the root filling to make room for a post. Hence, if it is known in advance that a post crown is to be made, it is advisable to seal the apical end of the canal alone, using a vertical condensation technique after softening the gutta percha with a heated spreader.

However, if the apical part of the canal is likely to be more or less round in cross section, it is possible after filing, to ream the canal to a size at which the apical 3-4mm has been cut in clean sound dentine. A root which tends to be wider bucco-lingually than mesio-distally may have a bifid or flattened canal which contra-indicates the use of a matched metal cone and sealer.

The apical tip technique thus can be used in any straight canal, the root of which has a circular cross section. It is contra-indicated in the following cases:

(a) curved canals
(b) very thin bifid roots
(c) flattened canals, eg upper lateral incisors or distal roots of lower molars.

The screw-off tips are available in silver or titanium in lengths of 3 or 6mm, and matched in shape to sizes 45-140 (ISO) reamers (**1070, 1071**).

Despite the assertion that the bio-degradability of silver precludes its use in endodontics, the author has used it as an apical root filling prior to crowning for fifteen years in hundreds of teeth with a failure rate of approximately two per cent. Successfully treated teeth which it has been necessary to remove subsequently because of root fracture or periodontal disease have shown no evidence of chemical degradation of the silver tip even when exposed to the periodontal environment through an apical extrusion (**1072**). If the tip fits the canal tightly, the periapical tissues can heal, with the development of a fibrous tissue sheath over the extruded foreign body at the apex.

In all cases reported, which showed chemical degradation of silver in root canals, the silver cone was lying loose in a canal from which any sealer had long since washed out and had been replaced by tissue fluids.

The technique for correct use of a silver cone entails very careful preparation of the canal and fitting of the cone so that a frictional fit is obtained at, or close to the apical constriction. Thus, a true lute of sealer can be used, making an analogy with the type of fit obtained, ideally, with a gold inlay.

1070

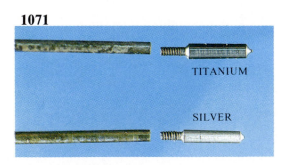

1071

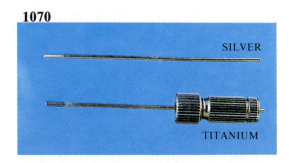

1072

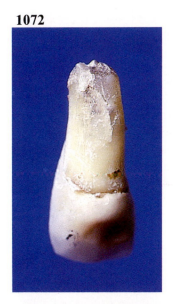

1072 This maxillary lateral incisor was root-treated and a silver cone was sealed in the resorbed apex. Healing was good with formation of intact lamina dura apically. However, the weakened root fractured vertically two years later and was extracted. There is no sign of chemical degradation of the silver.

TECHNIQUE FOR APICAL TIPS

File the canal until the dentine shavings are clean and the apical constriction has been reached but not breached. Ream 1-2 sizes further to produce a smooth, circular cross section. Irrigate and dry.

Affix a silver cone, on its holder, in the pin vice supplied, and adjust the length to the working length to which the canal was prepared. Gently insert the cone. If it reaches the constriction without binding, the canal has been over-prepared, therefore choose the next larger size, after the use of a reamer one size larger. When the cone binds short of the apex, ream a few turns gently with the same size of reamer, trying the cone at intervals until it is felt to bind at the correct length (tug-back) (**1073**). It is disengaged gently and, using a low viscosity mix of sealant, such as AH26, a reamer two sizes smaller is coated, placed in the canal, and turned counter-clockwise to paint a thin film of sealer over the walls. If too much sealer is inserted or a spiral filler is used, it is impossible to seat the apical tip, and the force needed can expel a quantity of sealer beyond the apex, resulting frequently in postoperative pain. The cone is advanced slowly along the canal, with a reaming action (reciprocatory) to allow the back-tracking of sealer and prevent it from being forced apically in sufficient quantity to exert back pressure. If the cone will not seat home, remove it, ream out some of the sealer, and replace the cone at the apex.

1073

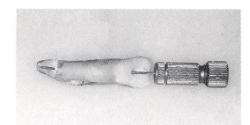

When the cone has been locked into place under pressure, the pin-vice is turned to unscrew it and is withdrawn. The space between the tip and the crown, already coated with sealer, is next filled with a matching gutta percha cone, shortened apically by the length of the apical tip. It is heated and softened with a spreader and condensed with pluggers. If a post is to be fitted in the foreseeable future, no condensation is necessary.

Great care must be exercised never to exert undue pressure when fitting an apical cone. If it becomes jammed in the canal, attempted removal could strip its screw thread, making its removal impossible and leaving it without a lute of sealant. If this occurs, place sealer in the canal and condense gutta percha to fill up the remainder of the canal. In the event that periapical pathosis develops, a surgical approach would be indicated but, if the canal has been well prepared and the cone is fairly close to the apex, it is likely to remain free from problems.

CASES IN WHICH SILVER APICAL TIPS HAVE BEEN USED (1074-1084)

1074

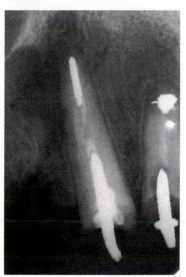

1075

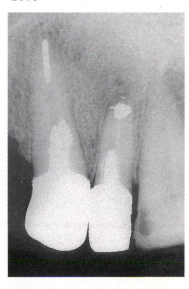

1074, 1075. Maxillary canine 3 years after root filling with a silver tip plus AH26.

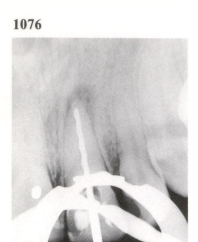

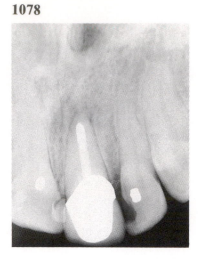

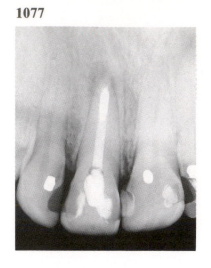

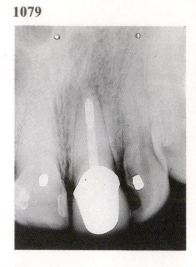

1076, 1077. Maxillary incisor canal root filled with a silver tip plus AH26.
1078, 1079. Follow up radiographs 6 months and 14 months postoperative.

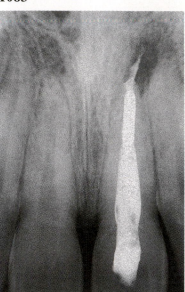

1083

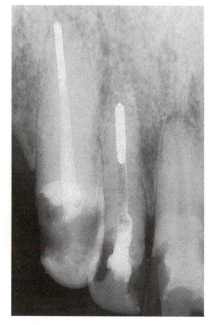

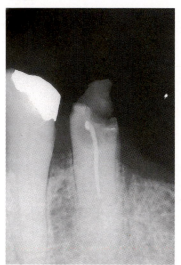

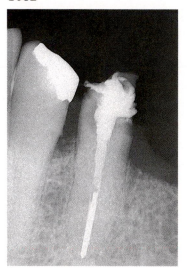

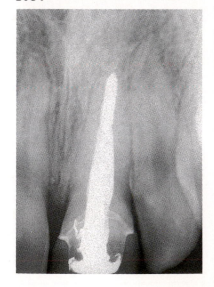

1084

1080. Maxillary incisor and canine 9 years after root filling with silver tip plus AH26.

1081, 1082. Mandibular premolar requiring a crown, but inadequately root-treated. Apical tip and AH26 inserted prior to preparation of the canal for a post.
1083, 1084. Healing and resorption of excess AH26 from the periapical region one year after placement of an apical silver tip.

1085

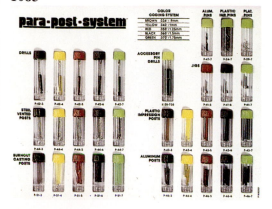

THE PARA-POST SYSTEM

This technique requires reduction of the root face close to the gingival margin. The canal is then prepared so that the post will be longer than the crown, and a paralleling jig, related in diameter to the drill used, is placed within the canal. This allows the cutting of an accessory pin channel, parallel with the root canal and distanced from it by the choice of hole in the jig. Plastic pins, placed in the canal and accessory channel are incorporated in the impression from which the post-core assembly may be constructed. The accessory pin (more than one can be inserted) acts to increase retention and provides an anti-torsion lock. Aluminium posts and pins are provided for incorporation in temporary restorations. As an alternative to casting the post and core, matched stainless steel posts are available, to be used in conjunction with accessory pins for the retention of an amalgam or composite resin core (**1085**).

1086

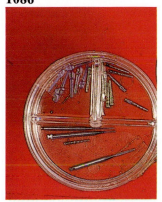

THE C.I. KIT

This is a simpler kit which supplies plastic post/core patterns matched to reamers, in addition to steel posts for the retention of amalgam cores (**1086**). The shape of the coronal end of the canal is modified to resist torsion and the plastic core is built up to contour with wax, cast and the gold post/core cemented.

1087

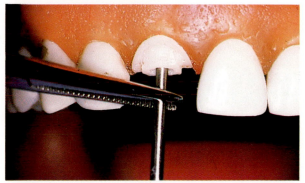

THE WIPTAM TECHNIQUE

The author has used chrome-cobalt wire as a post with a gold core cast on to it for about thirty years without problems. The technique is simple and economical. The canal is prepared, using a twist drill (1.0-1.5mm depending on the diameter of the root) and the matching size of wire (Wiptam) is fitted so that it projects to lie well within the proposed core build-up (**1087**). An anti-torsion lock is produced by cutting minimum lateral extensions in the coronal part of the canal. The tooth is lubricated and the projecting end of the post is notched to provide retention for the gold (**1088**). A thin mix of Duralay, a pattern acrylic, is coated over the wire and into the orifice of the canal (**1089**). As it starts to polymerize, it is shaped with a plastic instrument dipped in monomer and when it is slightly over-built, it is left to harden, (60-90 seconds).

1088   **1089**

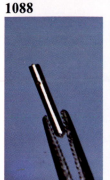
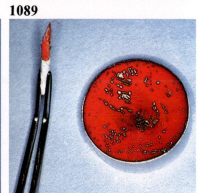

When hard, it is pulled out of the canal, shaped and re-inserted, checking the occlusion in all excursions to ensure sufficient room for the proposed restoration. Blue wax is then melted around the part of the wire and plastic which fits the coronal orifice and, while the wax is molten, the post/core is re-inserted and pressed home. Wax is thus forced into the prepared root canal and anti-torsion lock to obtain good retention (**1090**). After removal of the excess wax at the margins, the post/core is removed, sprued and invested, and the core is cast in hard gold.

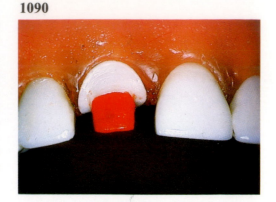

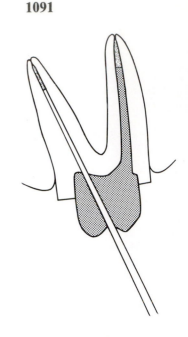

A DIRECT TECHNIQUE FOR A CAST CORE AND POSTS FOR A TOOTH WITH DIVERGENT ROOTS

The walls of the pulp chamber must be free from undercuts which should be obliterated with phosphate cement. If they interfere with the line of withdrawal, they should be eliminated by cutting back the dentine.

The canals are prepared, leaving a minimum of 3mm of root filling at the apex, thus ensuring maximum length for the posts. The canals are enlarged with the appropriate twist drill to a width which relates to the width of the root and the diameter to which the canal has been reamed (1.0-1.5mm).

One post is made retentive by cutting notches coronally and bending that end to lie within the confines of the projected core. The other post must be smooth and unbent and about 1.0cm longer.

The dentine surfaces and the smooth post are coated with a film of the lubricant supplied with Duralay, and the posts are placed in the canals. A fluid mix of Duralay is flowed around the posts and, when it begins to polymerize, it is moulded with a flat plastic instrument, dipped periodically in monomer.

When the acrylic is almost hard, the longer post is grasped lightly with pliers, twisted to detach it, withdrawn slightly, and replaced. Once the Duralay is hard, the longer post is removed so that the occlusal clearance can be checked. The core is ground to shape, using carborundum stones and abrasive discs. Finally, the post and core assembly is removed and the core is cast in precious metal. In order to ensure the patency of the hole in the wax, a length of stainless steel wire of equal diameter is inserted into it. After casting, the wire is removed with a twist and a pull.

The casting is placed in the tooth and the separate post is inserted into the canal through the hole in the core. After completing any necessary adjustments, the core and the second post are cemented in turn, cutting off the protruding excess of wire while the cement is still soft. The same technique may be used for a tooth with three canals.

To ensure success the following points should be noted. Removable posts must be smooth, straight and well lubricated, and they should be rotated at intervals while the acrylic is polymerizing.

It is possible to use an indirect technique for multi-rooted teeth, but it is more complicated and the author prefers and recommends the simplicity of the direct method (**1091**).

As an alternative to the use of Wiptam wire, prefabricated gold alloy posts are available which are matched to root canal instrument sizes (ISO).

Crowning of the tooth should be delayed for at least four weeks after endodontic treatment of a tooth without a periapical area. If a periapical area is present and there are signs of healing after 3-6 months, the crowning may be started. However, if the patient insists on an earlier cosmetic improvement, crowning can be done provided that the patient is informed that subsequent periapical breakdown would necessitate an apicectomy and retro-filling of the root. It is imperative that, during the waiting period prior to crowning, the tooth be ground free of the occlusion as an aid to healing and to minimise the risk of fracture of weak dentine.

It is axiomatic that no root-treated incisor or canine should be prepared for a permanent crown without the prior cementation of a post/core or, at least, a strengthening post (eg Kurer crown saver). Failure to observe this rule will often lead to fracture of the crown stump. Excessive widening of a canal will tend to predispose to vertical fracture of the root. Hence it is advisable to provide a full or three-quarter collar in gold to splint the walls of the root, where over-preparation of the canal has occurred.

PREFABRICATED POST/CORE SYSTEMS

The use of Charlton (**1092**) and Kurer (**1093**) post/core systems is limited to roots which are wide and long. The reason for this preference is dictated by the parallel-sided profile of the posts, and the tendency to over-prepare the apical dentine, which can predispose to fracture of the root. This is more likely to occur if the root is short or narrow (**1094, 1095**). However, when width and length are adequate, the use of prefabricated posts and cores allows a saving of chairside time and laboratory fees.

The chief precautions to be observed in their use are:
(a) avoidance of excessive force when preparing the canal;
(b) the post should occupy two-thirds of the length of the canal in order to minimise the risk of an excessive concentration of stresses that would occur at the apical end of a short post, increasing the risk of a vertical or oblique fracture of the root;
(c) avoidance of over-preparation of the diameter of the canal, thus removing the necessary frictional fit;
(d) provision of an anti-torsion lock (**1096**). This feature is embodied in the Charlton post technique but, when a Kurer post has been cemented, it is salutary to prepare a small cavity lingually, involving the brass head and the subjacent dentine, make it retentive, and fill it with amalgam or composite resin. This will prevent breakdown of the luting cement under torsional stress, which would permit a degree of movement with marginal leakage, although it would be necessary to remove the crown in order to unscrew the post.

1092

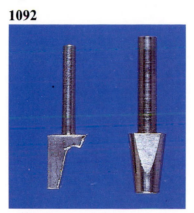

1093

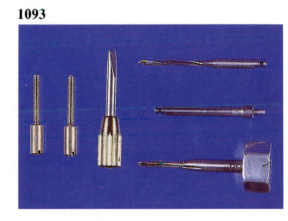

1094

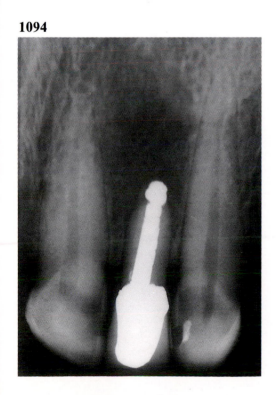

1095

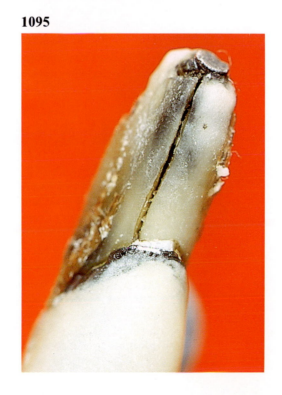

1096

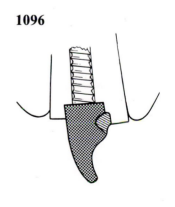

IMMEDIATE RESTORATION OF THE ROOT-FILLED TOOTH

On completion of the root filling, the coronal end of a large canal (eg palatal of upper molar) is left free from filling material, and either the pulp chamber and the canal extension are filled with silver amalgam, or a screw device (eg Dentatus screw **1097**) is cemented with phosphate cement,

1097

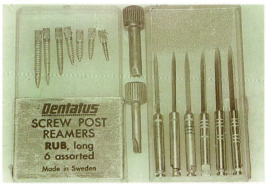

1098

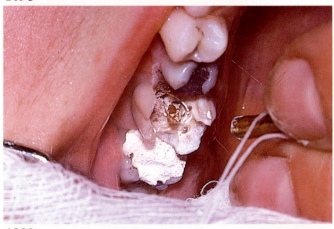

1099

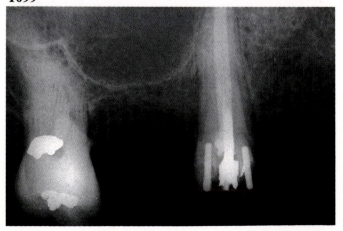

ensuring that it is not screwed tightly into the canal. The special engine reamers should be used to complete the screw space in the canal, thus providing a better fit for the appropriate screw (**1098**). The head of the screw is then locked to the surrounding composite or amalgam by insertion of the appropriate material. By uniting the core and the root, the risk of a fracture through the core and residual dentine within the crown is reduced.

With the exception of root-treated anterior teeth which, apart from the access cavity, are ostensibly sound, all root-filled teeth should be restored with cast restorations. Weakened cusps under stress tend to fracture when shearing forces are brought to bear on them when chewing tough foods, and the fracture line usually extends deeply sub-gingival or through the furcation area. Thus, the options lie between an onlay, a three-quarter crown and a full veneer crown. The deciding factors influencing the choice of restoration are: aesthetics; the extent of tooth loss; the retention available, eg the restoration of a short crown, especially where there is severe attrition.

Where there is gross tooth-loss, it is necessary to rebuild the contour initially, using amalgam or composite resin which is locked to the roots by means of retention pins and screws. Although without accepted scientific proof as to its effectiveness, as yet, there is a wealth of clinical evidence and popular acceptance of the Baldwin technique as an accessory means of retention. Amalgam is condensed on to a layer of sticky phosphate cement on the dentine of the floor and walls of the cavity, after initially condensing amalgam at the perimeter in order to avoid any extrusion of cement around the margins. The multiple retentive tags of amalgam which become cemented to the dentine ensure that the core does not break away during the crown preparation, while the retaining pins or screws lock the core firmly to the roots.

Alternative methods for restoring the lost tissue are either to condense amalgam into the coronal ends of the canals and the pulp chamber, filling up the crown with amalgam to rely on the bulk of metal for strength or bond a composite core, such as Clearfil (Cavex) or P10 (3M) to the dentine.

PROBLEMS RELATING TO THE USE OF PINS AND SCREWS

Retention screws should never be used in canals before the matching drill has been used to shape the canal. The screw is then checked to ensure its length will allow it to be enclosed within the core. It must not be so tight a fit that pressure is exerted on the walls of the canal. The canal is given a light coating of phosphate cement and the screw is rotated into it until it starts to bind. At that juncture, the screw is left until the cement has hardened. If the screw were forced home by excessive tightening of the spanner, the compression of dentine could lead to immediate or delayed fracture of the root. It is not a sound technique to leave the screw uncemented, because there is a risk that it may break loose with loss of the crown. More than one screw may be inserted if there is room, or a combination of screws, pins and undercuts may be adapted to fit each individual situation (**1099**). As a basic premise, as much dentine should be preserved as circumstances allow.

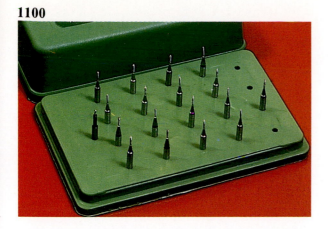

1100

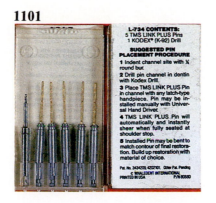

1101

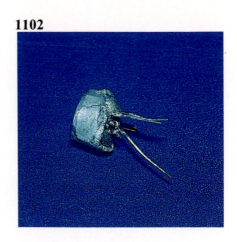

1102

Pins, when used, should be inserted over the roots, care being exercised to avoid furcations, through which perforations are apt to occur. As a useful rule of thumb, one pin should be inserted for each quadrant of a molar being restored and one for each cusp of a premolar (**1100, 1101**).

A non-vital tooth is weaker than one with a vital pulp. Self-shearing screw pins have been shown to produce crazing of the dentine surrounding the channel, leading to a risk of fracture of the root. For this reason it is safer to use threaded stainless steel wires (Markley) cemented into the channels. If a self-shearing pin is to be used, the channel should be made over-sized by prolonged preparation. The pin is dipped into phosphate cement, placed in the channel and fractured off by bending it from side to side. The handpiece, not attached to the unit, may be used as a convenient handle when placing pins in relatively inaccessible areas.

CORES OVER METAL CONES

Projecting ends of silver or titanium cones should be bent over and pressed firmly into the floor of the pulp chamber and embedded in a base of phosphate cement, in order to minimise the risk of subsequent disturbance, and to prevent thermal conduction to periodontal tissues through a metal coronal restoration.

1102 If amalgam were condensed around the cones, any subsequent disturbance of that amalgam could result in luxation of the whole root filling.

TYPES OF CORONAL RESTORATION

When the buccal face of a root-treated tooth is sound and aesthetically acceptable, a three-quarter or seven-eighths crown may be ideal. There must be sufficient coronal height to permit a retentive preparation and the crown, after root filling, should have been reinforced with amalgam or, if minimally defective, with composite resin, as described.

Should the lingual and buccal walls of the tooth be sound, an M.O.D. onlay will provide good protection against fracture, the final restoration being only slightly different from the three-quarter crown, with regard to the area of lingual enamel involved (**1103**).

1103

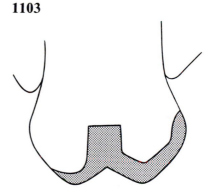

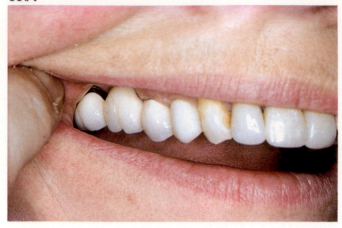

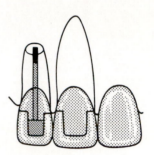

When there are buccal and lingual restorations present or the tooth has discoloured, a full veneer cast crown is the restoration of choice. It may be constructed in gold or, when aesthetic demands must be met, in porcelain bonded to gold. In the latter case, in order to preserve the strength of the residual coronal dentine, the margin should be chamfered and the metal built out to a small step, at which the porcelain is finished, short of the gingival margin. This will present a narrow gingival gold rim to the crown, acceptable when hidden by the lip (**1104**). However, if the edge of the crown is visible when the patient smiles, a 1.0-1.5mm step should be cut buccally so that the porcelain can be finished flush with the margin.

Access to sub-gingival margins may be improved by electrosurgical excision of hyperplastic tissue but, where crowns are short, they should be lengthened by gingivectomy and osseous reduction to maintain the zone of attached gingiva.

After surgical procedures such as root resection or hemisection, the final restoration must be designed to facilitate access for cleaning the margins and to minimise stress on the reduced radicular base. All stresses should fall within the area of the roots but, where this is not feasible, modification of the size and shape of the occlusal table will do much to reduce stress.

Teeth, shortened unduly by over-enthusiastic apicectomy, may not be suitable as major bridge abutments but, by joining them to neighbouring abutments by soldered joints or precision-attached retainers, reciprocal resistance to stress is provided (**1105**).

EMERGENCY RESTORATION FOLLOWING EXTRACTION OF AN ANTERIOR TOOTH

When an anterior tooth has to be extracted in an emergency as, for example, in **1106** when there had been a vertical fracture of the root, subsequent replacement by means of a fixed bridge must be delayed for several months, to allow the alveolus to become remodelled as the socket heals.

In such a case, the provision of a removable prosthesis is far from ideal, being uncomfortable, tending to interfere with the maintenance of gingival health, requiring modification at intervals and, sometimes being poorly tolerated.

1106

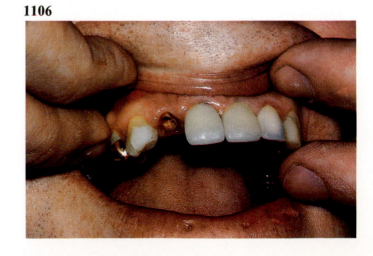

The following technique has proved to be an eminently satisfactory alternative:

The crown is replaced in the fractured root and a silicone matrix is formed by moulding a high viscosity material over it and its neighbours (**1107**). Fine detail can be reproduced by drying the matrix, coating it with a light bodied silicone wash and replacing it over the teeth (**1108**). The root is next extracted and the socket is covered with a strip of Stomahesive intra-oral bandage.

A crown preparation is now cut on one or more of the adjacent teeth and the prepared surfaces and the neighbouring teeth wiped over with petroleum jelly (**1109**).

A suitable temporary bridge material, such as 'Trim' is placed in the crown and pontic areas of the matrix, which is carried to place over the teeth and pressed home. Once the material has begun to polymerize, the matrix is eased a few millimetres off the teeth and replaced. When the plastic has hardened further, the matrix, with its temporary bridge, is removed carefully and placed in hot water (70°C-80°C) for about one minute, so that polymerization can be completed.

Any peripheral flash of plastic can be removed with crown scissors and the margins are then finished with sandpaper discs and rubber abrasive wheels to ensure as perfect a margin as can be obtained. The occlusion is adjusted to provide minimum stress on the retainer and the pontic is ground free from the bite and polished. The temporary bridge is cemented with phosphate or polycarboxylate cement (**1110**). Alternatively, when time is limited and the natural crown is available following extraction of the tooth, it is sectioned from the root at the gingival level, and both it and the enamel of the adjacent crowns are polished with pumice/water slurry, etched and coated with bonding resin and composite resin. The crown is then replaced, the occlusion being checked briefly, and held there until the resin has hardened.

The occlusion is re-checked and adjusted and, if necessary, further resin is added to increase bulk at the joints. Then, the resin is polished, using Soflex (3M) abrasive discs. Care must be taken to prevent encroachment of the resin on to the gingivae. If there is no usable crown, an acrylic denture tooth may be used. A wide groove is cut through the lingual surface in a mesio-distal direction. It is undercut and filled with composite resin, which is bonded proximally to the adjacent enamel surfaces (**1111, 1112**).

Should the bond to the adjacent teeth break down before the pontic area is ready for the bridge preparation, it is a simple matter to re-etch the enamel surfaces and re-attach the temporary pontic with a new mix of composite resin.

1107

1108

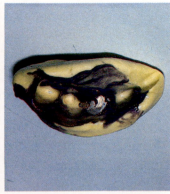

1109

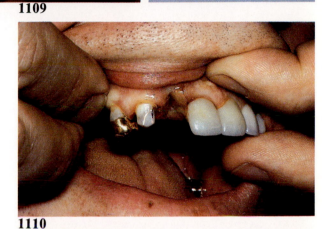

1110

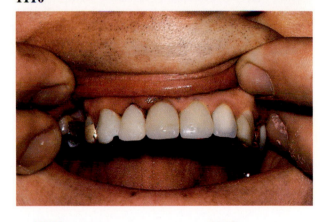

1111

1112

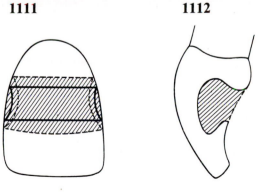

21   The Way Ahead

There has been a steady increase in the demand by patients for conservative dentistry rather than extraction. The provision of extensive restorative work, pinned amalgams, crowns and bridges, has resulted inevitably in some pulpal death. This has provoked a sudden and widespread interest in endodontic treatment, a subject until recently shrouded in mystique and ignorance, and often poorly taught in dental school. The response by clinicians, research workers and manufacturers has been to produce a plethora of new materials, instruments and techniques. The advances made in the last ten years have been considerable and the trend is likely to continue. In attempting to assess the future of endodontics, several emergent trends may be significant.

The present methods available for diagnosing the state of the pulp are crude and unreliable. Current research may well produce new ways of pulp testing: already sophisticated devices are about to become available which will allow measured quantities of both heat and cold to be applied to the tooth. Perhaps more relevant would be a test to measure the vascular supply to the tooth rather than the response by the nerve fibres.

The aims in endodontics are now understood with the emphasis firmly on cleaning, shaping and obturating the root canal system. The use of caustic drugs for canal medication, particularly formaldehydes, should be declining because the necessity of removing the contents of the root canal and not merely sterilising them, is realised. The advance in modern technology has produced new cutting instruments for the root canals which are sharper and more flexible. New methods have been introduced for the preparation of root canals, notably the step-back and crown-down pressureless techniques. Mechanical devices for preparing canals are currently changing with alternating handpieces being superseded by those with a subsonic vibratory movement. The most promising innovation is the use of ultrasound as a method of cleaning and preparing the root canal system.

The search for the ideal filling material continues and will surely do so for a long time. Gutta percha has outlived the metal cones despite its deficiencies. The present trend of applying heat to gutta percha to make it pliable enough to be adapted to the canal walls is perhaps reaching its climax with the electrically-heated spreaders and thermo-plasticised injection moulded techniques. The majority of the techniques, involving the placement of instruments within the root canal and condensation of the gutta percha, require an application of force which risks vertical fracture of the root. The incidence of vertical fracture as a direct result of endodontic treatment is sufficiently high to cause concern for the future of these techniques.

A paste which is injected into the canal, sets to a rubbery consistency and requires no sealer must be nearer to the ideal, provided it is an inert substance which either expands to fill the entire canal space or adheres to the canal wall. Two new filling materials Hydron, a hydrophilic chemical, and Lee endofill, a type of silicone impression material, both show a new ray of hope.

The sudden reduction in the caries rate will produce a lasting effect on the dental profession worldwide. The dentist has the chance to catch up with the treatment of oral disease in his patients. The general practitioner can now broaden his horizons and refer less and less to specialists. In the United States of America the endodontic specialist is receiving fewer referrals; and the patients who are being referred make greater use of his skills. The standard of endodontics taught in dental school is rising, with a more practical approach to classical techniques. The general practitioner of the future will require greater skills than his present-day counterpart as he provides total dental care for his patients.

The dissemination of endodontic knowledge and skill to all practitioners will produce a challenge to accepted techniques. Many of these techniques have claimed clinical success based mainly on in vitro research; few longitudinal clinical studies have been carried out, comparing the success rate of different techniques and materials. Computer technology will provide many answers in this field. It may be that a simple system already in use will prove as successful as a technique taking considerably longer to complete. The demand for simplified techniques will continue to grow and eventually one must be evolved which satisfies contemporary basic concepts of endodontics.

References

Chapter 11

Abou-Rass, M., Frank, A. L. and Glick, D. H. (1980) — The anticurvature filing method to prepare the curved root canal. *J.A.D.A.,* 101: 792-794.

Lim, S. S. and Stock, C. J. R. (1987) — The risk of perforation in the curved canal: anticurvature filing compared with the stepback technique. *Int. Endo. J.* 20: 33-39.

Cunningham, W. and Martin, H. (1982) — A scanning electron microscope evaluation of root canal debridement with the endosonic ultrasonic synergistic system. *Oral Surg.* 53: 401-404.

Martin, H., Cunningham, W., Norris, J. and Cotton, W. (1980) — Ultrasonic versus hand filing of dentin: a quantitative study. *Oral Surg.* 49: 79-81.

Caulk Dentsply. *The Endosonic system technique* (pub. 1984).

Chapter 12

Techniques in Clinical Endodontics edited by Gerstein. W. B. Saunders 1983 — Preparation of root canals and filling by lateral condensation techniques. pp.42-75 S. Patterson and C. Newton.

Techniques in Clinical Endodontics edited by Gerstein. W. B. Saunders 1983 — Vertical compaction of warm gutta percha. pp.76-98 H. Schilder.

Tagger, M., Tamse, A., Katj, A. and Korjen, B. M. Evaluation of the apical seal produced by a hybrid root canal filling method, combining lateral condensation and thermatic compaction. *J. of Endodontics* 10: 299-303 1984.

Trade references

Page 11

[1]Snap-a-Ray Hager und Werkhen GmbH, West Germany
[2]Eggin holder Sweden
[3]Rinn Rinn Corp., Elgin, Illinois, U.S.A.

Page 12

[1]Super X30 Phil-x, Italy
[2]Manumatic Westone Products Ltd., 104-112 Marylebone Lane, London W1M 5PV, England.

Page 13

[1]Velopex Medivance Instruments Ltd., 127 Acton Lane, Harlesden, London NW10 8UR, England
[2]Gimad 283 Unident S.A., 39 Rue Peillonnex, Ch-1225 Chene-Bourg, Geneva, Switzerland.

Page 14

[1]X-Ray Film Mount FM2 Westone Products Ltd., 104-112 Marylebone Lane, London W1M 5FV, England.
[2]Acetate Converters Ltd., Glebe House, Armfield Close, East Molesey, Surrey KT8 0RY, England. (Acetate sheet 190 Microns 9 in. × $5^5/_{18}$ in.).

Page 45

[1]W. Greenwood Electronic Ltd., 21 Germain Street, Chesham, Bucks., England.
[2]Analytic Technology, 3301 181ST PI. N.E. Redmond. WA 98052 U.S.A.

Page 64

[1]Amalgamated Dental Co. Ltd., 26-40 Broadwick Street, London W1A 2AD, England.
[2]DG16. Hu Friedy, 3232 North Rockwell Street, Chicago, Illinois 60618, U.S.A.
[3]Front surface mirror. Indian head. Union Branch Corporation, 36-40, 37th Street, Long Island City, N.Y. 11101 U.S.A.
[4]Marquis, Prima, 23 Faris Barn Drive, Woodham, Weybridge, Surrey, Engand.
[5]American pattern probe No. 3, Prima, 23 Faris Barn Drive, Woodham, Weybridge, Surrey, England
[6]Endolocking tweezers, Carl Martin, PO Box 170148, D565 Solingen 17, Hohscheid, West Germany.

Page 66

[1]K-Flex. Kerr Manufacturing Company, Detroit 8, Michigan, U.S.A.
[2]Flex-O-File. Les Fils D'Auguste, Maillefer S.A., Ballaigues, CH-1338, Switzerland.
[3]Unifile. Ransom and Randolf Dentsply, 324 Chestnut Street, Toledo, Ohio, 43604, U.S.A.
[4]Helifile, Micromega S.A., 5-2 Rue de Tunnel, Besançon 25006, France.

Page 68

[1]Giromatic, Micromega S.A., 5-2 Rue de Tunnel, Besançon 25006, France.
[2]Cursor.

Page 69

[1]Rispi, Micromega S.A., Rue de Tunnel, Besançon, 25006, France.
[2]Dynatrak, Ransom and Randolf Dentsply, 324 Chestnut Street, Toledo, Ohio 43604, U.S.A.
[3]Heligiro, Micromega.
[4]Hawes-Neos root filler, 6925 Gentillino, Lugano 3, Switzerland.
[5]Micromega.

Page 70

[1]Goose neck or Muller bur. Hager and Meisinger GmbH., Kronprinzenstrasse 5-11, D-4000 Düsseldorf 1, West Germany.
[2]Peeso reamer. Meisinger.
[3]Gates Glidden. Meisinger.
[4]Whaledent Inc., 236 Fifth Avenue, New York, N.Y. 10001, U.S.A.
[5]IFG 701 Jet carbide bur. Beaver Dental Products Ltd., Morrisburg, Ontario, Canada.
[6]FG 332/018 Horico. Hopf. Ringleb & Co. GmbH & Cie., Gardeschutzenweg 82, D-1000 Berlin 45, West Germany.

Page 71

[1]Test tubes Solmedia Ltd., 31 Orford Road, London E17 9NL, England.
[2]Cap-o-Test tops Solmedia Ltd.
[3]Kerr endo-module Kerr Division of Sybron (Europe) AG, Aeschengrabenio, CH-4010 Basle, Switzerland.

Page 72

[1]Kerr endo-module, Kerr Division of Sybron (Europe) AG, Aeschengrabenio, CH-4010, Basle, Switzerland.
[2]RAF Tray J. & S. Davis Ltd., Cordent House, 34/36 Friern Park, London N12 9DQ England.
[3]Double Tray (DT) J. & S. Davis Ltd.

Page 73

[1]Sonicleaner Dawe Instruments, Concord Road, Western Avenue, London W3 0SD, England.
[2]Sporicidin The Sporicidin Co., 4000 Massachusetts Avenue NW., Washington D.C., U.S.A.
[3]Cidex Johnson & Johnson Ltd., 260 Bath Road, Slough, Bucks. SL1 4EA, England.
[4]Roccal Winthrop Laboratories, Surbiton upon Thames, Surrey, England.
[5]Hot air Steriliser Elektrolux AD., P.O. Box 12, S-441, 01 Alingsas 1, Sweden.

Page 74

[1]Bead Steriliser National Keystone Products Co., 2nd and Noble Street, Philadelphia, Pa 19123, U.S.A.
[2]Browne's tube Albert Browne Ltd., Chancery House, Abbey Gate, Leicester LE4 0AA, England.
[3]Sterilisation bags—DRG Hospital Supplies. Supplied by Jon Dron Ltd., Devonshire House, 4 The Broadway Crouch End, London N8, England.

Page 75

[1]Endoguyd Scalatron, 57 Lee High Road, Lewisham, London SE13 5NS, England.
[2]Neosono D Amadent, P.O. Box 3422, Cherry Hill, N.J. 08034, U.S.A.

Page 76

[1]Endodontic ruler. Union Broach Corp., 36-40 37th Street, Long Island City, N.Y. 11101, U.S.A.
[2]Endogauge. K.R.D., Manchester M3 2AD, England.
[3]Endostops Silicone. Polydent S.A., CH 6607, Taverne, Switzerland.
(Left). White Silicone stops—Maillefer. Les Fils D'Auguste, Maillefer S.A., Ballaigues CH 1338, Switzerland.
(Right). Red rubber. Micromega S.A., 5-12 Rue de Tunnel, Besançon 25006, France.

Page 77

[1]Vari-fix stops and gauge. Vereinigte, Dental Werke, Zdarsky Ehrler K.G., D8 Munich 70, West Germany.
[2]Test handle system. Vereinigte, Dental Werke, Antaeos Beutelroc, Zipperer, Zdarsky Ehrler K.G., D8 Munich 70, West Germany.

Page 78

[1]Endodontic syringe and needle, Monojet, 503 ED, Sherwood (Medical), St. Louis MO 63103, U.S.A.
[2]Paper points. Dental Supply and Engineering Co. Ltd., High Path, London SW19 2LW England.

Page 79

[1]Cresatin. Interdent, 391 Steelcase Road W., Unit 16, Markham, Ontario, L3R 3V9, Canada.
[2]Ledermix. Lederle Laboratories, Cyanamid of G.B. Ltd., Bush House, Aldwych, London WC2B 4PU, England.
[3]Reogan-rapid. Vivadent, Schaan, Liechtenstein.
[4]Hypocal. Ellman International Mfg. Inc., Hewlett, N.Y. 11557, U.S.A.
[5]Messing Gun. Messing endodontic amalgam carrier, Produits Dentaires, Vevey, Switzerland.

Page 80

[1]Kerr pulp canal sealer. Kerr Manufacturing Co., Detroit 8, Michigan, U.S.A.
[2]Tubliseal. Kerr Manufacturing Co.
[3]Diaket. Espe GmbH, Seefeld, Oberbayern, West Germany.

Page 81

[1]AH26. DeTrey Dentsply Ltd., Weybridge, Surrey, England.
[2]N2 Normal & Apical and Universal Indrag AGSA S.A., CH-6616, Lausanne, Switzerland.
[3]Endomethasone Specialities Septodont, 58 Rue de Pont de Creteil, 94100 Saint-Maur, France.

Page 82

[1]Endofill Lee Pharmaceuticals, South El Monte, California, U.S.A.

Page 83

[1]Spreaders D11 and D11T Hu Friedy, 3232 North Rockwell Street, Chicago, Illinois 60618, U.S.A.
[2]RC 25S Premier Dental Products, Philadelphia, P.A., U.S.A.
[3]Finger Spreaders & Pluggers Kerr Manufacturing Co., Detroit 8, Michigan, U.S.A.
[4]Prima Plugger Prima, 23 Faris Barn Drive, Woodham, Weybridge, Surrey, England.
[5]5/7 Plugger Hu Friedy, 3232 North Rockwell Street, Chicago, Illinois 60618, U.S.A.
[6]No. 3 Spreader Kerr Manufacturing Co., Detroit 8, Michigan, U.S.A.
[7]PCA D4 Pulpdent Corporation of America, 75 Boylston Street, Brooklyn, Mass. 02147, U.S.A.

Page 107

[1]Paraffin Gauze dressing. Code No. 7404. T. J. Smyth & Nephew Ltd, Welwyn Garden City, England.

Page 114

[1]Binocular loops. Carl Zeiss, P.O. Box 78, Woodfield Road, Welwyn Garden City, Herts AL7 1LV England.

Page 135

[1]Copper Ring. Dentatus A.B., Jakobsdalsvagen 14-16, S-126 53 Hagersten, Sweden.
[2]Orthodontic band. Hawley Russell & Baker Ltd., Leyton House, 35 Darks Lane, Potters Bar, Herts, England.
[3]Aluminium Crown form. Produits Dentaires, S.A., Vevey, Switzerland.
[4]Isoform temporary crown, 3 M, 225 East Baker Avenue, Costa Mesa, California 92626, U.S.A.

Page 138

Tempobond. Kerr Manufacturing Co., Detroit 8, Michigan, U.S.A.

Page 141

[1]Endo-Vu's. Richard W. Pecina & Associates Inc., 2348 North Lewis, Waukegan, Illinois 60085, U.S.A.

Page 143

[1]RC Prep Premier Dental Products, Philadelphia, Pa U.S.A.
[2]Hibiscrub ICI Ltd., Alderley Park, Macclesfield, Cheshire, England.

Page 159

[1]P.D. Apical tips. Produits Dentaires S.A., Vevey, Switzerland.

Page 169

[1]McSpadden Ransom and Randolf Dentsply, 324 Chestnut Street, Toledo, Ohio 43604, U.S.A.
[2]Engine Plugger Vereinigte Dental Werke, Zdarsky, Ehrler, GmbH & Co, KG, Munchen 70, West Germany.
[3]Compactor Les Fils D'Auguste, Maillefer S.A., Ballaigues CH 1338, Switzerland.

Page 170

[1]Hypocal Ellman International Mfg. Inc., Hewlett, N.Y. 11557, U.S.A.
[2]Reogan-rapid Vivadent, Schaan, Liechtenstein
[3]Dycal Caulk-Dentsply International
[4]Procal 3M
[5]Life Kerr Manufacturing Co., Detroit 8, Michigan, U.S.A.

Page 171

[1]Dycal Caulk-Dentsply International
[2]Life Kerr Manufacturing Co., Detroit 8, Michigan, U.S.A.

Page 172

[1]Ellman Int. Mfg. Inc., New York, U.S.A.
[2]Rower
[3]Septodont Paris, France.

Page 173

[1]Septomixine Septodont Paris, France

Page 178

[1]Bernard, P.D. 1967 Therapie Ocalexique, Maloine, Paris, France.

INDEX

Numbers refer to pages.

Abscess, periapical 97,98
Access cavities 108,109,110,111
— — faults with 116,117,118,250
— — through bridges 140
— — through crowns 138,139
Acetone 261
Acrylic 258
Adrenaline - 1/1000 203
Alloy (zinc free) 206
Aluminium crown form 135
Amalgam 58,155,196,203,213,235,236
— core 224,268
— effect of zinc 203
— plugger 64
Anaesthesia, anaesthetic solutions 59
— with devitalising paste 63
— failure of 62,63,96
— general 198
— local 59,198,199
— pain free technique 63
Anaesthetic, topical 87,198
Analgesia, for incising abscess 62
— relative 63
Analgesics 97,99
Anastomosis, of canals 122
Ankylosis 173,174,215,238
Antibiotic 40,58,97,99,173,198
— amoxycillin (oral) 40,97
— — (intramuscular) 40
— demethylchlortetracycline 79
— erythromycin (oral) 40
Anti-tetanus injection 173
Anti-torsion lock 266,267
Apexification 176
Apical amalgam carrier 206,224
— — seal 195,235,236
— cavity 202
— curettage 207
— delta 122,201
— flaring (see zipping) 141
— foramen 119,144,145
— seal 196,262
— silver tips 262
— stop 145
— titanium tips 262
— — — (technique) 263
Apicectomy 194
Artery forceps 64
Auto-transplanted 238
Avulsed teeth 106,173,248

Baldwin burnisher 259
— technique 268
Barbed broach 66,143
Barium sulphate 177
Benzalkonium chloride 73
Beutelrock drill 261
Bicuspidisation 218,222
Bijou bottle 195
Binocular loops 114
Biocalex 178,179,180-183,251
Biogradability of silver 262
Bisphenol diglycidyl ether 81
Bleaching 257
— agent 258
— lamp 257,258
Bone, labial cortex plate 199
Briault probe, 64,201
Browne's tubes 74
Bruxism 241
Buccal object rule 146
Burs, Gates-Glidden 70,149,235,250,256,261,
— goose neck, round 70
— long shank 70
— standard 70

Calcific repair tissue 171
Calcification (dystrophic) 172,178,194
Calcinosis 237
Calcium carbonate 179
— eugenolate 180
— hydroxide 79,96,104,170-179,245
— oxide 179
Canal orifices 114,115
— probe 64
Canals, lateral 225
Cardiac disease 194
Case history 38
Cavity 58
Cement, calcium sulphate 203
— glass ionomer 203,248
— polycarboxylate 203
— zinc eugenolate 203
Charlton post 267
Chelation 180
Chloral hydrate 258,259
Chlorhexidine 90
Chloroform 167,256,258,261
Chloropercha 80
Chorea 194
CI Kit 265
Cingulum groove 231
Clamps (rubber dam) 86,87
— wingless 87
Clove hitch 89
Cocaine 62,63,199
Coepak 222

Colour coding 65,150
— — micromega 65
Composite resin 86,93,268
Copper band 85,95,135
Core/post 222,260,261
Cortico steroid 79,81,170
Cotton wool (sterile) 64
Cracked tooth 101
Creosote (beechwood) 188,189
Crown bonded porcelain 222
— form 92
— full 260,270
— gold 222
— lengthening procedure 134
— temporary acrylic 223
— — construction 91-93
— three-quarter 269
Curettage 195,200
Curette (spoon) 200
Cusps, reducing weakened 135
Cyst 190,199,200

Debilitating diseases 194
Debridement of bone wound 207
Dehiscence 196
Dentatus screw 268
Dentine, bridge 171
— dento-cemental junction 36
— dento-enamel junction 36
— demineralised 170,171
— elasticity of 36,260
— reparative 36
— secondary 36,123
— tubules 36
— — sclerosis of 36,171
Devitalising paste 187
Diagnosis 38
— with local anaesthetic 47,60
— mobility 45
— palpation 44
— with test cavity 48
— with transillumination 48
— with wooden stick 48
Diazepam (I-V) 59
Dilaceration 193
Discoloration 193
Drain (rubber dam) 98
Drainage 198
Duralay 265,266

Electro-surgery 134,270
Electronic measurement of canal 144,145
Emergency 86
Endodontic amalgam carrier 196
Endo-locking tweezers 64
Endo-perio lesion 225

Endosonics 151,152
Epithelial attachment 196
Epithelium, lined sinus track 200
Ether 258
Ethylenediaminetetracetic acid 143
Ethylene glycol 179
Eucalyptus oil 167
Eugenol 80
Excavator, long shank 64
Exposure of dentine 103
—— pulp 103

Face, asymmetry of 41
Facial scarring 194
Fenestration 200
Ferric sulphide 257
Ferrous oxide 257
Fibreoptic light 48
Fibrous repair tissue 197
File 65,66,249
— diamond 151
— flexofile 66
— Hedstroem 66
— helifile 66
— K flex 66
— K type 66
— unifile 66
Filing technique 146,147,148,249
—— anticurvature 149
—— circumferential 149
Finger spreaders 83
Flaps design of 196
— envelope 196
— Ochsenbein-Luebke 196
— semilunar 196
— trapezoidal 196,197
Floss threader 222
Formaldehyde 81
Formolcresol (Buckley's) 185,187
— saline 195,200
Fracture, hairline 48
— of instrument in canal 56,218,250,251
— of tooth 100,136,191,218,268
— vertical 218,229,261
Furcal arch 222
Furcation involvement 218,225

Gagging 95
Gates-Gidden bur 70,149,235,250,256,261
Gaucher's disease 237
Gingiva, hyperplastic 95
Gingival retraction 223
Gingivectomy 270
Glass ionomer cement 248
Glutaraldehyde 73
Gold collar 266
Granulation tissue 195
Granuloma 199
Groove, palatal 233
Guttapercha 82,137,150
— cone 196
— removal from canals 256

Haemoglobin 252
Haemorrhagic diseases 194
Haemostasis 203
Handpiece (pedodontic) 202
— micro (kavo) 202
Heat carrier 82
—— (battery operated) 83
Hemisection 218-220,223,228
— instruments for 224
Hexachlorophene 81
History, case 38
— medical 38
Hollenback carver 212
Horsley's bone wax 203,204
Hunt's syringe 207
Hydrogen peroxide (30%) 258
Hydron 82
Hypercementosis 237
Hyperparathyroidism 237
Hypoparathyroidism 237

Idiosyncracy to iodine 221
Infective endocarditis 38,39,51
Inferior dental canal 194,195
Inflammation, periapical 37
Injectable silicone resin 82
Injection, infiltration 59
— intraligamental 60
— intraosseous 60-62
— intrapapillary 59,199
— palatal 199
— submucous 199
Instructions to patient after surgery 209
——— icepacks 209
——— mouthwashes 209
Instrument, cursor 68
— flat plastic 64
— fracture 67,249
— giromatic 68
— ingestion of 95
— inhalation of 95
— marking paste stops 77
— metal stops 77
— mishandling 249
— power assisted 68
— rubber stops 76
— spiral root canal fillers 69
— sterilisation of 249
— storage 71
Intrusion 248
Iodine, strong solution 250
Iodoform 177,221,224
— paste 82
Irrigation 78,150
— of bone 195
— with sodium hypochlorite 78
— with syringe
Isotonic saline 212

'Jiffy' tube 178

Kurer crown saver 266
— post/core system 267

Ledermix 79,96
Ligature (dental floss) 89
Luxated teeth 106,191,237

Malassez, cell rests 37
Marginal gingivitis 194
Masseran kit 252
— technique 251,253
Matrix band 85
Maxillary antrum 194,195
McSpadden compactor 168
Mechanical amalgam condensor 196
Medication 150,178
Mental nerve 194
Mepivacaine 59
Messing gun 79
Metacresyl acetate 79,96
Methyl methacrylate in chloroform 259
Microleakage 203
Milk 173
Mirror, front surface 64
Mitchell's trimmer 204
Mouthwash, chlorhexidine 215
Mucoperiosteum 196
Mucoperiosteal flap 200

Nickel-chrome crown 187
Nylon sutures 207

Occlusion 151
Onlay 260,269
Open drainage 98
Oral hygiene instruction 133,134
Orthodontic band 135
Orthograde 196
Osteitis, alveolar 221
— chronic periapical 173
Osteoclastic activity 237
Overdenture 49

Paget's disease 237,242
Pain control, psychology of 198
— post operative 99,100,101
— pulpal 40
— spontaneous 96
Paper points 78
Parachlorphenol 79
Parachute 84
Para post system 265
Perforations iatrogenic 178
— through bifurcation 118
— through crown 118
— through roots 29,118

Periapical lesion 290
Periodontal condition 133
— disease 237
— fibre, transeptal 218
— infrabony 218
— pack 215
— pocket, infection from 123
— pocketing 196
— problem 55
— support 52
Perio-endo lesion 58,225-236
Periosteal elevator 197
Peripheral resorption 173
Phosphatase, acid 173
— alkaline 172,173
Phosphoric acid 258
Pink spot 243
— — pseudo 242
Plastic points 154
Plaque control 222
Pluggers 82,83
Polyketone 80
Poor oral hygiene 194
Post crown 138
— removal of 254
— remover (Eggler) 254
— space 49
Post-surgical palatal defect 210
Povidone-iodine 90,212
Pregnancy 194
Premaxillary area of palate
Pre-operative medication 198
Prilocaine 59
Pulp, anatomy 33
— calcification 36
— capping 103,104,170,171,185
— chamber, floor 109
— — roof 108
— exposure 170
— extirpation 96
— histology 31
— inflammation 37
— innervation 35
— necrosis 37,225,236
— plexus of Raschkow 35
— remnants (vital) 62,99
— response to injury 33
— sclerosis 50
— stones 36
— testers, electrical 45,46
— tests 45,46
— — thermal 46,47
Pulp theory of sensitivity (hydrodynamic) 35
— trauma 50
— vascular supply 35
— zones of cells 34
Pulpectomy 104,188,189
Pulpitis, irreversible 40,41,96,102
— reversible 40,41,96
Pulpotomy 50,81,103,104,170-172,185,189
Pus, discharge of 97

Radiation therapy 237
Radiograph, use of 43
Radiographic control of surgery 209,210
— landmarks, anterior nasal spine 23
— — bone 22
— — cementum 22
— — dentine 22
— — enamel 22
— — incisive foramen 24
— — lingual foramen 25
— — mandibular canal 24
— — maxillary antrum 23
— — median suture 23
— — mental foramen 25
— — nasal septum 23
— — nose and lip lines 23
— — nutrient canal 25
— — periodontal ligament 22
— — pulp 22
— — stones 22
Radiographic techniques, bisecting angle 19,20,21
— — coning off 17,20
— — paralleling 19,21,110
— — periapical 19-20
— — Rinn holder and ring 19
Radiolucency, of dental origin 26
— furcation involvement 28
— lateral areas 28
— non-dental 30
— periapical 27
— — early changes 28
Radiopacifier 177
Radiopacity, cementoma 30
— condensing osteitis 29
Reamer 65,66
— (Peeso) 70,250
Reattachment 215
Recapitulation 148
Remineralization 170
Removal of pulp 143
— — sutures 209
Replacement resorption 215,238,239
Replantation 106,173,211,212
— planned 224
Resection of apex 201
Resorbable paste 188
Resorption, burrowing 242
— idiopathic 214
— inflammatory 237
— lacunae 237
— peripheral cervical 242
— pressure 240
— surface 237
Restoration, initial 58
Retention pins 269
— screws 268
Retrofilling with Kalzinol 206
Retrograde approach 196,203,236
Rheumatic fever 194
Root, bifid 201
— canals, accessory 201
— — anatomy 119,120(124-132)
— — apical delta 122,201

— — filling paste 81,82
— — fin-like grooves 120
— — lateral 122.201.226
— — lateral, formation of 133,
— — measurement 75,143
— — medication 79
— — obstructed 55
— — perforation 57,58,194,218
— — preparation of 141
— — — ultrasonic 151,152
— — probe 64
— — removal of obstructions 249
— filling with amalgam 155,159,160
— — the canal 153
— — by cold lateral condensation 161-164
— — — custom-made point 166
— — with Gutta percha 153,159
— — — — with solvents 167
— — by hot vertical condensation 165,166
— — with Messing apical amalgam carrier 157,158
— — — paste alone 169
— — — precision titanium tips 159
— — sectional technique 159
— — with single cone and sealer 161
— — by thermal compaction 168,245-246
— — — warm lateral condensation 164
— fractured, diagnosis of 28
— fractures 52,105
— with necrotic pulp 106
— planing 232
— section of 218,235
— resorption, external 53,178,218,237,244,247
— — internal 53,104,178,218,226,237,243,244,245
— — of, post-orthodontic 178
Rubber dam 84-88
— — clamp 84-89
— — — forceps 90
— — frames 90
— — punch 90
— — techniques 88,89,94
Ruler, metal 64

Safety chain 95
Scrubbing up 198
Self-shearing screw pins 269
Sharpey's fibres 173
Silico-phosphate cement 178
Silver cones 154
Simon's classification 234
Sinus-tract 43,44,55,223
— discharging 179,181,192,
Sodium carbonate 73
— nitrite 73
— perborate 258
Splinting 107,174,215
Spreaders 82,83,272
Stainless steel orthodontic band 85
Steiglitz forceps 251
Step-back technique 142,146,147,148,149

Sterile box 72
— double tray 72
— R.A.F. tray 72
— tray 72
Sterilization 73
— bags 74
— dry heat 73
— moist heat 74
Sterilizer, glass bead 71,74
— hot air oven 72,73
Stomahesive 208,221,271
Stop, apical 147
— rubber 147
Stress to alveolar bone 219
Subluxation 248
Superoxol 258
Surgeon's twist 89

Teeth, immature 172
— induction of apical closure 176
Temporary bridge with acrylic tooth 271
— — material 271
— — matrix 271
— — with natural crown 271
— seal 150
Test cavity 227
— handle system 77
Tetanus prophylaxis 106
Tetracycline staining 257
Thermoplasticised injection moulding 272
Throat pack 95
Time gaps 48
Titanium 256
— cones 154
Tooth, ameloblasts 32
— the bell 32
— cell rests of Malassez 33,37
— dental lamina 31
— — papilla 32
— development 31
— — of root 33
— enamel organ 31
— Hertwig's sheath 33
— inner and outer enamel epithelium 31
— odontoblasts 32
— stellate reticulum 31
— Von Korff's fibres 32
Toxaemia 97
Transillumination 255
Transplantation 248
Trauma 102,103,191
Treatment planning 38,49
Trismus 194
Tug-back 263
Turner's syndrome 237

Ultrasound 151

Varnish (copal-Ether) 172,213
Vaso-constrictor 203
Vitality check-up 209

Walking bleach 258
Wiptam technique 258

Xeroradiography 14
X-ray, collimation 9
— cone 10
— — in buccal object rule 146
— exposure (Roentgen) 15
— — Rad 15
— — Rem 15
— film 10
— — badge 15
— — holders 10,11,15
— kilovolt peak 9
— lead apron 14
— machine 9
— Masel paralleling instruments 11
— in pregnancy 15
— processing 16
— — faults 16,17,18
— processors 12
— — automatic 13
— — — Velopex 13
— — Gimad 13
— — manual 12
— — Westone Manumatic 12
— safety 14
— viewer 13
Xylol 256

Zinc eugenolate cement 90,170
— — — polystyrene bonded 215
— oxide 179
Zipping 141